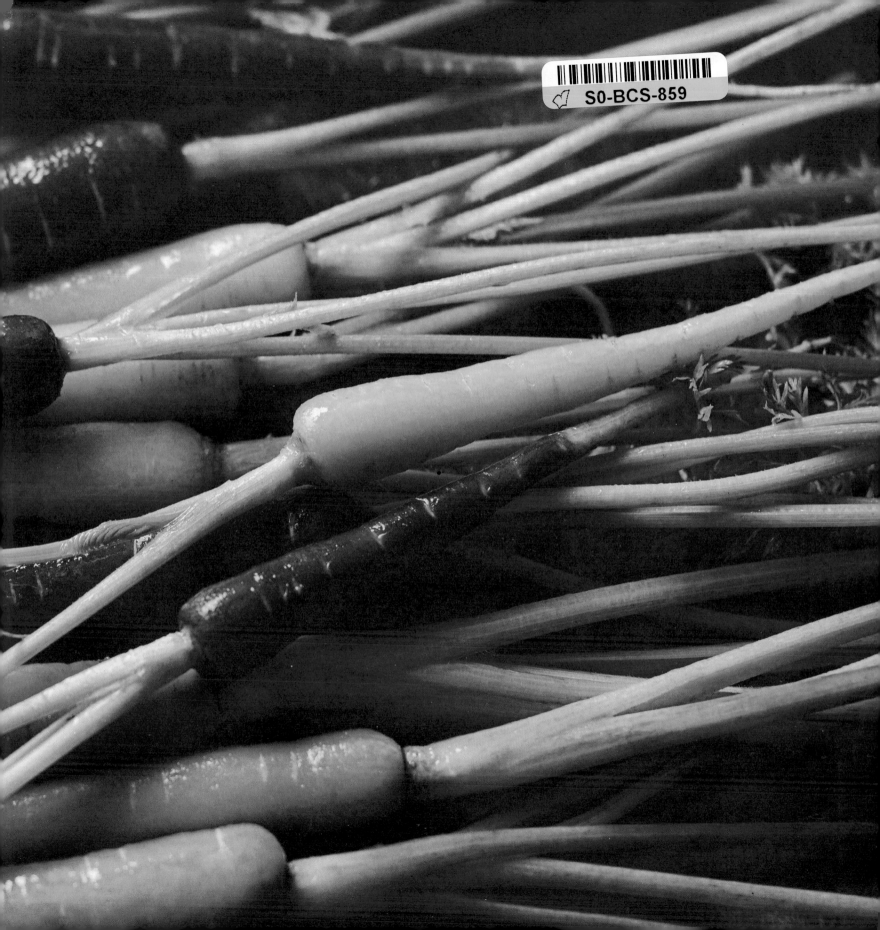

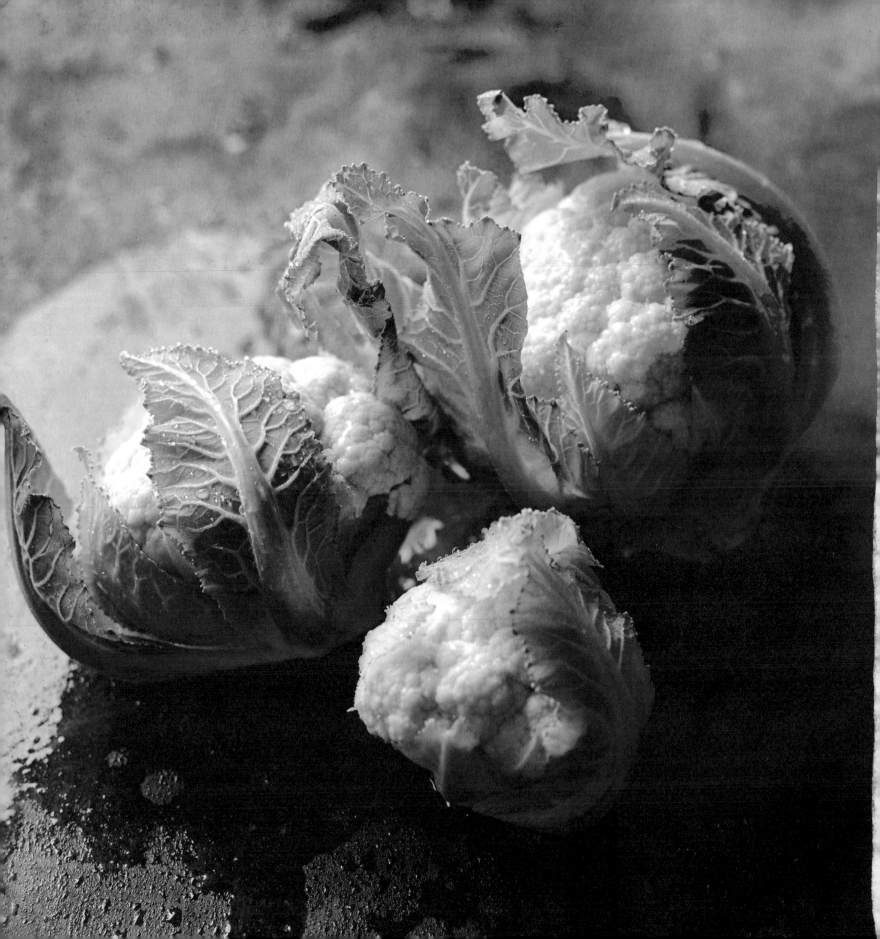

life in balance

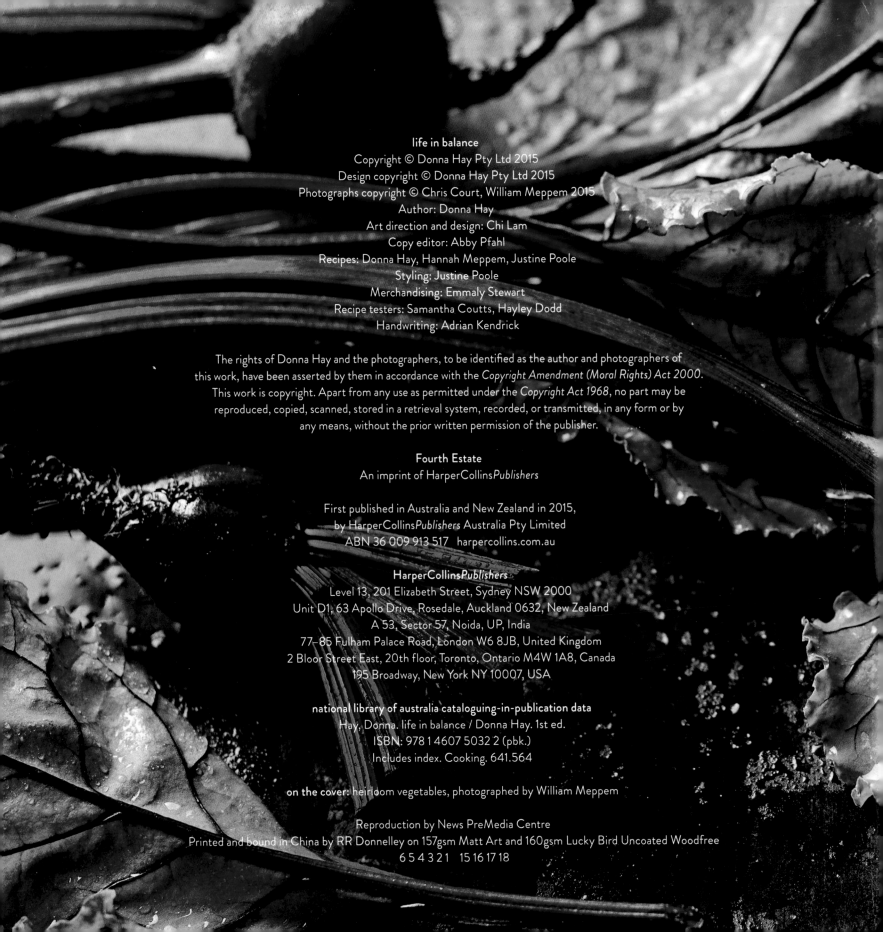

life in balance

Copyright © Donna Hay Pty Ltd 2015
Design copyright © Donna Hay Pty Ltd 2015
Photographs copyright © Chris Court, William Meppem 2015
Author: Donna Hay
Art direction and design: Chi Lam
Copy editor: Abby Pfahl
Recipes: Donna Hay, Hannah Meppem, Justine Poole
Styling: Justine Poole
Merchandising: Emmaly Stewart
Recipe testers: Samantha Coutts, Hayley Dodd
Handwriting: Adrian Kendrick

Fourth Estate
An imprint of HarperCollins*Publishers*

First published in Australia and New Zealand in 2015,
by HarperCollins*Publishers* Australia Pty Limited
ABN 36 009 913 517   harpercollins.com.au

HarperCollins*Publishers*
Level 13, 201 Elizabeth Street, Sydney NSW 2000
Unit D1, 63 Apollo Drive, Rosedale, Auckland 0632, New Zealand
A 53, Sector 57, Noida, UP, India
77–85 Fulham Palace Road, London W6 8JB, United Kingdom
2 Bloor Street East, 20th floor, Toronto, Ontario M4W 1A8, Canada
195 Broadway, New York NY 10007, USA

national library of australia cataloguing-in-publication data
Hay, Donna. life in balance / Donna Hay. 1st ed.
ISBN: 978 1 4607 5032 2 (pbk.)
Includes index. Cooking. 641.564

on the cover: heirloom vegetables, photographed by William Meppem

Reproduction by News PreMedia Centre
Printed and bound in China by RR Donnelley on 157gsm Matt Art and 160gsm Lucky Bird Uncoated Woodfree
6 5 4 3 2 1   15 16 17 18

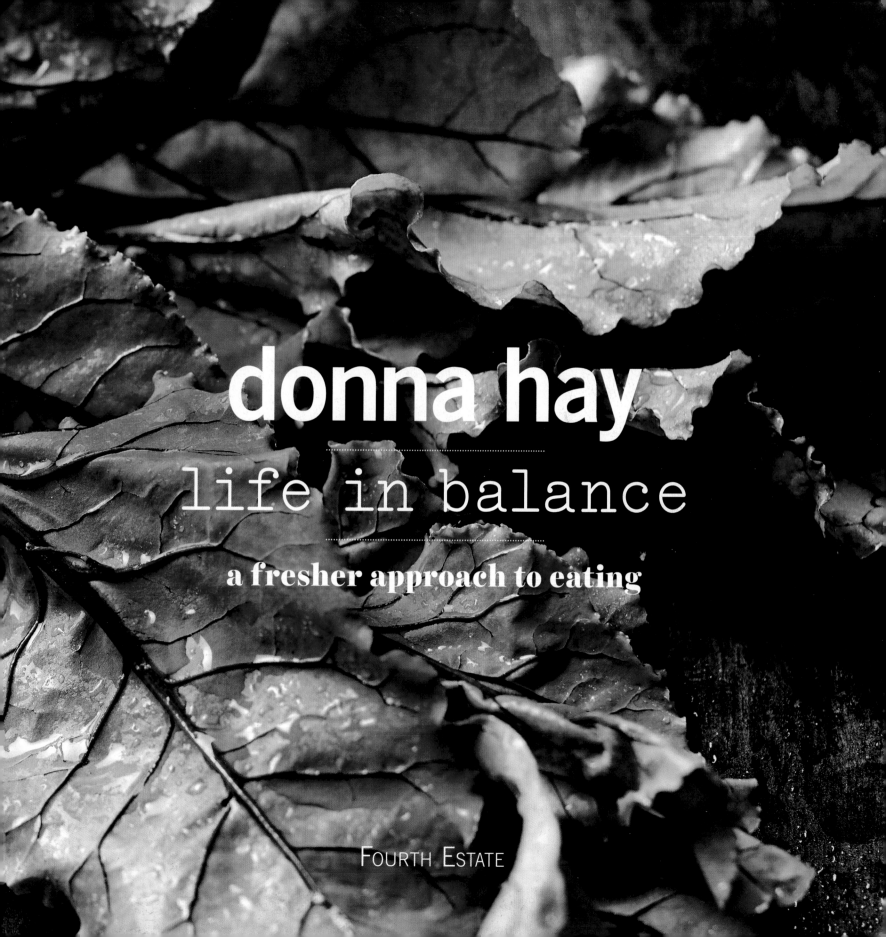

donna hay

life in balance

a fresher approach to eating

FOURTH ESTATE

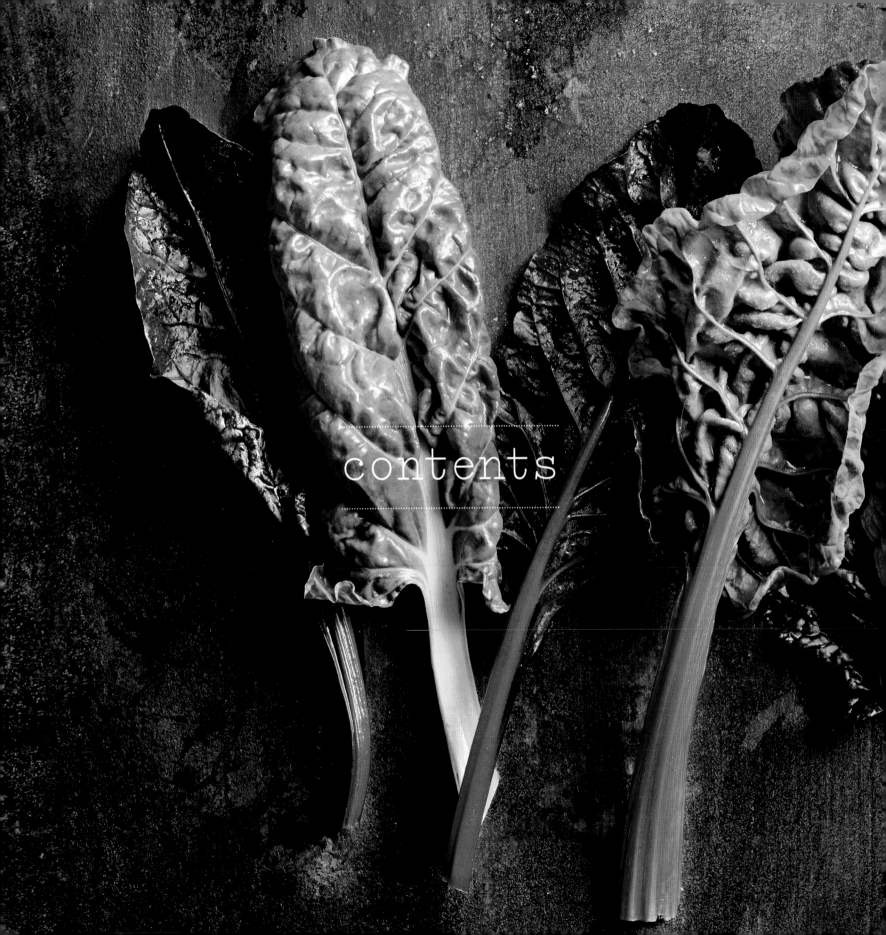

contents

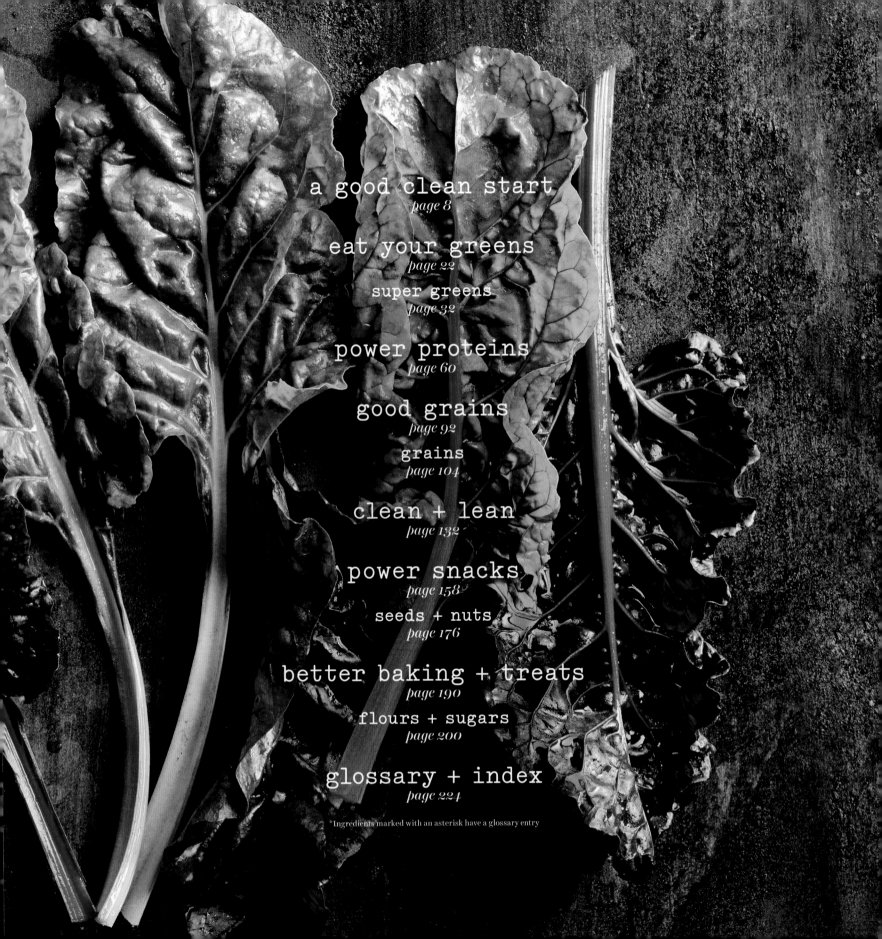

*Ingredients marked with an asterisk have a glossary entry

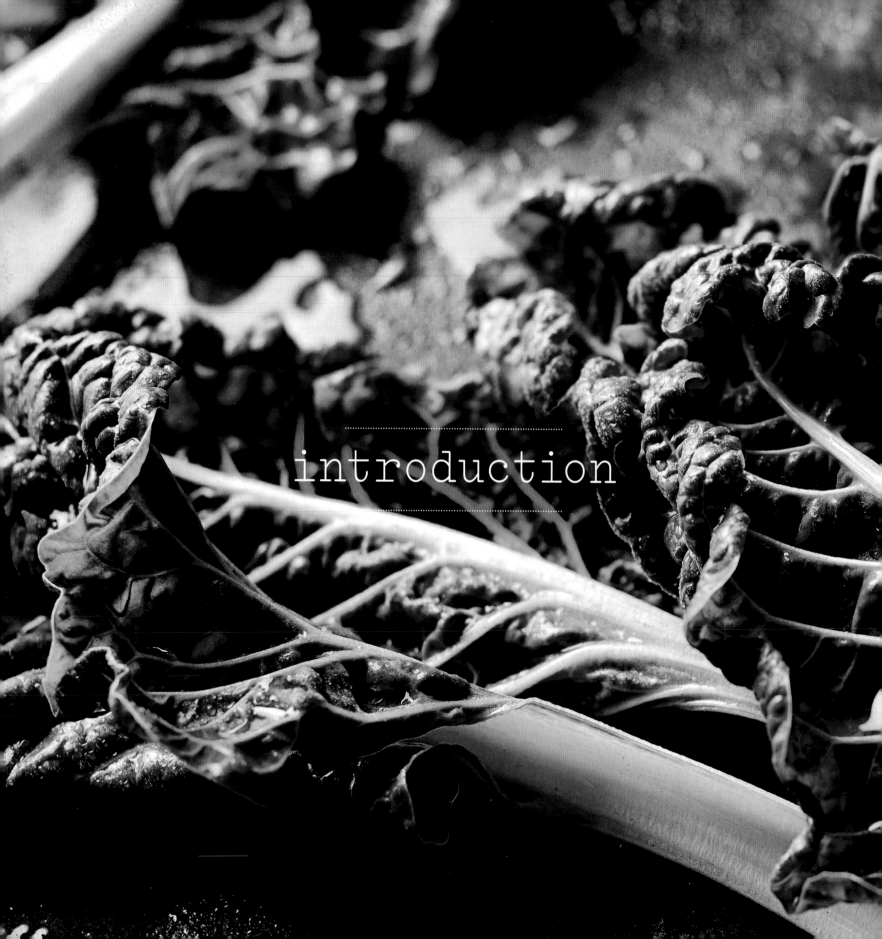

introduction

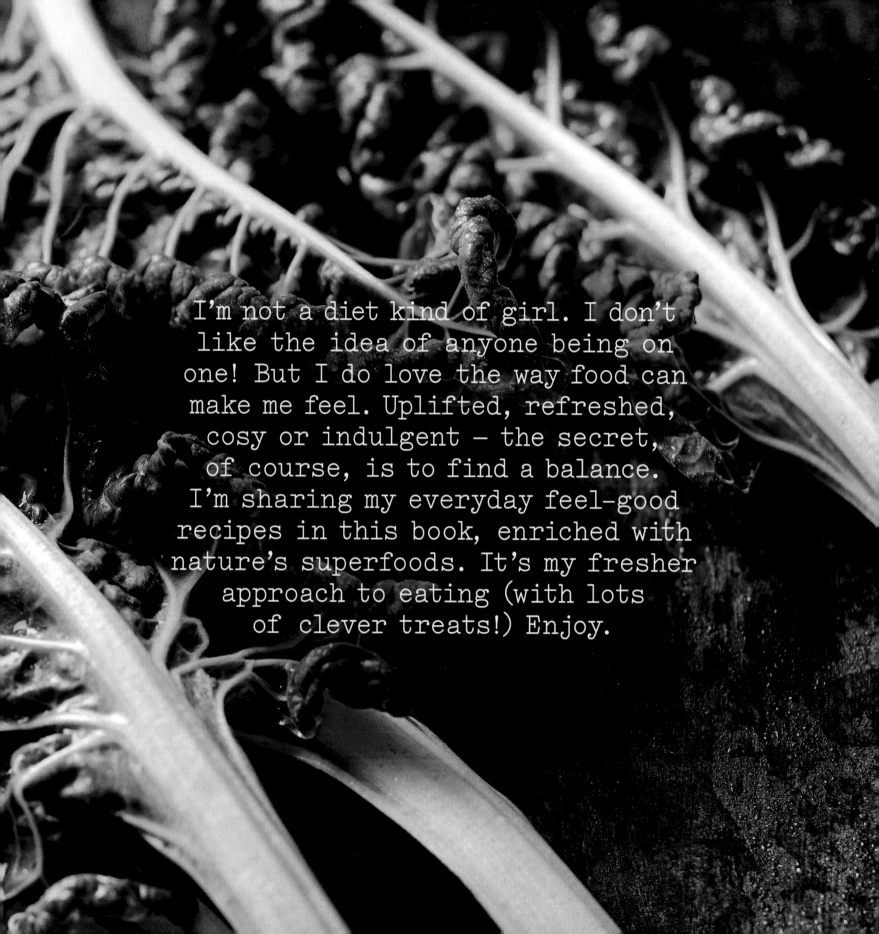

I'm not a diet kind of girl. I don't like the idea of anyone being on one! But I do love the way food can make me feel. Uplifted, refreshed, cosy or indulgent – the secret, of course, is to find a balance. I'm sharing my everyday feel-good recipes in this book, enriched with nature's superfoods. It's my fresher approach to eating (with lots of clever treats!) Enjoy.

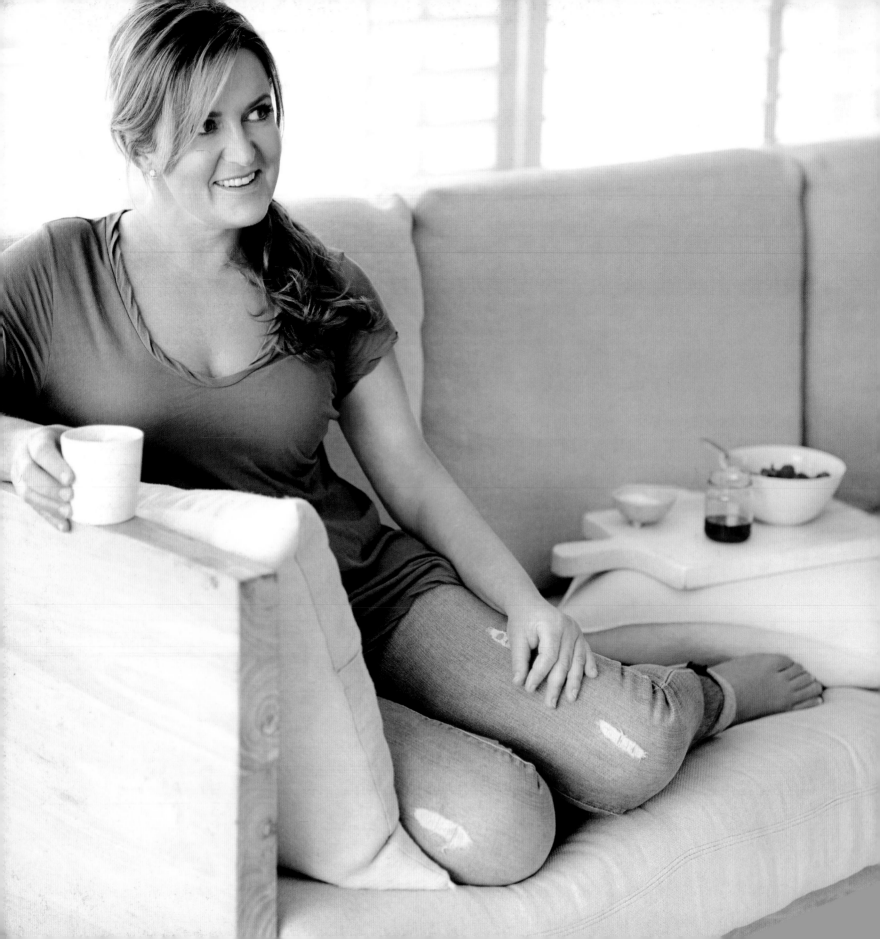

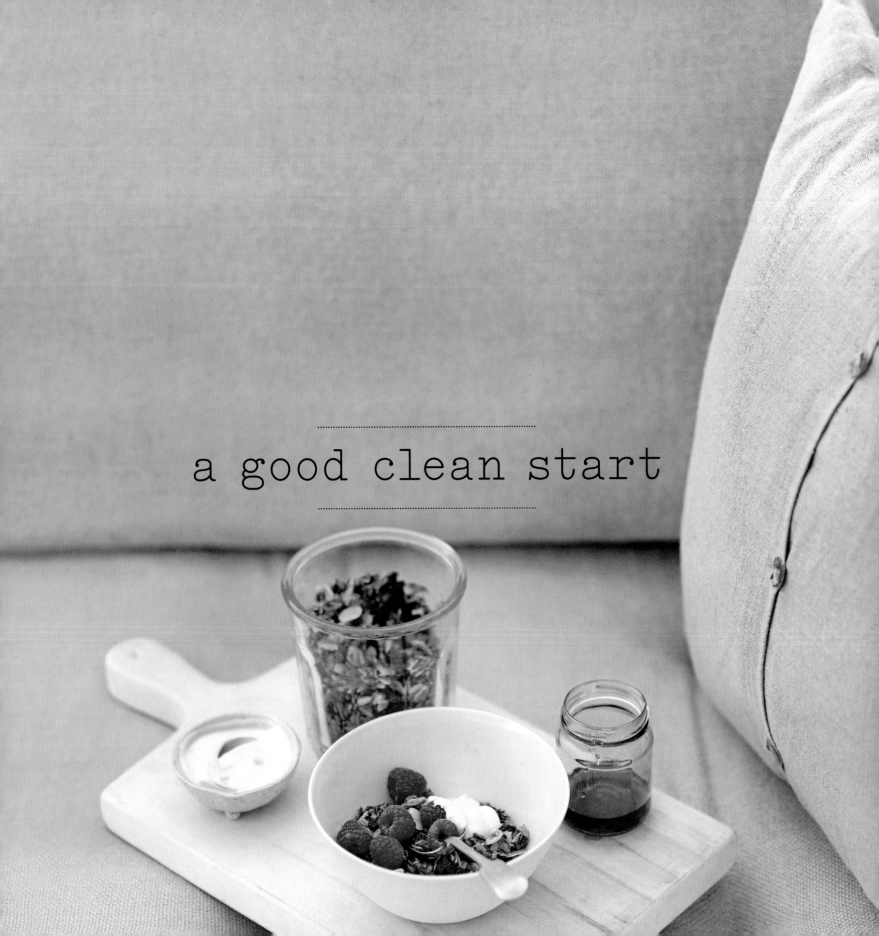

a good clean start

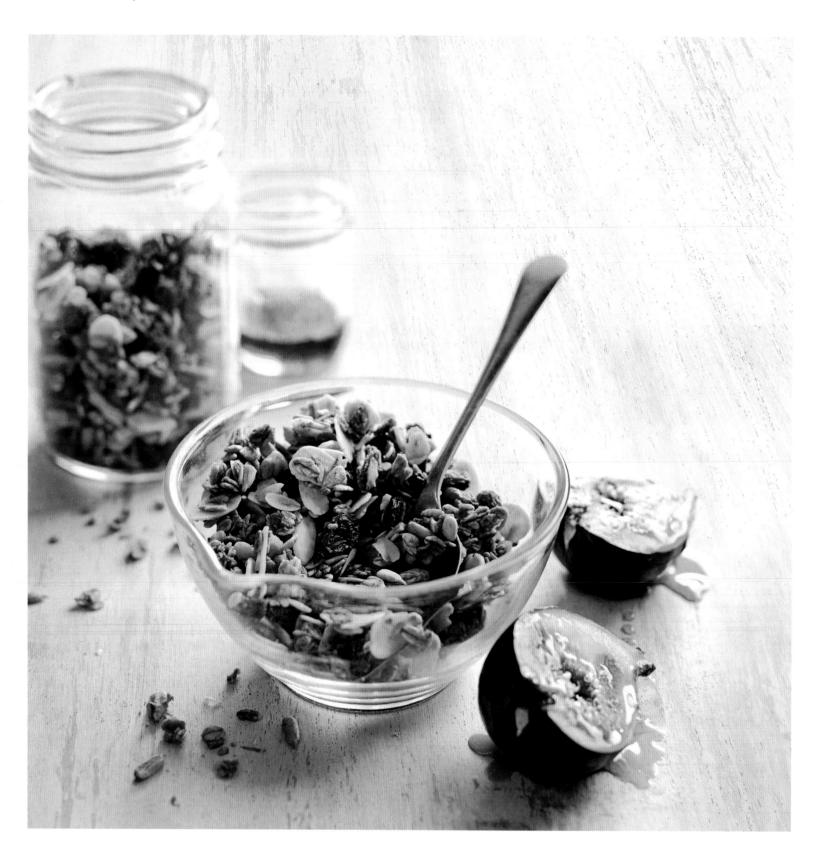

espresso granola

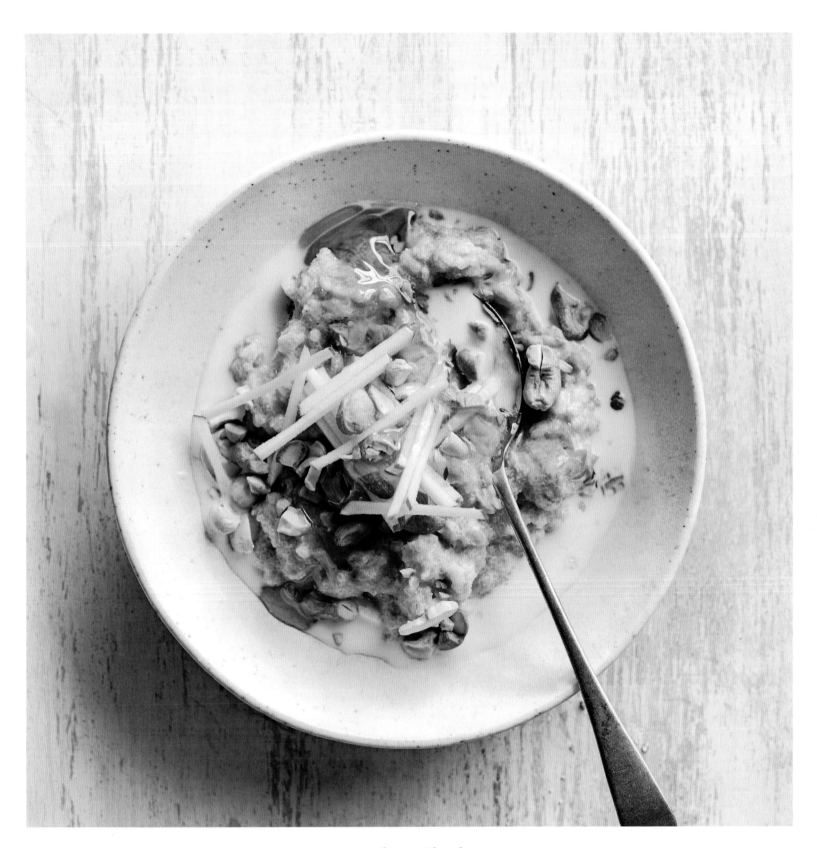

amaranth oats with cashews

espresso granola

4 x 30ml shots espresso or strong brewed coffee
½ cup (125ml) hot water
2 cups (240g) rolled oats
⅔ cup (100g) raisins
⅓ cup (80ml) maple syrup, plus extra to serve
⅔ cup (100g) sunflower seeds*
⅔ cup (50g) flaked almonds
milk or nut milk, to serve
figs, halved, to serve

Preheat oven to 120°C (250°F). Place the espresso and water in a medium bowl and stir to combine. Add the oats and raisins, mix to combine and allow to stand for 20 minutes or until the liquid is absorbed. Add the maple syrup, sunflower seeds and almonds and mix to combine. Spread the mixture onto 2 baking trays lined with non-stick baking paper and bake, tossing occasionally, for 45 minutes or until the oats are crisp. Allow to cool on trays. Store granola in an airtight container for up to 2 weeks. To serve, divide between bowls and top with milk, fig and extra maple syrup. SERVES 4

amaranth oats with cashews

1½ cups (180g) rolled oats
½ teaspoon sea salt flakes
2 cups (500ml) milk, plus extra to serve
1 cup (250ml) water
½ cup (60g) amaranth flakes*
1 tablespoon honey, plus extra to serve
½ teaspoon ground cinnamon
1 apple, cored and cut into matchsticks, to serve
toasted cashews, to serve

enrich your breakfast bowl with nourishing amaranth for energy and essential minerals

Place the oats, salt, milk and water in a saucepan over medium heat. Cook, stirring occasionally, for 10 minutes or until the oats are beginning to soften. Add the amaranth and cook, stirring, for a further 2–3 minutes or until soft. Add the honey and cinnamon and stir to combine. Spoon the oats into serving bowls and top with extra milk and honey. Sprinkle with the apple and cashews to serve. SERVES 4

banana buckwheat pancakes

¾ cup (120g) buckwheat flour*
¾ cup (95g) white spelt flour*
3 teaspoons baking powder
1 teaspoon ground cinnamon
¾ cup (200g) mashed banana (about 3 bananas)
1 egg
¼ cup (60ml) maple syrup, plus extra to serve
¾ cup (180ml) milk
unsalted butter, to grease the pan
store-bought vanilla bean yoghurt, to serve
extra banana, sliced, to serve

Buckwheat flour adds fluffiness and a warm, nutty flavour to pancakes

Place both the flours, the baking powder and cinnamon in a large bowl and mix to combine. Add the banana, egg, maple syrup and milk and whisk until smooth.

Heat a little of the butter in a non-stick frying pan over medium heat. Add ⅓ cup (80ml) of the batter to the pan and cook for 2–3 minutes each side or until golden. Set aside and keep warm. Repeat with the butter and remaining batter. Divide pancakes between serving plates and top with yoghurt and extra banana. Drizzle with extra maple syrup to serve. SERVES 4

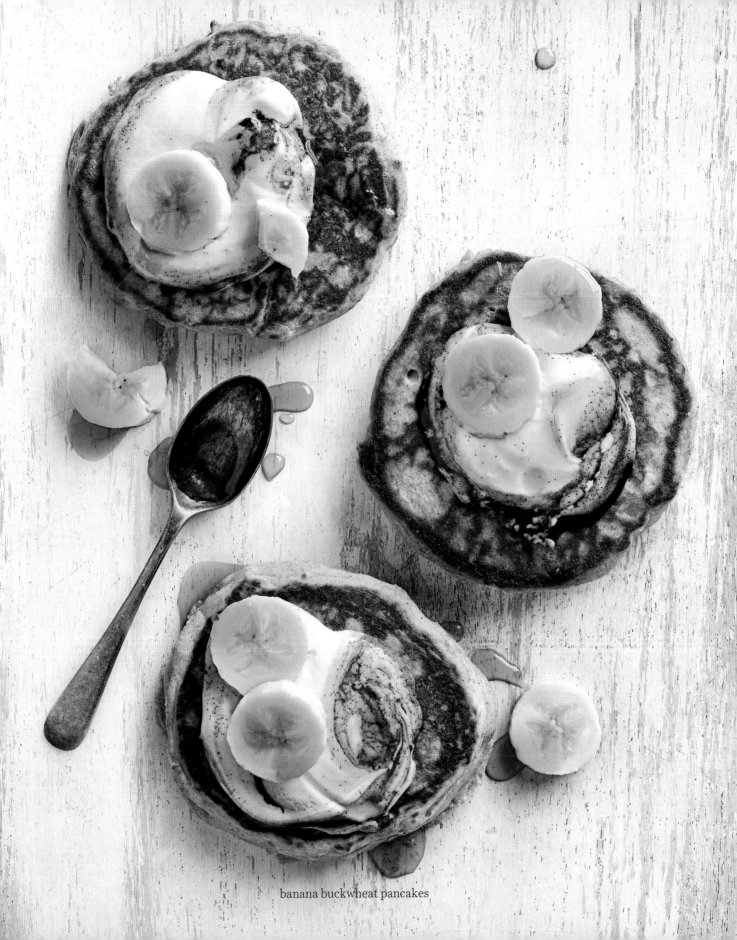

banana buckwheat pancakes

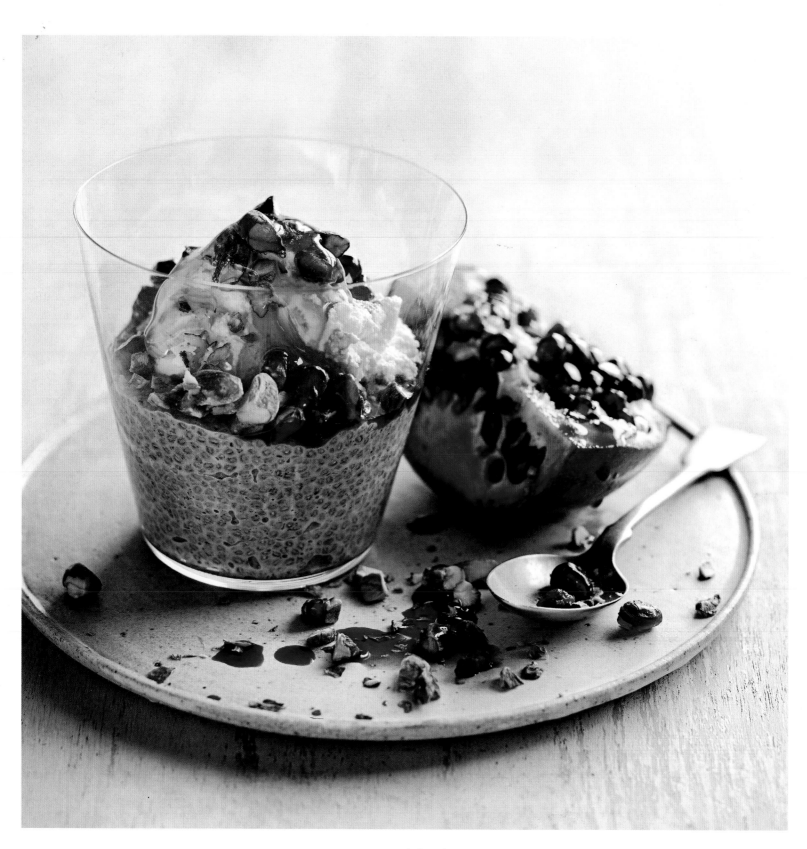

coconut and chai chia

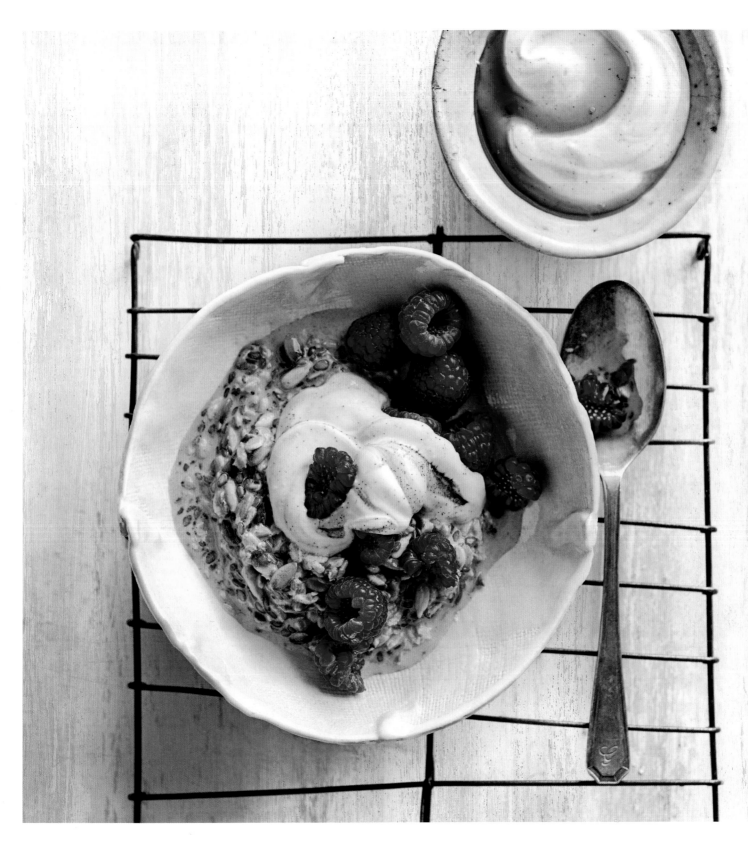

power seed bircher with maple vanilla yoghurt

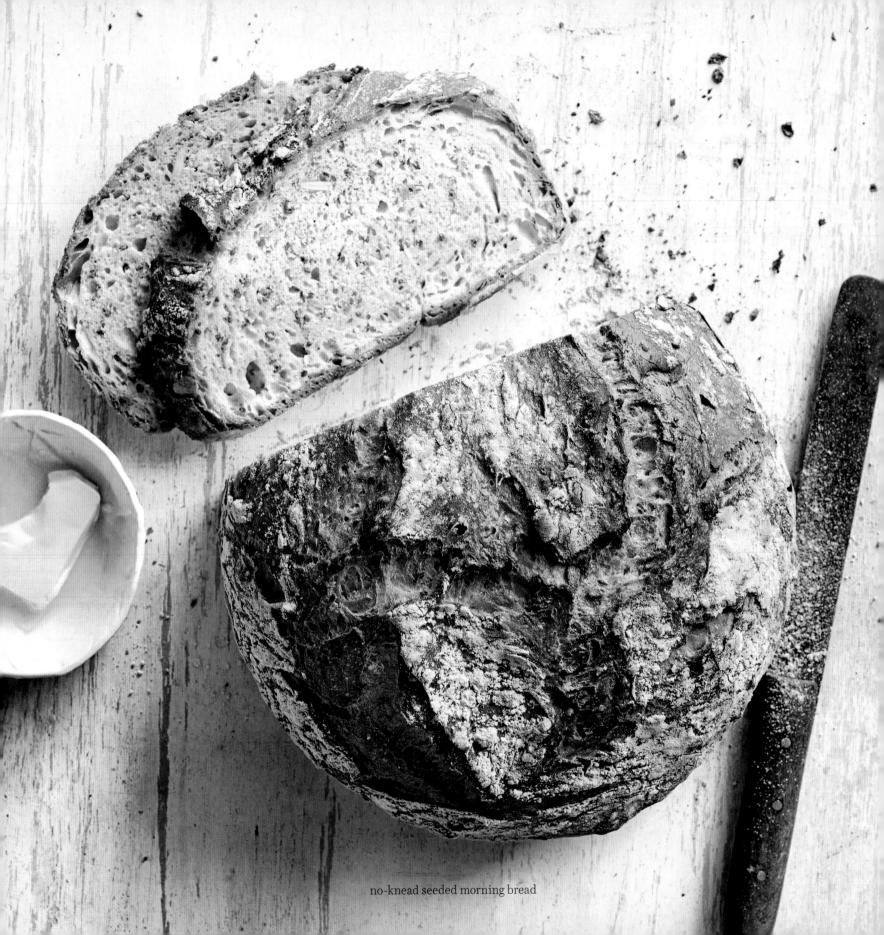

no-knead seeded morning bread

coconut and chai chia

3 tablespoons chai tea
1½ cups (375ml) coconut milk
1½ cups (375ml) milk or nut milk
3 tablespoons raw honey*, plus extra to serve
½ cup (100g) white chia seeds*
coconut yoghurt*, chopped pistachios
    and pomegranate seeds, to serve

Place the tea and coconut milk in a saucepan over medium
heat. Bring to a gentle simmer and cook for 2 minutes. Strain
the mixture into a medium bowl, discarding the solids. Add the
milk, honey and chia seeds, mix to combine and refrigerate for
20 minutes or until the liquid is absorbed and the chia is soft.

Divide chia between glasses and top with yoghurt, pistachio,
pomegranate and extra honey to serve. SERVES 4–6

power seed bircher with maple vanilla yoghurt

⅓ cup (55g) sunflower seeds*
⅓ cup (55g) pepitas (pumpkin seeds)*
⅓ cup (60g) linseeds (flaxseeds)*
½ cup (60g) rolled spelt oats*
1½ cups (375ml) milk or nut milk
½ teaspoon ground cinnamon
1 tablespoon honey
1 firm pear, grated
raspberries, to serve
maple vanilla yoghurt
1 cup (280g) plain Greek-style (thick) yoghurt
2 tablespoons maple syrup
1 teaspoon vanilla bean paste

Place the sunflower seeds, pepitas, linseeds and oats
in a large bowl. Add the milk, cinnamon and honey and
mix to combine. Refrigerate for 4 hours or overnight.

To make the maple vanilla yoghurt, place the yoghurt,
maple syrup and vanilla in a bowl and mix to combine.

Add the pear to the bircher and stir to combine.
Spoon the bircher into serving bowls or jars and top
with the yoghurt and raspberries to serve. SERVES 4

no-knead seeded morning bread

3⅓ cups (830ml) water
1 teaspoon dry yeast
1 tablespoon maple syrup
3 teaspoons sea salt flakes
6 cups (780g) white spelt flour*, plus extra for dusting
½ cup (90g) linseeds (flaxseeds)*
½ cup (80g) sunflower seeds*
butter, to serve

spelt is an ancient grain that's high in protein and easy to digest ✓

Place the water, yeast, maple syrup and salt in a large bowl and
mix to combine. Add the flour, linseeds and sunflower seeds and
mix until a sticky dough forms. Turn out the dough onto a surface
dusted with flour and fold over the edges to form a rough round
loaf. Place the dough in a clean bowl dusted with flour. Dust the
top of the dough with flour and cover with a clean tea towel.
Allow to stand for 8 hours or overnight.

Preheat oven to 250°C (480°F). Heat a large heavy-based
cast-iron saucepan in the oven for 30 minutes or until very hot.
Carefully remove the pan from the oven and dust with flour.
Slide the dough into the hot pan. Using a small sharp knife,
score the top of the dough with a cross pattern. Cover with a
tight-fitting lid and bake for 40–45 minutes. Reduce the oven
temperature to 220°C (425°F), remove the lid and bake, uncovered,
for a further 20 minutes or until the bread sounds hollow when
tapped. Slice the bread and serve warm with butter. MAKES 1 LOAF

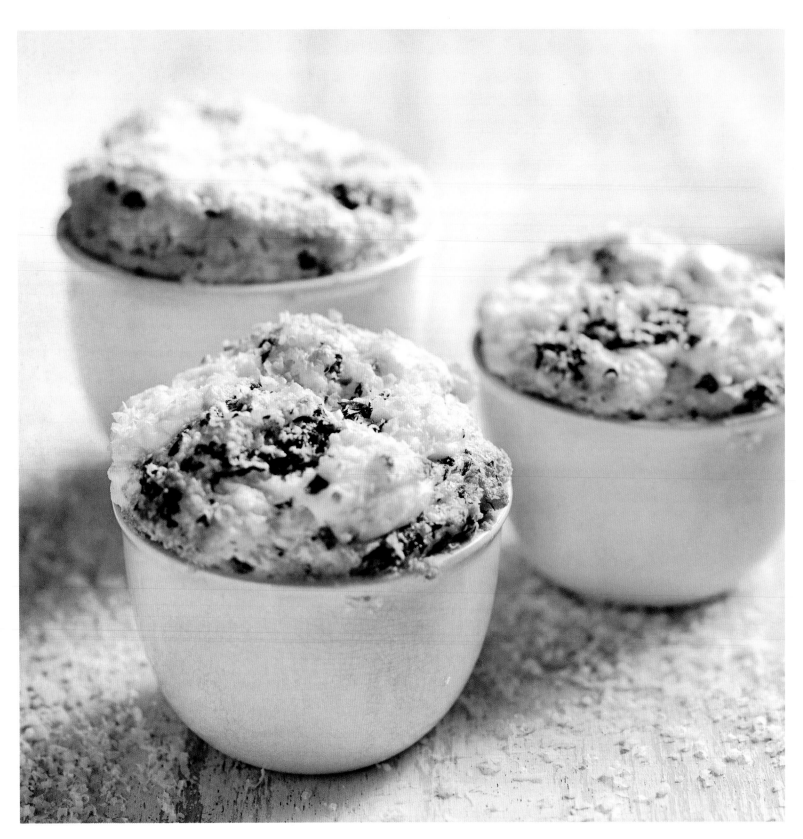

baked spinach and parmesan eggwhite soufflés

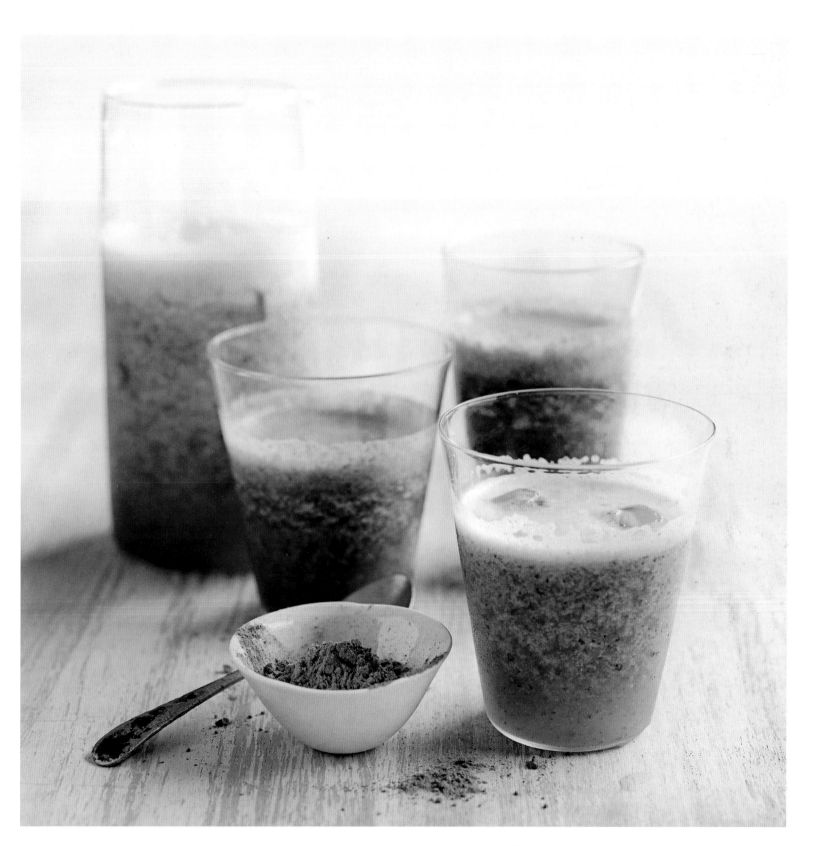

the smoothest of green smoothies + cool smoothies

baked spinach and parmesan eggwhite soufflés

20g unsalted butter, melted
2 tablespoons finely grated parmesan
2 cups (50g) baby spinach leaves
6 eggwhites
1 teaspoon finely chopped tarragon
¾ cup (60g) finely grated parmesan, extra
½ cup (120g) fresh ricotta
sea salt and cracked white pepper

Preheat oven to 180°C (350°F). Brush 4 x ¾-cup-capacity (180ml)
ovenproof ramekins with the butter. Divide the parmesan between
the ramekins and shake to coat.
   Place the spinach in a bowl, cover with boiling water and drain
immediately. Transfer to layers of paper towel, dry and chop finely.
   Place the eggwhites in a large bowl and whisk until soft peaks
form. Add the spinach and tarragon, ¼ cup (40g) of the extra
parmesan, the ricotta, salt and pepper and gently fold to combine.
Spoon the mixture into the ramekins and place on a baking tray.
Bake for 12–14 minutes or until puffed and lightly golden. Top
with the remaining parmesan and serve immediately. **SERVES 4**

the smoothest of green smoothies

1 banana, peeled
1 cup (25g) baby spinach leaves
1 stalk silverbeet (Swiss chard) or kale, trimmed
    and leaves chopped
2 tablespoons flat-leaf parsley leaves
2 tablespoons mint leaves
2 cups (500ml) coconut water
1 cup ice cubes

Place the banana, spinach, silverbeet, parsley, mint, coconut
water and ice in a blender and blend until smooth. Divide
between glasses to serve. **SERVES 2**

cool smoothies

2 Lebanese cucumbers (260g), roughly chopped
¼ cup mint leaves
½ teaspoon matcha green tea powder*
2 cups (500ml) coconut water

pick up this power tea at health food shops or asian grocers

Place the cucumber, mint, matcha and coconut water in
a blender and blend until smooth. Divide between glasses,
over ice, to serve. **SERVES 2**

breakfast fritters

4 cups (400g) cauliflower florets, finely chopped
1 cup (120g) coarsely grated eggplant (aubergine) cheeks
    (about 1 medium eggplant)
2 cups (360g) coarsely grated zucchini (courgette)
    (about 3 zucchinis)
¾ cup (70g) coarsely grated firm goat's cheese
2 eggwhites
¼ cup (45g) white rice flour*
1 tablespoon finely grated lemon rind
¼ cup chopped flat-leaf parsley
extra virgin olive oil, for frying
labne (yoghurt cheese), to serve
poached eggs (optional), to serve
baby (micro) mint leaves (optional), ground sumac*
    and lemon wedges, to serve

add a poached egg to each plate for an extra sunny start to the day

Place the cauliflower, eggplant, zucchini, goat's cheese, eggwhites,
flour, lemon rind and parsley in a bowl and mix well to combine.
Heat a little of the oil in a non-stick frying pan over medium heat.
Add ½ cup (60ml) of the mixture to the pan and flatten slightly.
Cook for 3 minutes each side or until golden. Set aside and keep
warm. Repeat with the oil and remaining mixture. Divide fritters
between serving plates and top with labne, poached eggs and
mint. Sprinkle with sumac and serve with lemon wedges. **SERVES 4**

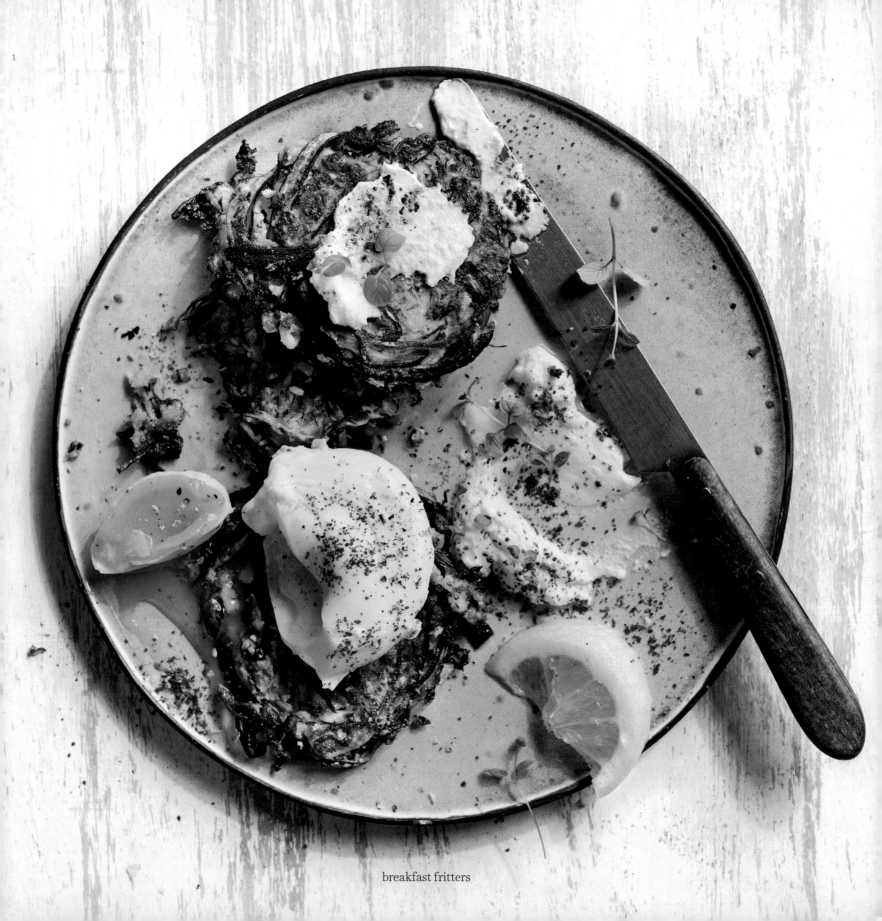

breakfast fritters

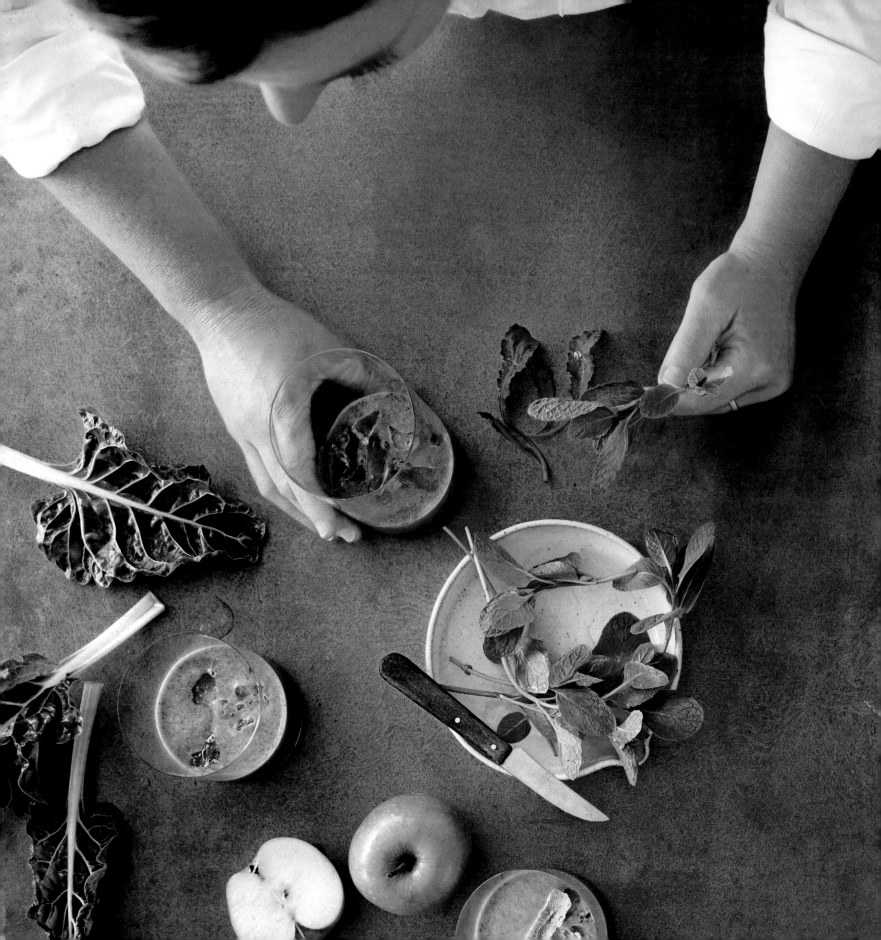

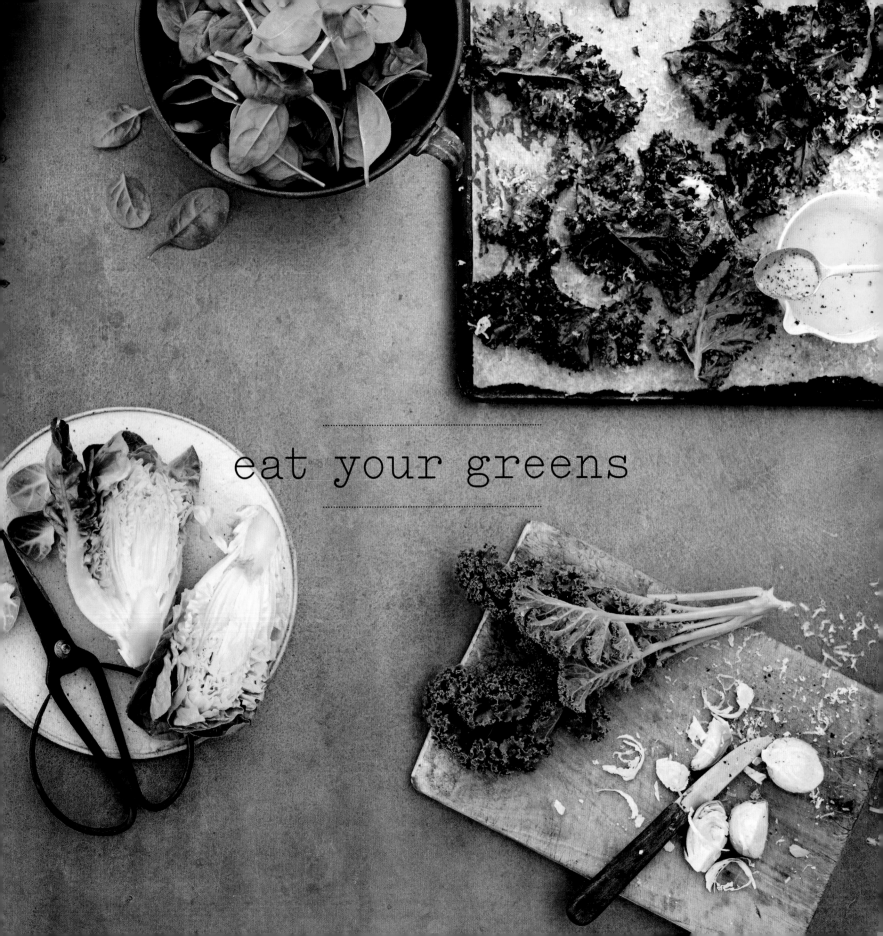

eat your greens

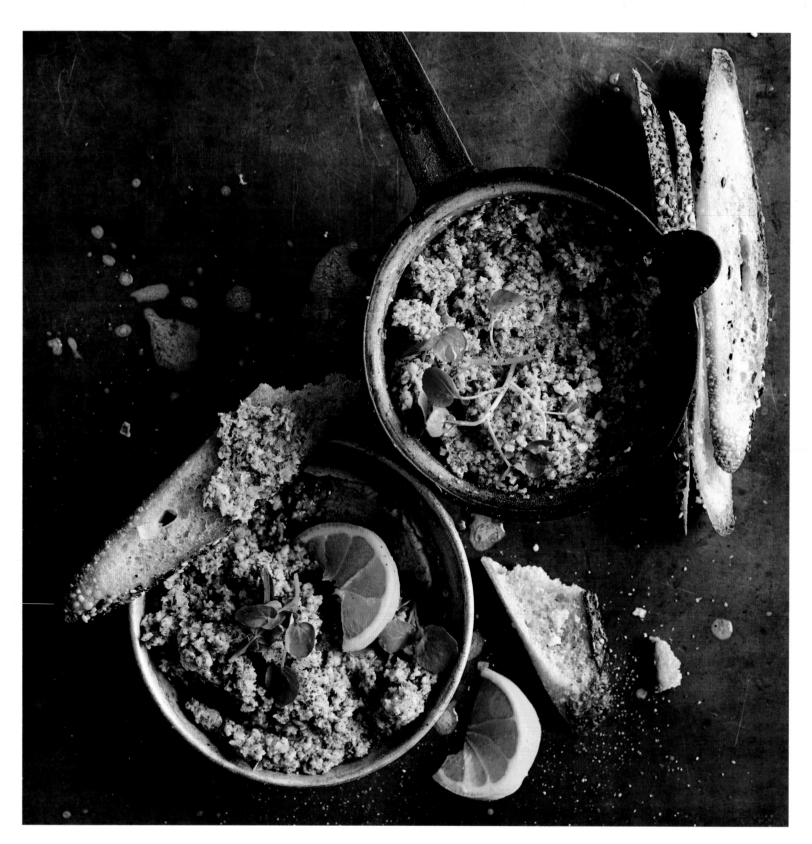

watercress, broccoli and roasted garlic pesto

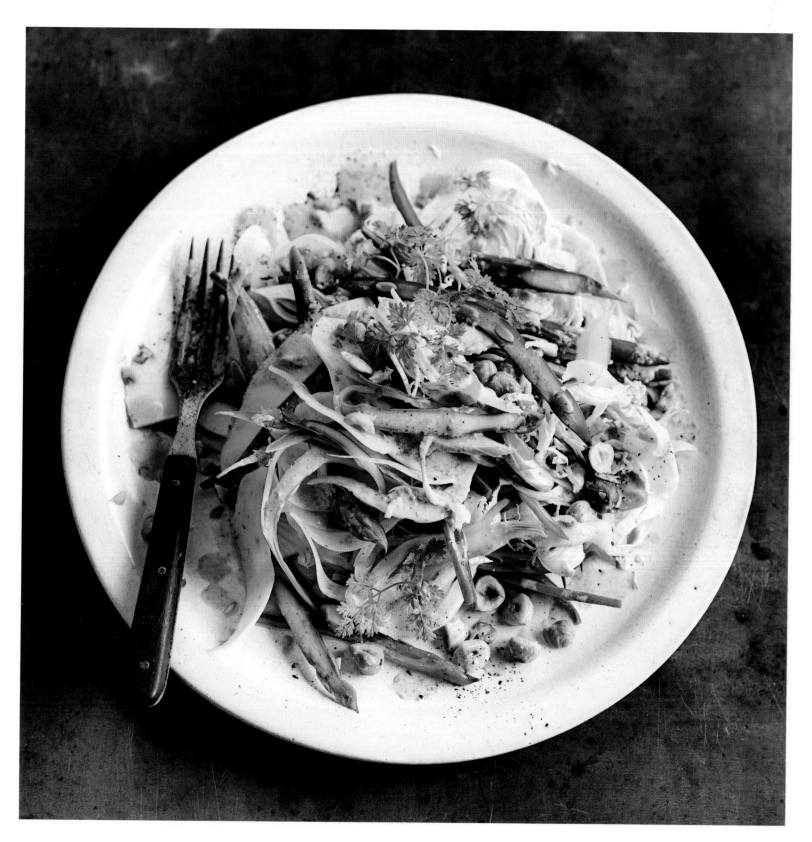

green vegetable salad

watercress, broccoli and roasted garlic pesto

head garlic
½ tablespoons extra virgin olive oil, for drizzling
cups (360g) broccoli florets
2 cups (30g) watercress sprigs, plus extra to serve
½ cup (80g) roasted almonds
2 teaspoons finely grated lemon rind
2 tablespoons lemon juice
½ cup (40g) finely grated parmesan
cup (180ml) extra virgin olive oil, extra
char-grilled bread and lemon wedges, to serve

Preheat oven to 180°C (350°F). Place the garlic on a sheet
of aluminium foil, drizzle with the oil and wrap to enclose.
Roast for 30 minutes or until golden and soft. Allow to cool
and squeeze the cloves from their skin into a food processor.
Add the broccoli, watercress, almonds, lemon rind and juice,
parmesan and extra oil and process to a coarse paste. Serve
with bread, lemon wedges and extra watercress. **MAKES 3 CUPS**

green vegetable salad

200g Brussels sprouts, blanched and sliced
bunch asparagus (150g), blanched and sliced
50g green beans, trimmed, blanched and shredded
small fennel bulb (180g), trimmed and thinly sliced
50g ricotta salata*, shaved
½ cup chervil sprigs
⅓ cup (45g) roasted hazelnuts, skins removed and chopped
green dressing
¼ cup (70g) plain Greek-style (thick) yoghurt
¼ cup (60ml) buttermilk
2 tablespoons each chopped tarragon and chopped chives
2 tablespoons lemon juice
clove garlic, crushed
anchovies, finely chopped
sea salt and cracked black pepper

To make the green dressing, place all the ingredients in a jug and,
using a hand-held stick blender, blend until smooth.
    Place the vegetables in a large bowl and toss to combine. Divide
between serving plates and top with the ricotta salata. Drizzle with
the dressing and top with the chervil and hazelnuts to serve. **SERVES 4**

kale and spinach omelette

2 stalks kale, trimmed and chopped
250g frozen spinach, thawed and drained
4 eggs, separated
⅓ cup (80ml) milk
sea salt and cracked black pepper
¼ cup (20g) finely grated parmesan, plus extra to serve
¼ cup (30g) grated cheddar
¼ cup (60g) soft goat's cheese
½ cup (120g) fresh ricotta
1 tablespoon chopped chives
20g unsalted butter
frozen peas, cooked and crushed, to serve

Place the kale and spinach in a food processor and process until
finely chopped. Place the egg yolks, milk, salt and pepper in a
large bowl and whisk to combine. Add the kale mixture, parmesan
and cheddar and mix to combine. Place the eggwhites in a bowl
and whisk until stiff peaks form. Add to the yolk mixture and
gently fold to combine. Place the goat's cheese, ricotta and chives
in a small bowl and mix to combine.
    Melt half the butter in a 20cm non-stick frying pan over
medium heat. Add half the egg mixture and cook for 5–6 minutes
or until just set. Spoon half the goat's cheese mixture onto one
side of the omelette and, using a spatula, carefully fold to enclose.
Cook for a further 1 minute, remove from the pan, set aside and
keep warm. Repeat with the remaining butter, egg mixture and
goat's cheese mixture. Place the omelettes on serving plates, top
with the peas and sprinkle with extra parmesan to serve. **SERVES 2**

to trim kale, run a small sharp knife along each side of the firm stem and discard

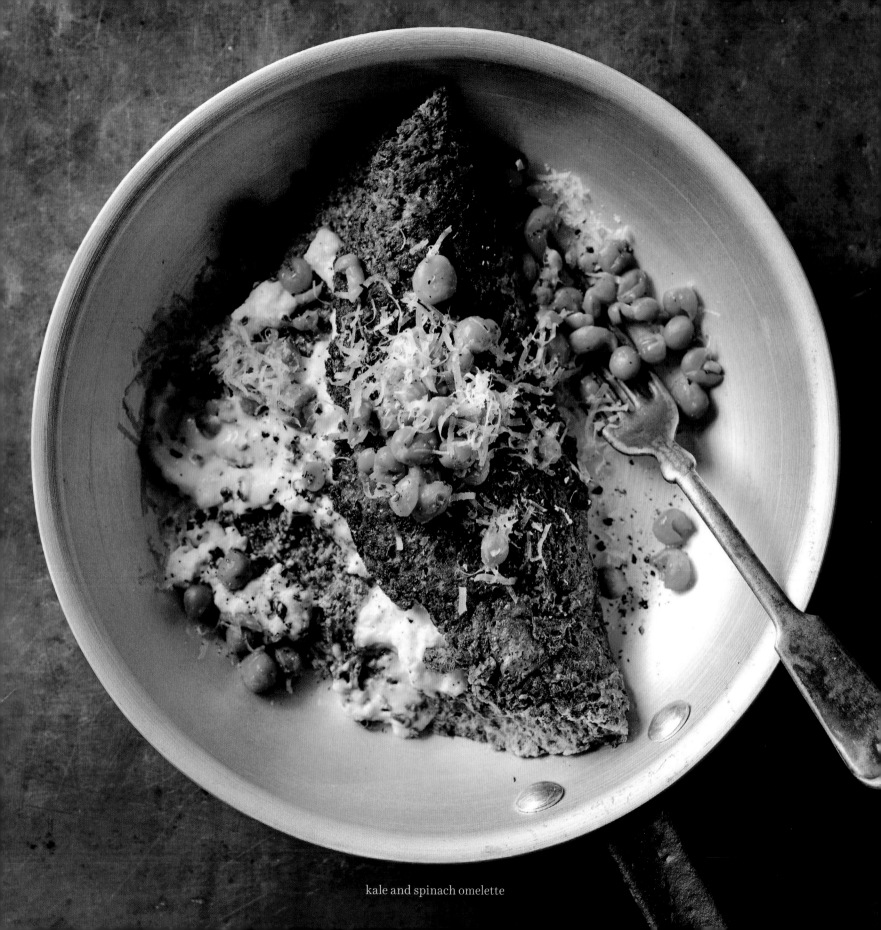

kale and spinach omelette

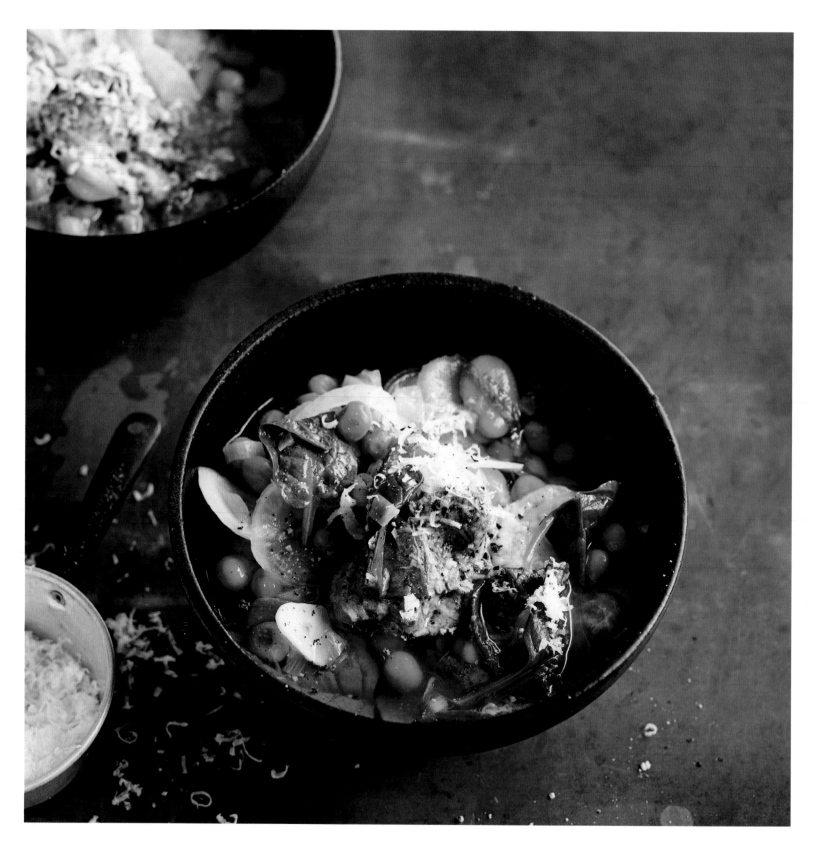

green minestrone

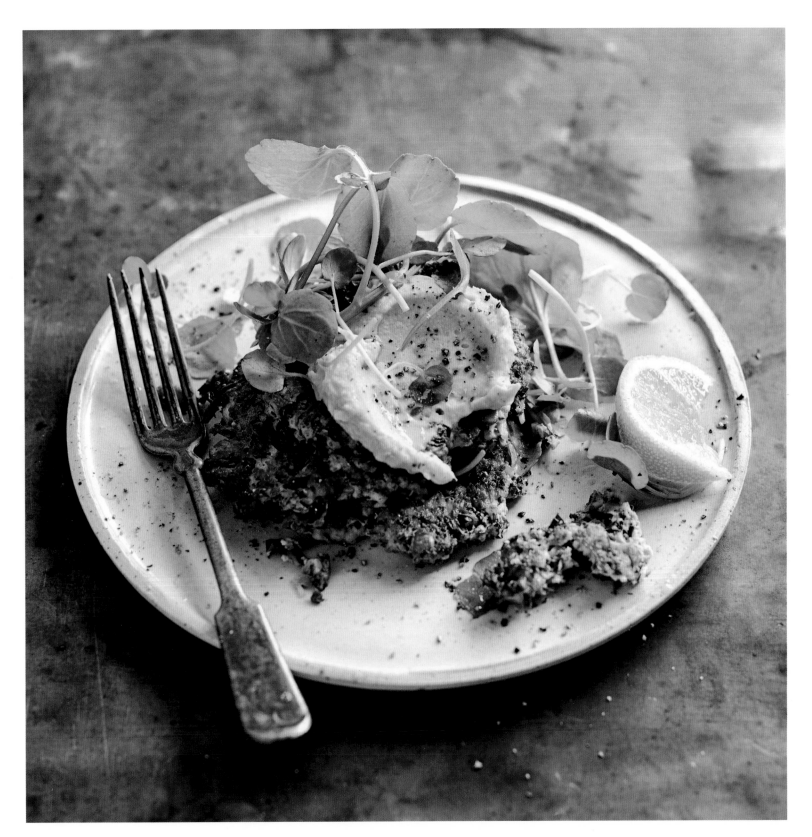

kale, pea and ricotta fritters

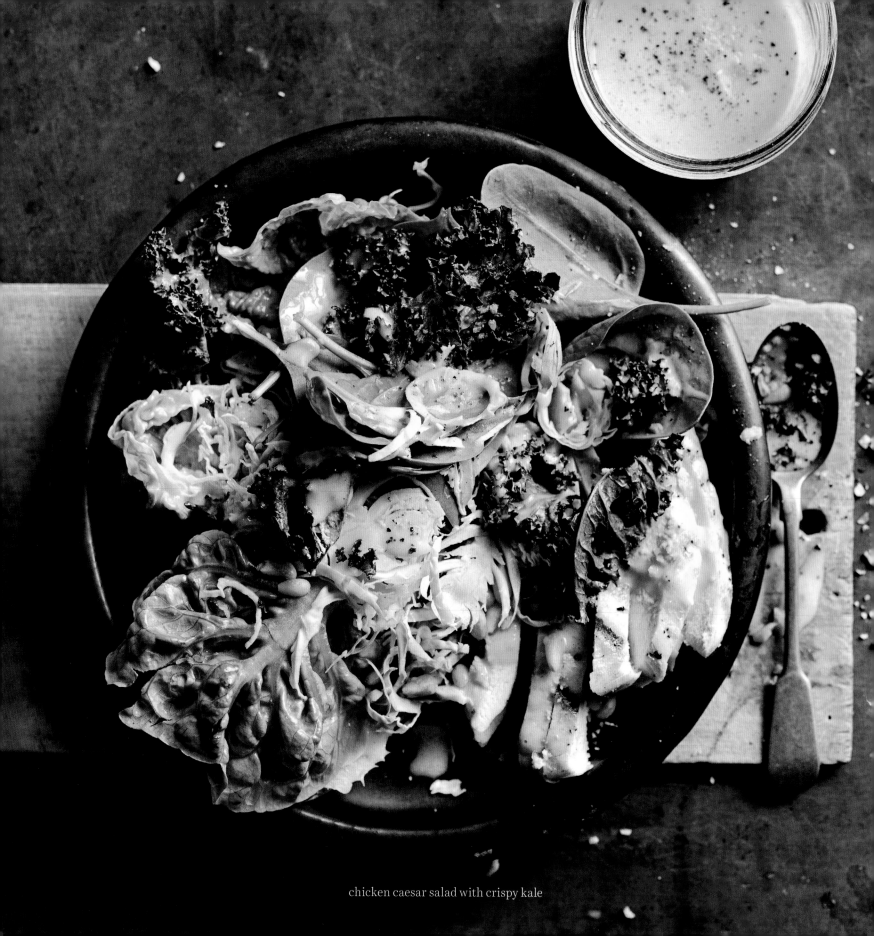

chicken caesar salad with crispy kale

green minestrone

2 tablespoons extra virgin olive oil
3 cloves garlic, thinly sliced
1 white onion, finely chopped
1 leek, white part only, finely chopped
1.5 litres chicken or vegetable stock
1 small fennel bulb (180g), trimmed and thinly sliced
2 stalks celery, sliced
2 cups (240g) frozen peas
1 cup (150g) peeled broad beans
4 cups (100g) baby spinach leaves
sea salt and cracked black pepper
¾ cup (195g) store-bought kale or basil pesto
finely grated parmesan, to serve

Heat the oil in a large saucepan over high heat. Add the garlic, onion and leek and cook, stirring, for 5–7 minutes or until softened. Add the stock and bring to the boil. Add the fennel, celery, peas and broad beans and cook for a further 5 minutes or until the vegetables are tender. Add the spinach, salt and pepper and stir to combine. Divide between serving bowls and top with the pesto and parmesan to serve. **SERVES 4**

kale, pea and ricotta fritters

1 cup (120g) frozen peas, thawed and crushed
3 cups (150g) finely shredded kale leaves
1 cup (240g) fresh ricotta
3 eggs
⅓ cup (50g) chia seeds*
1 tablespoon finely grated lemon rind
2 tablespoons chopped mint leaves
sea salt and cracked black pepper
2 tablespoons extra virgin olive oil
baba ganoush, watercress sprigs and lemon wedges, to serve

Place the peas, kale, ricotta, eggs, chia seeds, lemon rind, mint, salt and pepper in a bowl, mix to combine and allow to stand for 20 minutes.
Heat a little of the oil in a large non-stick frying pan over medium heat. Shape the mixture into 2-tablespoon patties and flatten slightly. Cook, in batches, for 2–3 minutes each side or until golden, adding more oil as necessary. Divide between serving plates and top with baba ganoush. Serve with watercress and lemon wedges. **MAKES 16**

chicken caesar salad with crispy kale

4 x 200g chicken breast fillets, trimmed
extra virgin olive oil, for brushing
sea salt and cracked black pepper
1 cup (200g) shredded Brussels sprouts
2 baby cos (romaine) lettuces (360g),
  trimmed and leaves separated
3 cups (75g) baby spinach leaves
½ cup (80g) pine nuts
crispy kale
8 stalks kale, trimmed
2 tablespoons extra virgin olive oil
⅓ cup (25g) finely grated parmesan
sea salt and cracked black pepper
dressing
3 egg yolks
3 cloves garlic, crushed
1 tablespoon Dijon mustard
¼ cup (60ml) extra virgin olive oil
1 tablespoon apple cider vinegar

To make the dressing, place the egg yolks, garlic and mustard in a bowl and whisk until thick and creamy. Gradually add half the oil, whisking continuously until combined. Gradually add the vinegar and the remaining oil, whisking to combine. Set aside.
To make the crispy kale, preheat oven to 150°C (300°F). Place the kale, oil, parmesan, salt and pepper in a bowl and toss to coat. Place in a single layer on baking trays lined with non-stick baking paper. Bake for 15–20 minutes or until crisp, and set aside.
Brush the chicken with oil and sprinkle with salt and pepper. Heat a char-grill pan or barbecue over high heat. Cook the chicken for 2–3 minutes each side or until cooked through. Slice the chicken and place in a large bowl. Add the Brussels sprout, lettuce, spinach and pine nuts and toss to combine. Divide between serving plates and top with crispy kale and the dressing to serve. **SERVES 4**

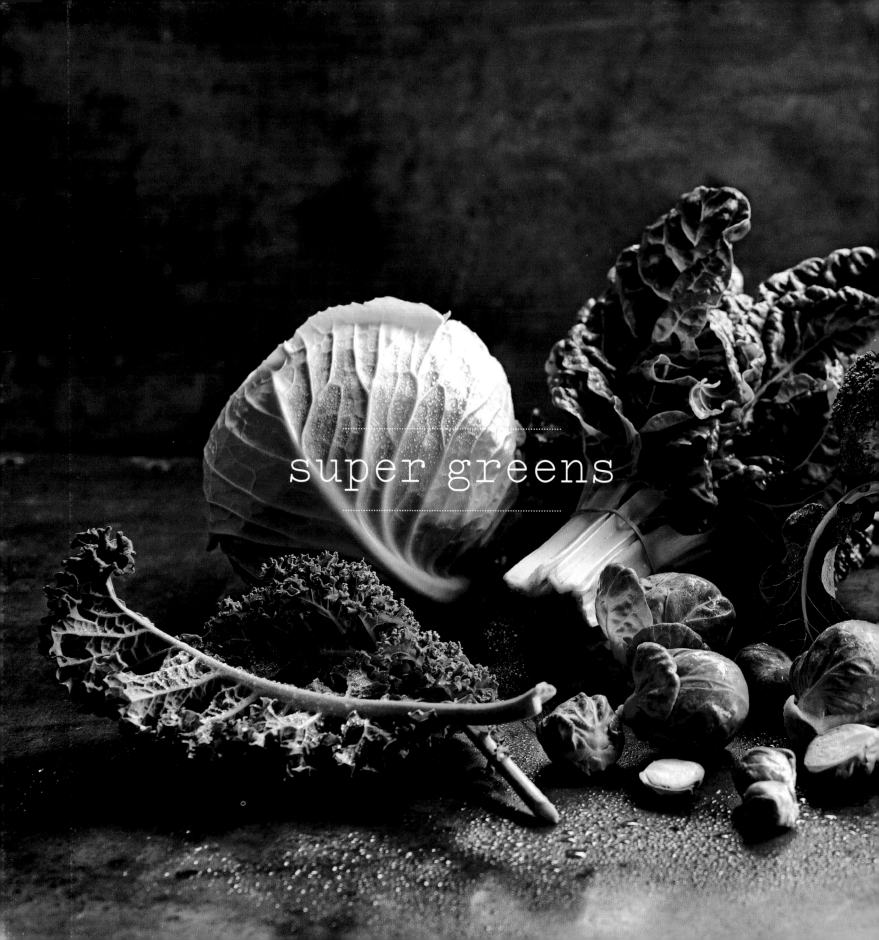

super greens

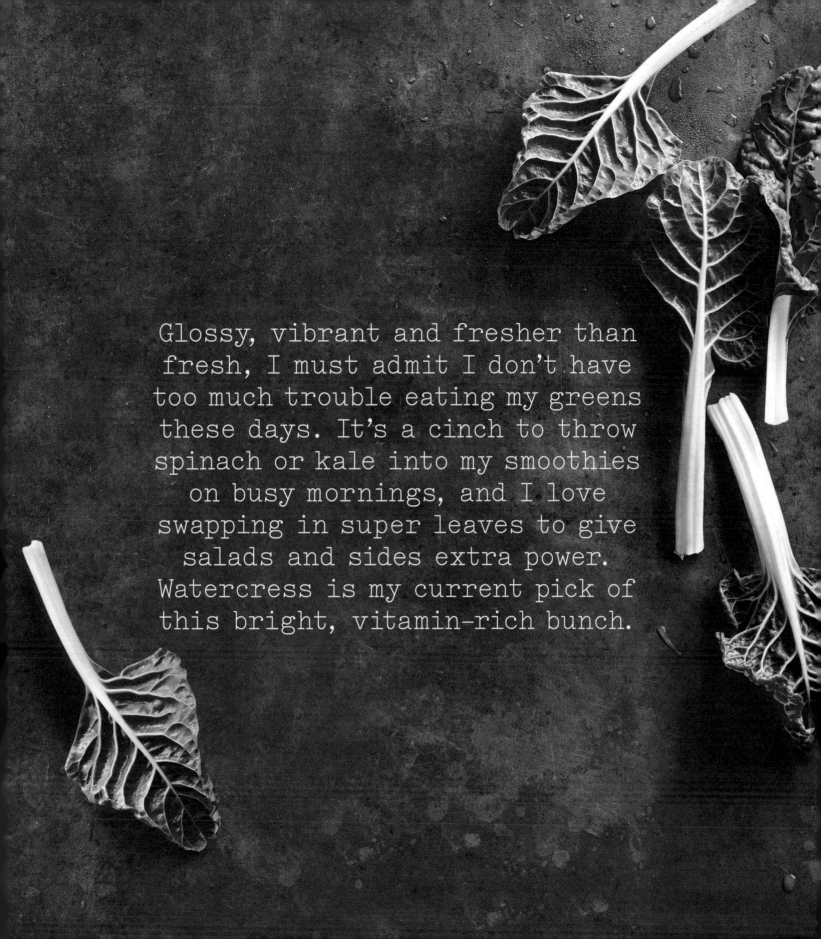

Glossy, vibrant and fresher than fresh, I must admit I don't have too much trouble eating my greens these days. It's a cinch to throw spinach or kale into my smoothies on busy mornings, and I love swapping in super leaves to give salads and sides extra power. Watercress is my current pick of this bright, vitamin-rich bunch.

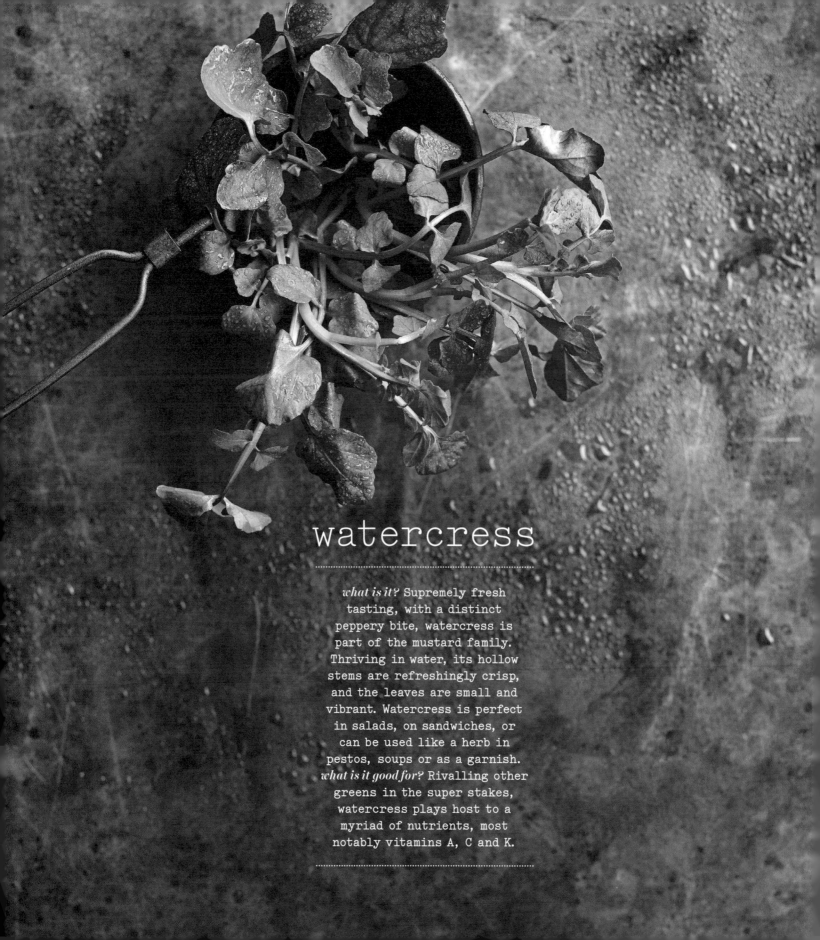

watercress

·······································

what is it? Supremely fresh
tasting, with a distinct
peppery bite, watercress is
part of the mustard family.
Thriving in water, its hollow
stems are refreshingly crisp,
and the leaves are small and
vibrant. Watercress is perfect
in salads, on sandwiches, or
can be used like a herb in
pestos, soups or as a garnish.
what is it good for? Rivalling other
greens in the super stakes,
watercress plays host to a
myriad of nutrients, most
notably vitamins A, C and K.

·······································

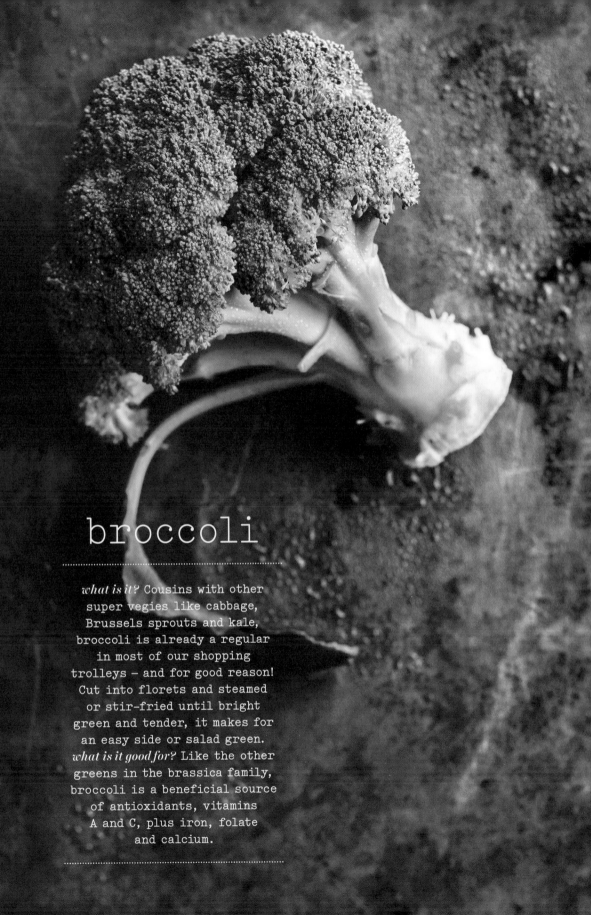

broccoli

what is it? Cousins with other
super vegies like cabbage,
Brussels sprouts and kale,
broccoli is already a regular
in most of our shopping
trolleys – and for good reason!
Cut into florets and steamed
or stir-fried until bright
green and tender, it makes for
an easy side or salad green.
what is it good for? Like the other
greens in the brassica family,
broccoli is a beneficial source
of antioxidants, vitamins
A and C, plus iron, folate
and calcium.

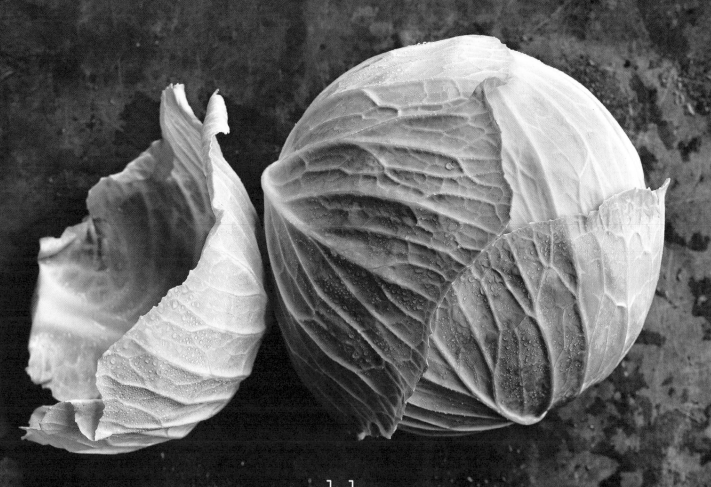

cabbage

· ·

what is it? In all its different
shapes, sizes and varieties,
– such as green, white, Savoy
and Chinese (wombok) – cabbage
is characterised by its waxy
layered leaves and crunchy
texture. Whether shredded into
crisp tangy slaws, cooked into
soft creamy sides, or pickled
into sauerkraut or kimchi,
this member of the brassicas
boasts plenty of goodness.
what is it good for? Vitamins A,
C and K, plus antioxidants and
minerals, make humble cabbage
a super smart choice.

· ·

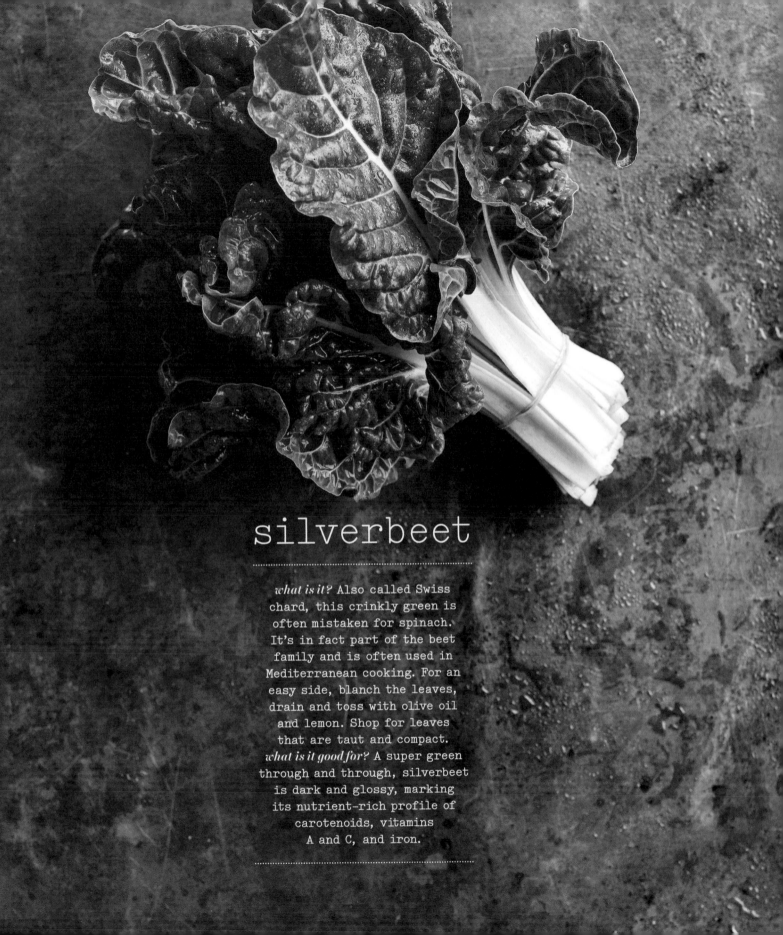

silverbeet

what is it? Also called Swiss
chard, this crinkly green is
often mistaken for spinach.
It's in fact part of the beet
family and is often used in
Mediterranean cooking. For an
easy side, blanch the leaves,
drain and toss with olive oil
and lemon. Shop for leaves
that are taut and compact.

what is it good for? A super green
through and through, silverbeet
is dark and glossy, marking
its nutrient-rich profile of
carotenoids, vitamins
A and C, and iron.

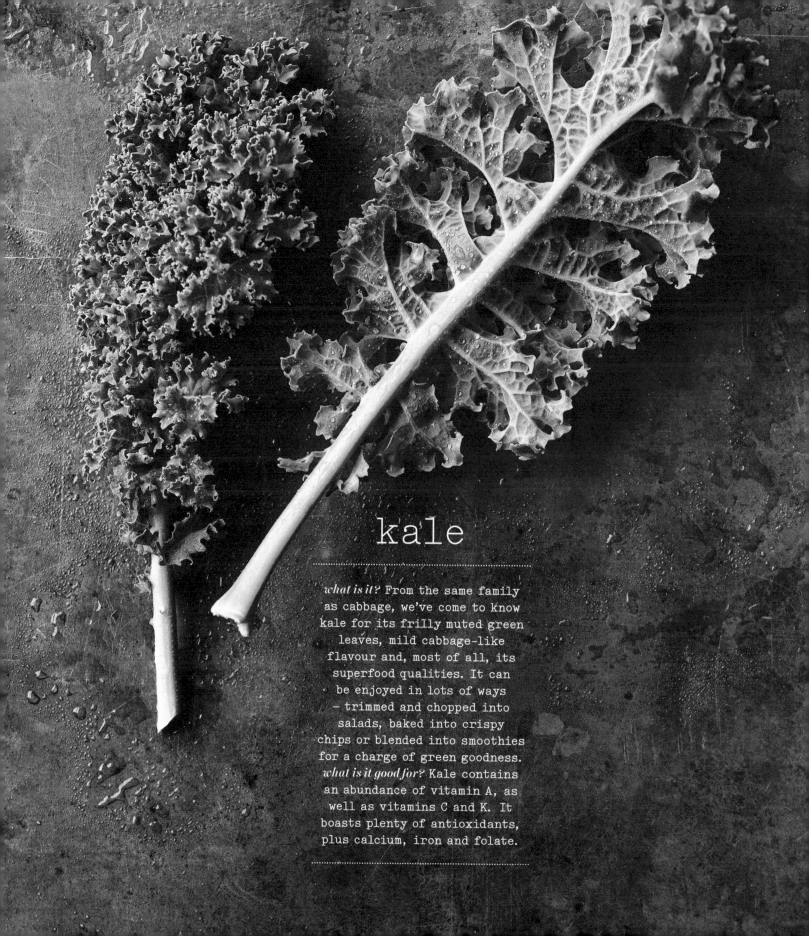

kale

what is it? From the same family as cabbage, we've come to know kale for its frilly muted green leaves, mild cabbage-like flavour and, most of all, its superfood qualities. It can be enjoyed in lots of ways – trimmed and chopped into salads, baked into crispy chips or blended into smoothies for a charge of green goodness. *what is it good for?* Kale contains an abundance of vitamin A, as well as vitamins C and K. It boasts plenty of antioxidants, plus calcium, iron and folate.

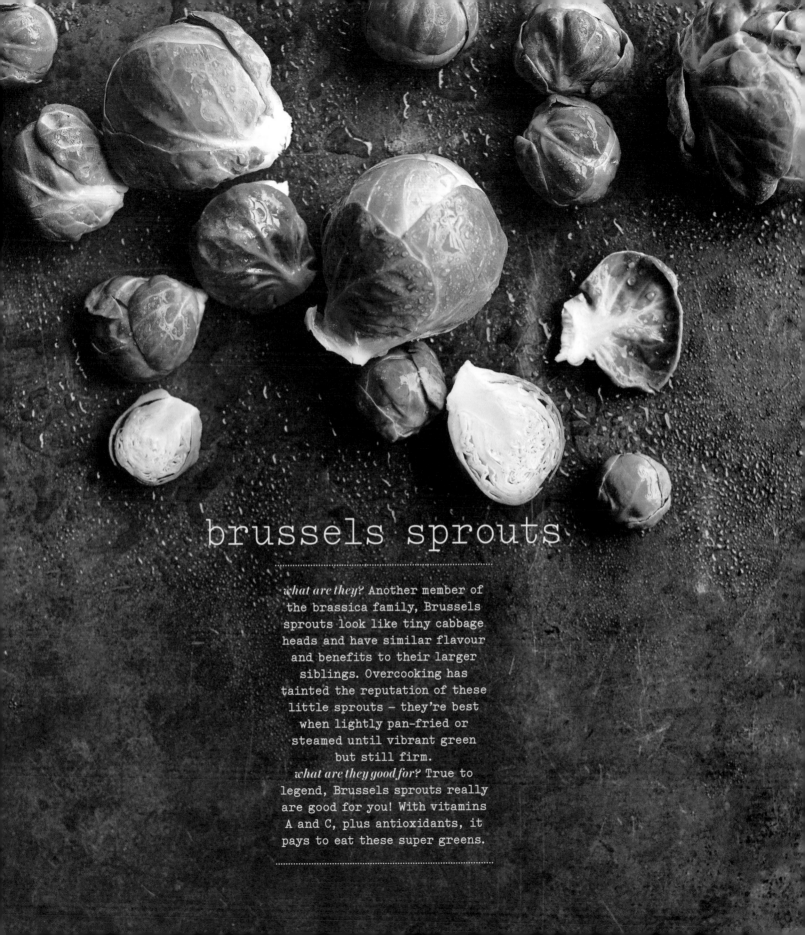

brussels sprouts

what are they? Another member of the brassica family, Brussels sprouts look like tiny cabbage heads and have similar flavour and benefits to their larger siblings. Overcooking has tainted the reputation of these little sprouts – they're best when lightly pan-fried or steamed until vibrant green but still firm.

what are they good for? True to legend, Brussels sprouts really are good for you! With vitamins A and C, plus antioxidants, it pays to eat these super greens.

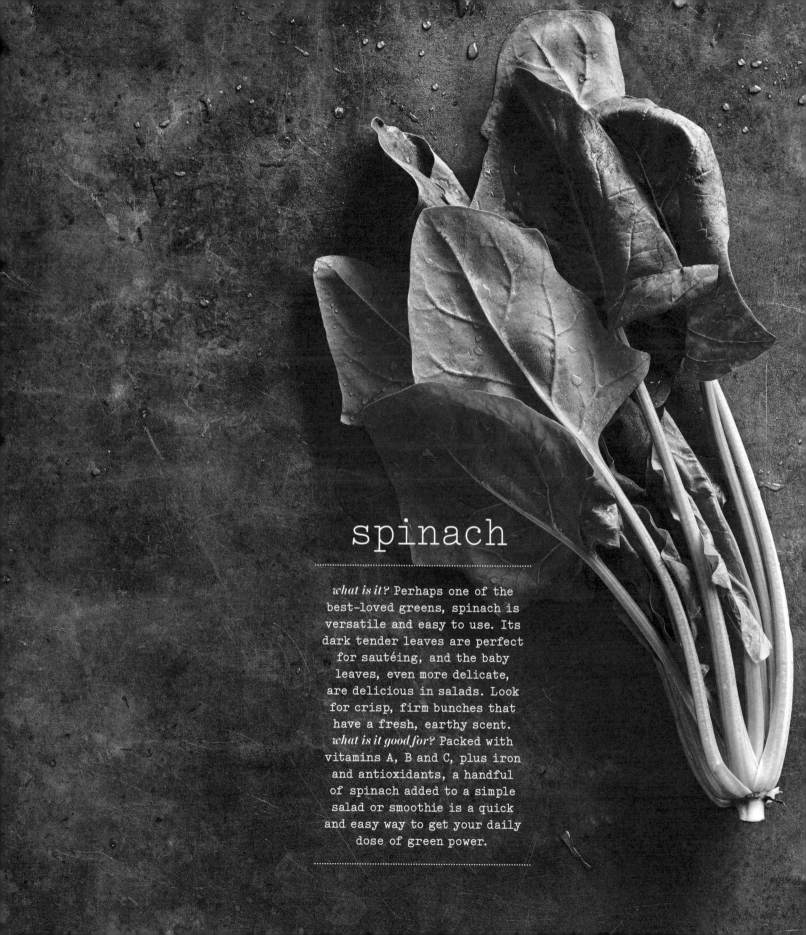

spinach

what is it? Perhaps one of the best-loved greens, spinach is versatile and easy to use. Its dark tender leaves are perfect for sautéing, and the baby leaves, even more delicate, are delicious in salads. Look for crisp, firm bunches that have a fresh, earthy scent. *what is it good for?* Packed with vitamins A, B and C, plus iron and antioxidants, a handful of spinach added to a simple salad or smoothie is a quick and easy way to get your daily dose of green power.

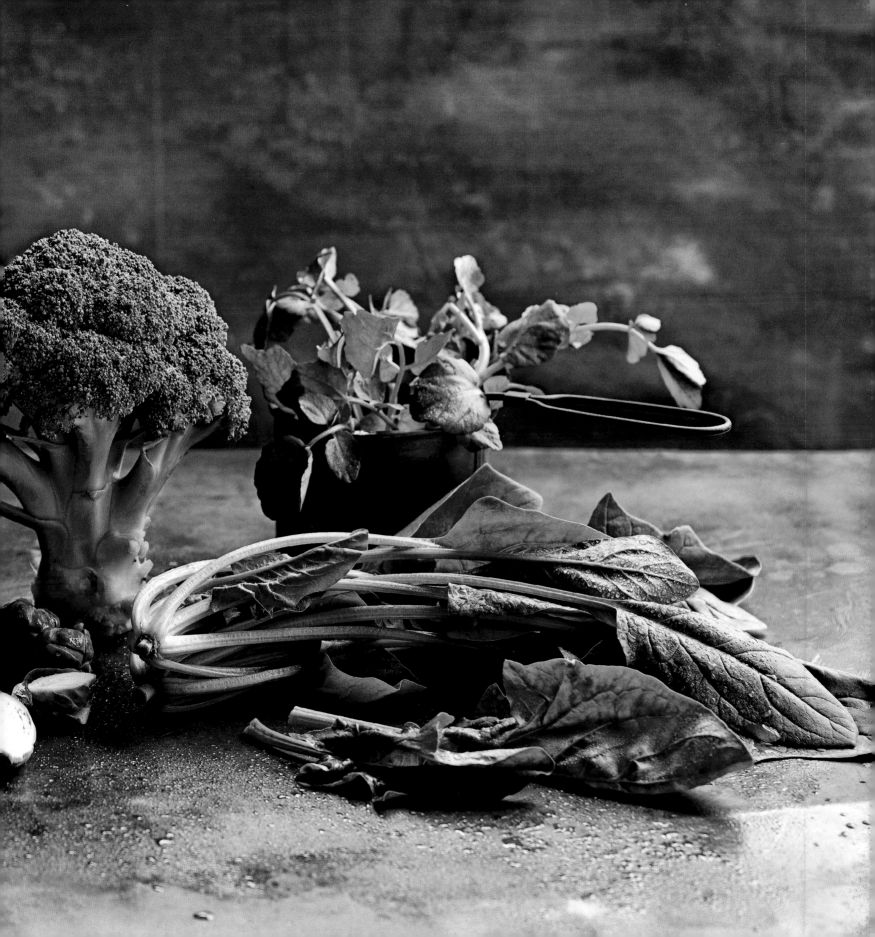

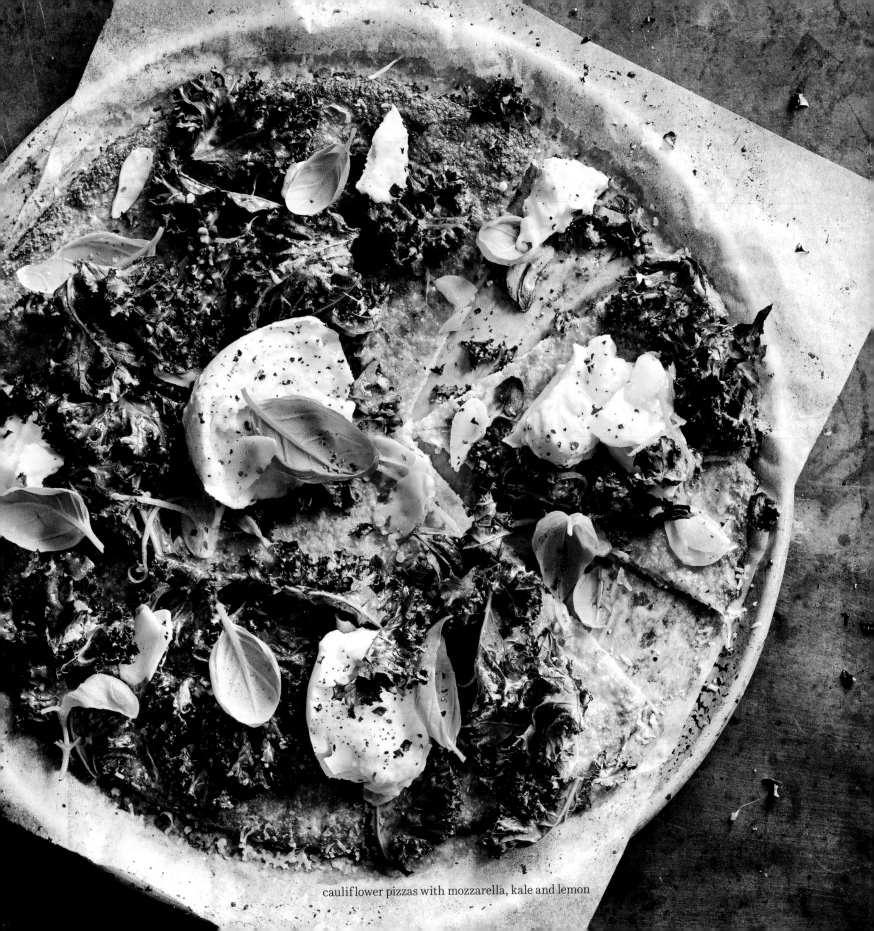

cauliflower pizzas with mozzarella, kale and lemon

cauliflower pizzas with mozzarella, kale and lemon

8 stalks kale, trimmed
2 tablespoons extra virgin olive oil
3 cloves garlic, sliced
½ teaspoon dried chilli flakes
1 tablespoon lemon zest
¼ cup (20g) finely grated parmesan
1 x 125g buffalo mozzarella, torn
⅓ cup small basil leaves
cauliflower pizza bases
6 cups (600g) cauliflower florets, roughly chopped
¾ cup (90g) almond meal (ground almonds)
½ cup (40g) finely grated parmesan
3 eggs, lightly beaten
sea salt and cracked black pepper

Preheat oven to 200°C (400°F). To make the cauliflower pizza bases, lightly grease 2 x 30cm round pizza trays and line with non-stick baking paper. Place the cauliflower, in batches, in a food processor and process until the mixture resembles fine crumbs. Transfer to a large bowl, add the almond meal, parmesan, egg, salt and pepper and mix until a soft dough forms. Divide the mixture in half and press into the prepared trays. Bake for 20–25 minutes or until golden and crisp.

Place the kale, oil, garlic, chilli and lemon zest in a bowl and toss to coat. Divide the mixture between the bases and top with the parmesan. Bake for 8–10 minutes or until the kale is crisp. Top each pizza with mozzarella and basil to serve. **SERVES 4**

kale, snow pea and pork dumplings

2½ cups (125g) finely shredded kale leaves
100g snow peas (mange tout), trimmed and finely chopped
2 tablespoons finely chopped water chestnuts*
½ cup coriander (cilantro) leaves, chopped
2 tablespoons chopped garlic chives
1 teaspoon finely grated ginger
1 tablespoon mirin (Japanese rice wine)
1 teaspoon sesame oil
150g pork mince
sea salt and cracked black pepper
30 gow gee wrappers
green onions (scallions), thinly sliced, to serve
chilli sauce and Chinese black vinegar, to serve

snow peas and water chestnuts add a little fresh crunch to these tasty dumplings

Place the kale, snow pea, water chestnut, coriander, chive, ginger, mirin, oil, pork, salt and pepper in a large bowl and mix well to combine.

Place the gow gee wrappers on a clean benchtop and brush the edges with water. Place 1 teaspoon of the kale mixture in the centre of each wrapper. Fold the edges of the wrappers over and press together to seal.

Place a steamer lined with non-stick baking paper over a saucepan of simmering water. Steam the dumplings, in batches, for 10–12 minutes or until cooked through. Top with the onion and serve with chilli sauce and black vinegar. **MAKES 30**

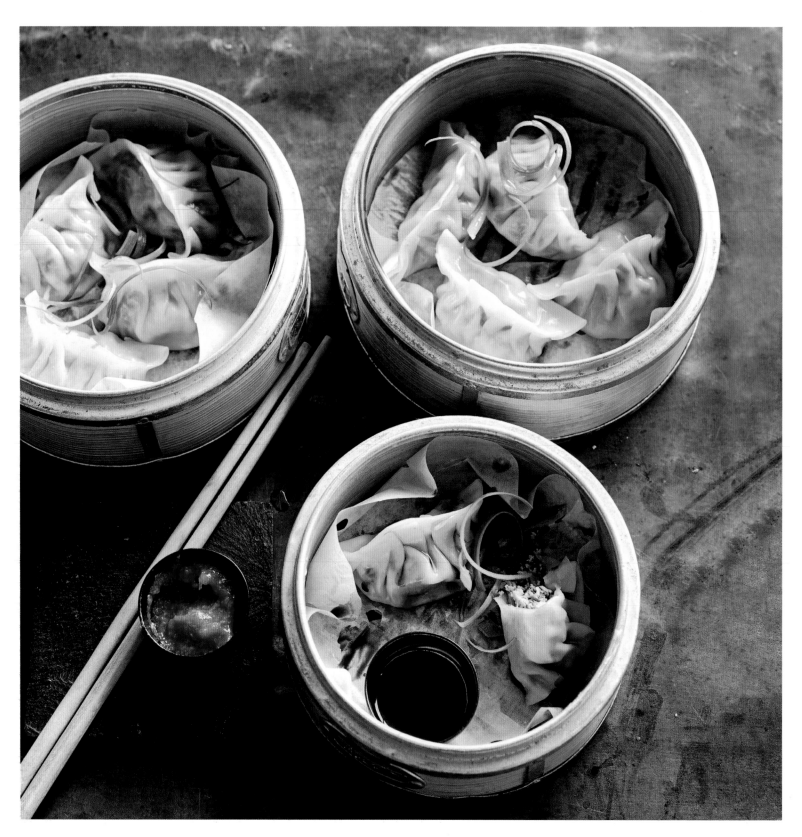

kale, snow pea and pork dumplings

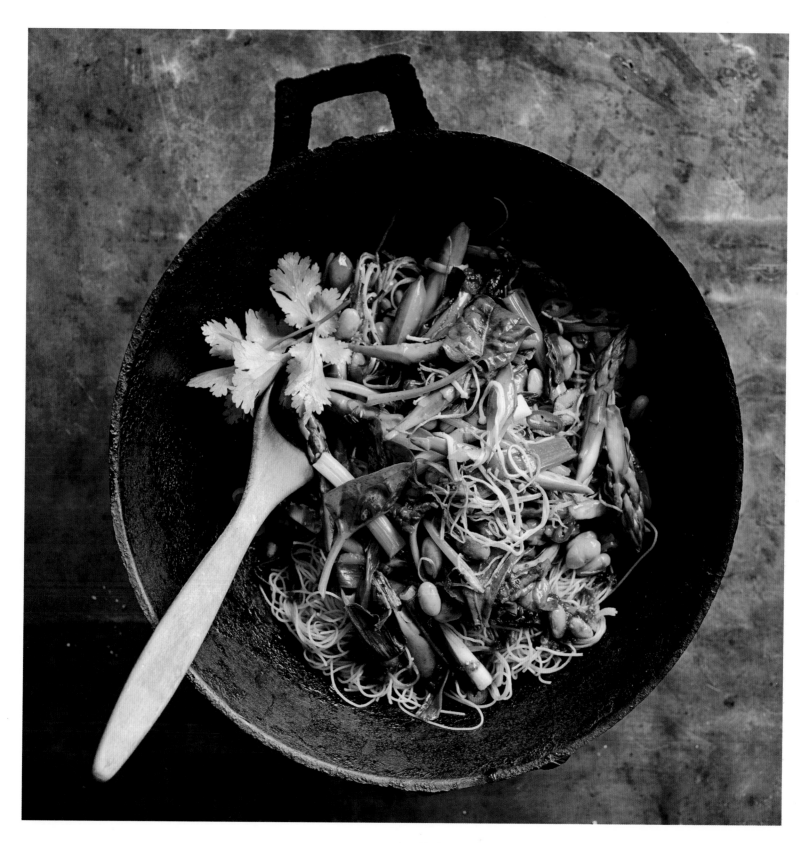

super green stir-fry

super green stir-fry

2 tablespoons peanut oil
1 tablespoon finely shredded ginger
2 cloves garlic, thinly sliced
2 bunches asparagus (300g), sliced
2 green onions (scallions), sliced
200g sugar snap peas, trimmed and halved
2 tablespoons chilli bean paste*
2 tablespoons light soy sauce
2 teaspoons water
1 cup (140g) podded edamame*
200g enoki mushrooms
250g English spinach, trimmed
250g thin brown rice noodles, cooked and drained
thinly sliced small red chilli or store-bought
    Asian chilli jam, to serve
coriander (cilantro) leaves, to serve

find edamame in the freezer section of your supermarket or at asian grocers

Heat the oil in a large non-stick frying pan or wok over high heat. Add the ginger and garlic and cook for 1 minute. Add the asparagus, onion and peas and cook, stirring, for a further 1 minute. Add the chilli bean paste, soy sauce and water and cook, stirring, for 1–2 minutes or until combined. Add the edamame, enoki, spinach and noodles, toss to combine and cook for 1 minute or until warmed through. Top with the chilli and coriander to serve. **SERVES 4**

silverbeet and cavolo nero whole-wheat pies

2 tablespoons extra virgin olive oil
2 cloves garlic, crushed
1 small celeriac (celery root) (500g), peeled and grated
2 tablespoons lemon thyme leaves
3 stalks silverbeet (Swiss chard), trimmed and shredded
3 stalks cavolo nero (Tuscan kale), trimmed and shredded
1 tablespoon chopped dill
1 cup (240g) fresh ricotta
sea salt and cracked black pepper
100g soft goat's cheese, sliced into 4 rounds
1 egg, lightly beaten
poppyseeds and extra lemon thyme sprigs, for sprinkling
whole-wheat pastry
1 cup (140g) wholemeal spelt flour*
2 cups (300g) whole-wheat flour*, plus extra for dusting
½ cup (40g) psyllium husk powder*
1 teaspoon sea salt flakes
300g cold unsalted butter, chopped
2 egg yolks
2 tablespoons iced water

To make the whole-wheat pastry, place both the flours, the psyllium husk power, salt and butter in a food processor and process until the mixture resembles coarse crumbs. Add the egg yolks and water and process until a soft dough forms. Turn out onto a lightly floured surface, divide in half and shape into 2 discs. Wrap in plastic wrap and refrigerate for 30 minutes.

Preheat oven to 190°C (375°F). Heat the oil in a large non-stick frying pan over medium heat. Add the garlic, celeriac and lemon thyme and cook, stirring, for 8–10 minutes or until the celeriac is soft. Add the silverbeet and cavolo nero and cook, stirring, for 1 minute or until the greens are wilted. Remove from the heat, transfer to a large bowl and allow to cool. Add the dill, ricotta, salt and pepper and mix to combine.

Roll out the dough between 2 sheets of non-stick baking paper to 4mm thick. Using a sharp knife, cut 4 x 12cm rounds and 4 x 15cm rounds from the pastry. Arrange the small rounds on a baking tray lined with non-stick baking paper. Divide the ricotta mixture between them and top with the goat's cheese. Brush the edges with egg and top with the larger pastry rounds. Press the edges with a fork to seal, brush pies with egg and sprinkle with poppyseeds and extra thyme. Bake for 25–30 minutes or until golden and crisp. **MAKES 4**

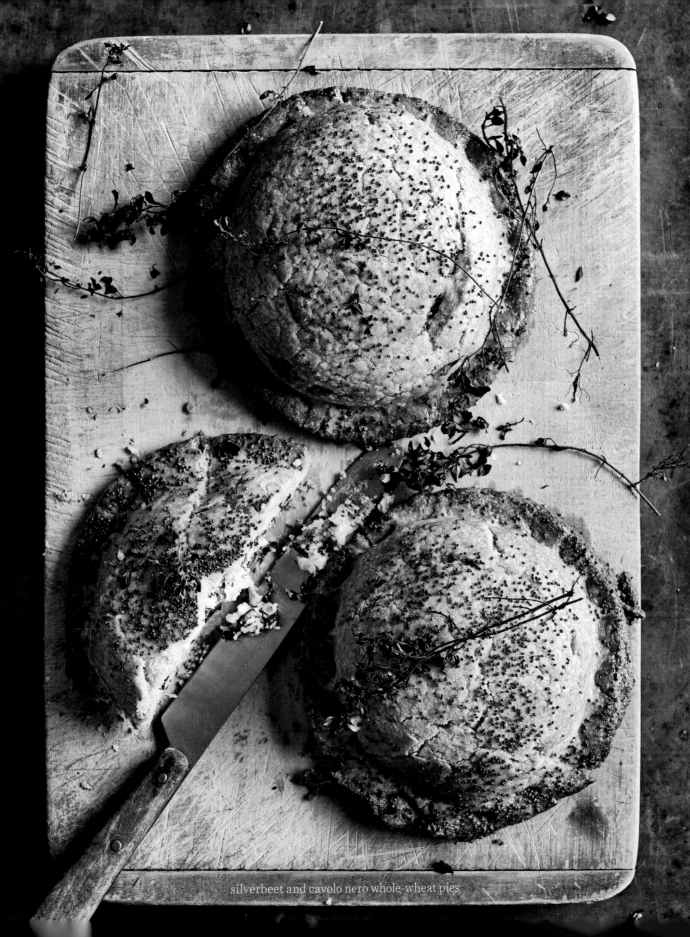

silverbeet and cavolo nero whole-wheat pies

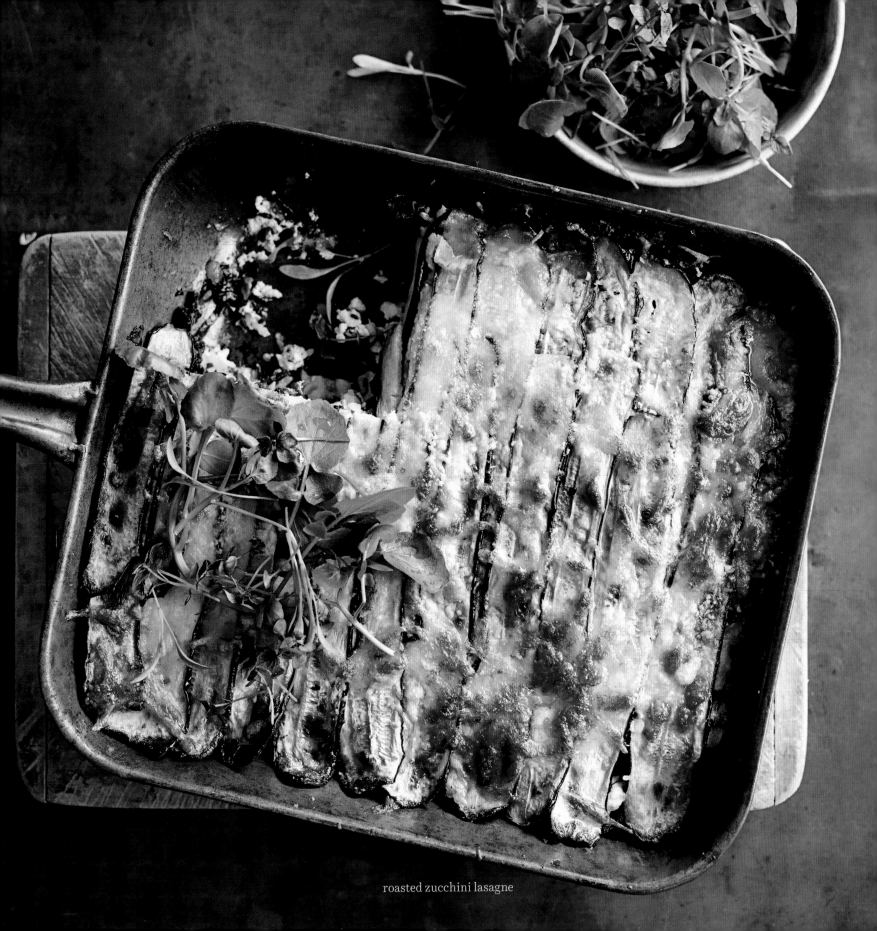

roasted zucchini lasagne

roasted zucchini lasagne

8 medium zucchinis (courgettes) (1kg), sliced into 4mm ribbons
extra virgin olive oil, for brushing, plus 2 tablespoons extra
sea salt and cracked black pepper
1 small onion, chopped
2 cloves garlic, crushed
2 tablespoons chopped oregano
1 bunch kale (500g), trimmed and blanched
1 bunch English spinach (375g), trimmed and blanched
2¼ cups (540g) fresh ricotta
1 tablespoon finely grated lemon rind
1 cup flat-leaf parsley, finely chopped
¾ cup (75g) grated mozzarella
¾ cup (60g) finely grated parmesan
baby (micro) salad mix (optional), to serve

Preheat oven to 220°C (425°F). Place the zucchini in a single layer on baking trays lined with non-stick baking paper. Brush both sides of the ribbons with oil and sprinkle with salt. Roast for 12–14 minutes or until golden.

Heat the extra oil in a medium non-stick frying pan over medium heat. Add the onion, garlic and oregano and cook for 4–5 minutes or until softened. Allow to cool slightly. Place the kale and spinach in paper towel or a clean tea towel and squeeze to remove any excess liquid. Roughly chop, add to the onion mixture and stir to combine. Place the ricotta, lemon rind, parsley, salt and pepper in a bowl and mix to combine.

Line the base of a lightly greased 2.25-litre-capacity baking dish with one-third of the roasted zucchini. Top with half the ricotta mixture and half the kale mixture. Sprinkle with one-third of the mozzarella and parmesan. Top with half the remaining zucchini, and the remaining ricotta and kale mixtures. Sprinkle with half the remaining mozzarella and parmesan. Top with the remaining zucchini and sprinkle with the remaining mozzarella and parmesan. Bake for 10–15 minutes or until crisp and golden. Slice and serve with the baby salad mix. **SERVES 4**

baked broccolini and mushroom tempura

1 cup (160g) sesame seeds, toasted
⅔ cup (120g) white rice flour*
2 teaspoons each sea salt flakes and cracked black pepper
3 bunches broccolini (525g), trimmed and blanched
2 eschalots (French shallots), thinly sliced
150g enoki mushrooms
150g oyster mushrooms
6 eggwhites, lightly whisked
vegetable oil, for drizzling
soy dressing
2 tablespoons soy sauce
1 tablespoon mirin (Japanese rice wine)
1 small red chilli, seeded and finely chopped
1 tablespoon lime juice

← *mushrooms are a great source of vitamins B and D, plus antioxidants*

Preheat oven to 220°C (425°F). To make the soy dressing, place the soy sauce, mirin, chilli and lime juice in a bowl. Whisk to combine and set aside.

Place the sesame seeds in a mortar and lightly crush with a pestle. Transfer to a bowl, add the flour, salt and pepper and mix to combine. Working in batches, dip the broccolini, eschalot and mushrooms in the eggwhite and dust with the sesame flour, shaking to remove any excess. Place in a single layer on 2 baking trays lined with non-stick baking paper. Drizzle with oil and bake for 10 minutes, turning halfway, until crisp and golden. Serve with the soy dressing. **SERVES 4**

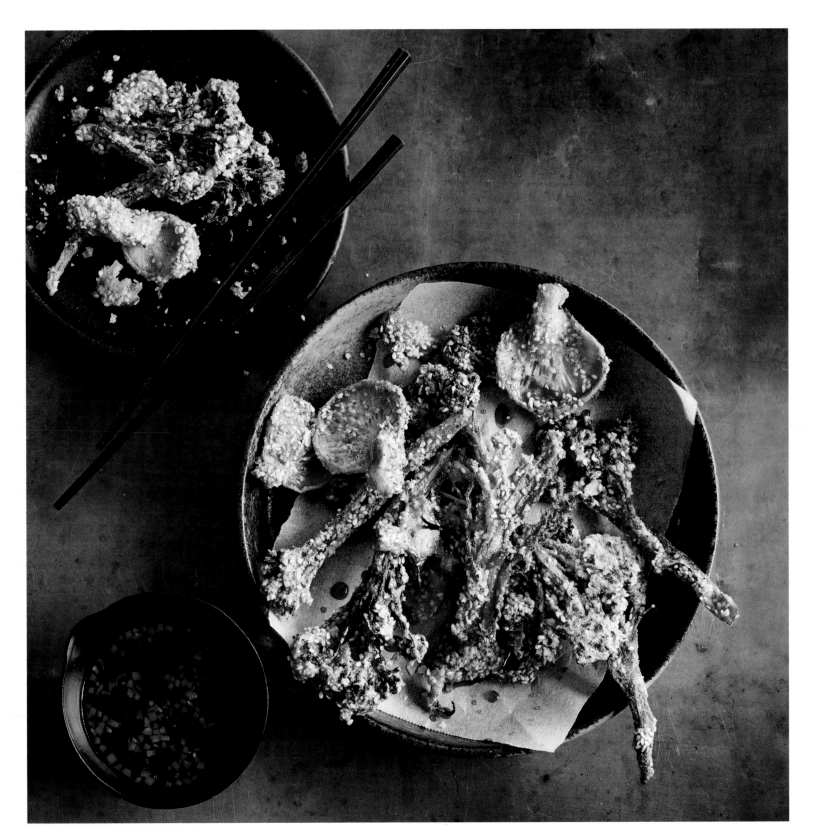

baked broccolini and mushroom tempura

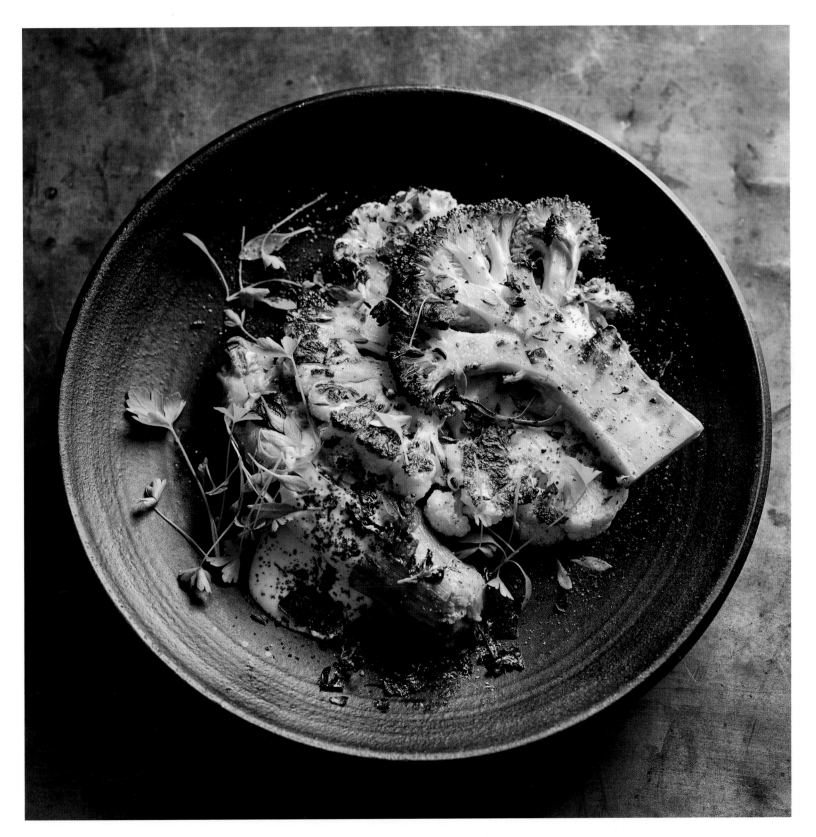

grilled cauliflower and broccoli steaks with smoky eggplant

grilled cauliflower and broccoli steaks with smoky eggplant

½ cup (125ml) extra virgin olive oil
3 cloves garlic, crushed
¼ cup oregano leaves
1 tablespoon fennel seeds, crushed
sea salt and cracked black pepper
4 x 1cm-thick slices broccoli (about 1 medium broccoli)
4 x 1cm-thick slices cauliflower (about 1 medium cauliflower)
4 small eggplants (aubergines) (800g)
baby (micro) parsley leaves (optional), to serve
ground sumac*, to serve
dressing
2 tablespoons tahini*
½ cup (140g) plain Greek-style (thick) yoghurt
⅓ cup (80ml) lemon juice
sea salt and cracked black pepper

To make the dressing, place the tahini, yoghurt, lemon juice, salt and pepper in a bowl. Mix to combine and set aside.

Place the oil, garlic, oregano, fennel seeds, salt and pepper in a bowl and mix to combine. Place the broccoli and cauliflower on a large tray lined with non-stick baking paper. Brush both sides of the steaks with the oil mixture and set aside.

Preheat a char-grill pan or barbecue over medium heat. Cook the eggplants, turning every 5–10 minutes, for 35–40 minutes or until the skins are charred and blackened. Set aside to cool slightly. Add the broccoli and cauliflower to the grill and cook for 2–3 minutes each side or until just tender.

Remove and discard the skins from the eggplants and spoon the flesh onto serving plates. Drizzle with the dressing and top with the broccoli and cauliflower. Sprinkle with parsley and sumac to serve. **SERVES 4**

brussels sprout and goat's cheese galettes

300g Brussels sprouts, blanched and quartered
2 tablespoons extra virgin olive oil
1 tablespoon finely grated lemon rind
¼ cup oregano leaves, plus extra for sprinkling
sea salt and cracked black pepper
2 tablespoons store-bought caramelised onion
50g soft goat's cheese
¼ cup (60g) fresh ricotta
1 egg, lightly beaten
whole-wheat pastry
½ cup (70g) wholemeal spelt flour*
1 cup (150g) whole-wheat flour*, plus extra for dusting
¼ cup (20g) psyllium husk powder*
150g unsalted butter, chopped
½ teaspoon sea salt flakes
1 egg yolk
1 tablespoon iced water

To make the whole-wheat pastry, place both the flours, the psyllium husk powder, butter and salt in a food processor and process until the mixture resembles coarse crumbs. Add the egg yolk and water and process until a soft dough forms. Turn out onto a lightly floured surface, divide in half and shape into 2 discs. Wrap in plastic wrap and refrigerate for 30 minutes.

Preheat oven to 190°C (375°F). Place the Brussels sprout, oil, lemon rind, oregano, salt and pepper in a bowl and toss to coat. Roll out each piece of dough between 2 sheets of non-stick baking paper to form 2 x 20cm rounds. Place on 2 baking trays and remove the top sheets of paper. Divide the caramelised onion between the pastry rounds and top with the Brussels sprout mixture, goat's cheese and ricotta. Fold in the edges of the pastry to slightly enclose and brush the edges with egg. Sprinkle the galettes with the extra oregano and bake for 25–30 minutes or until golden. **SERVES 4**

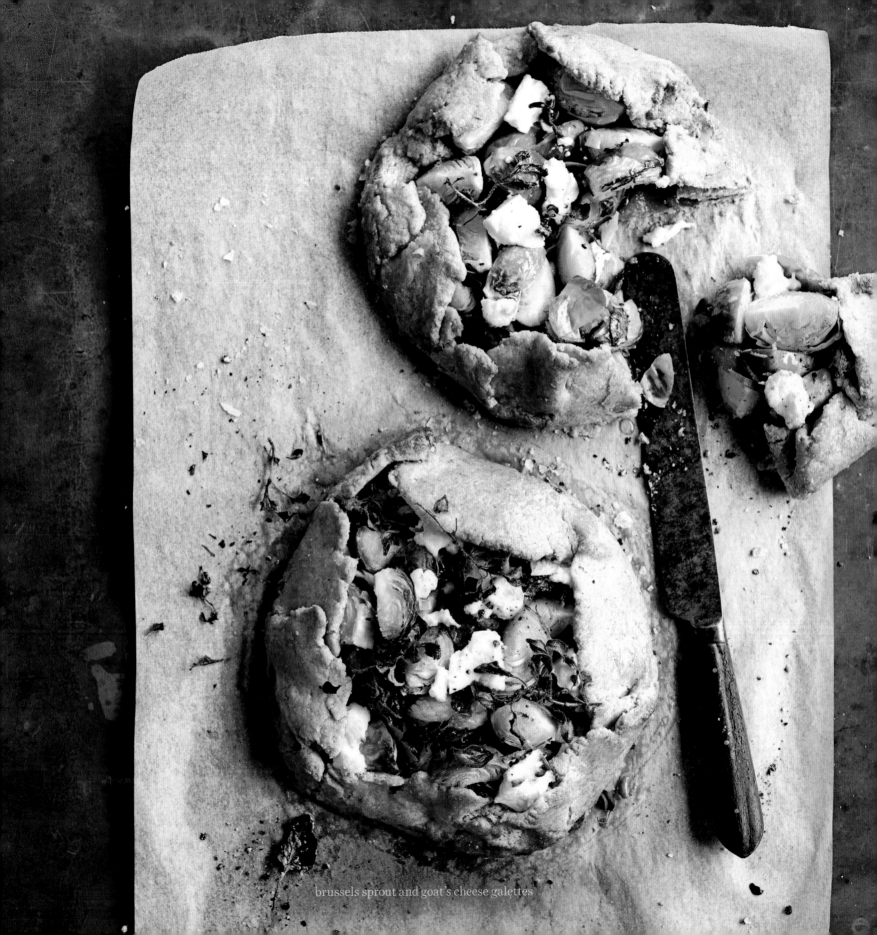

brussels sprout and goat's cheese galettes

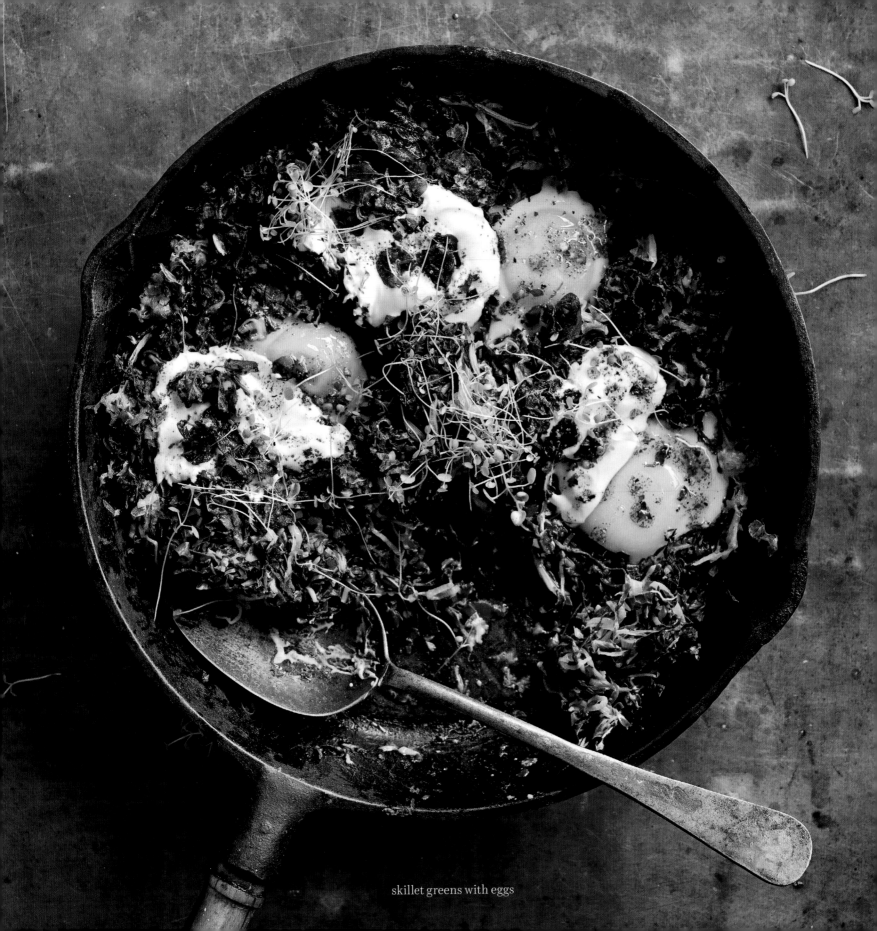

skillet greens with eggs

skillet greens with eggs

¼ cup (60ml) extra virgin olive oil
1 leek, white part only, thinly sliced
2 green onions (scallions), thinly sliced
1 bunch silverbeet (Swiss chard) (1kg), trimmed
  and shredded
1 tablespoon lemon juice
4 eggs
sea salt and cracked black pepper
½ cup (140g) plain Greek-style (thick) yoghurt
1 clove garlic, crushed
½ teaspoon dried chilli flakes
½ teaspoon ground sumac*
2 tablespoons oregano leaves
baby (micro) cress (optional), to serve

a sprinkling of sumac adds a pop of colour and zesty flavour

Preheat oven to 160°C (320°F). Heat 1 tablespoon of the oil
in a large ovenproof frying pan over medium heat. Add the leek
and onion and cook, stirring, for 10 minutes or until soft and
golden. Add the silverbeet and cook for 2–3 minutes or until
just wilted. Add the lemon juice and 1 tablespoon of the oil and
stir to combine. Make four spaces in the greens and carefully
add the eggs. Sprinkle with salt and pepper, transfer to the
oven and bake for 10–15 minutes or until the eggs are just set.

Place the yoghurt and garlic in a bowl, mix to combine and
set aside. Heat the remaining oil in a small non-stick frying
pan over low heat. Add the chilli, sumac, oregano, salt and
pepper and cook, stirring, for 3–4 minutes or until fragrant
and the oregano is crisp. Sprinkle the oregano mixture over
the greens and eggs and top with the garlic yoghurt and baby
cress to serve. **SERVES 4**

roasted cabbage and brussels sprouts with crispy herbs and tahini dressing

2 small cabbages (1.3kg), quartered
1kg Brussels sprouts, trimmed and halved
1 tablespoon honey
¼ cup (60ml) extra virgin olive oil,
  plus extra for drizzling
1 tablespoon finely grated lemon rind
1 tablespoon lemon juice
sea salt and cracked black pepper
1 bunch each sage, oregano and marjoram
lemon wedges, to serve
tahini dressing
1 cup (280g) plain Greek-style (thick) yoghurt
¼ cup (70g) tahini*
2 tablespoons lemon juice
sea salt and cracked black pepper

To make the tahini dressing, place the yoghurt, tahini,
lemon juice, salt and pepper in a small bowl and mix to
combine. Refrigerate until ready to serve.

Preheat oven to 180°C (350°F). Place the cabbage and
Brussels sprout in a large roasting pan lined with non-stick
baking paper. Place the honey, oil, lemon rind and juice,
salt and pepper in a small bowl and mix to combine. Pour
over the vegetables and roast for 30 minutes or until tender
and just beginning to brown.

Increase the oven temperature to 200°C (400°F). Add
the herbs to the pan and drizzle with the extra oil. Roast
for a further 10–15 minutes or until the vegetables are golden
and the herbs are crisp. Serve with the tahini dressing
and lemon wedges. **SERVES 4**

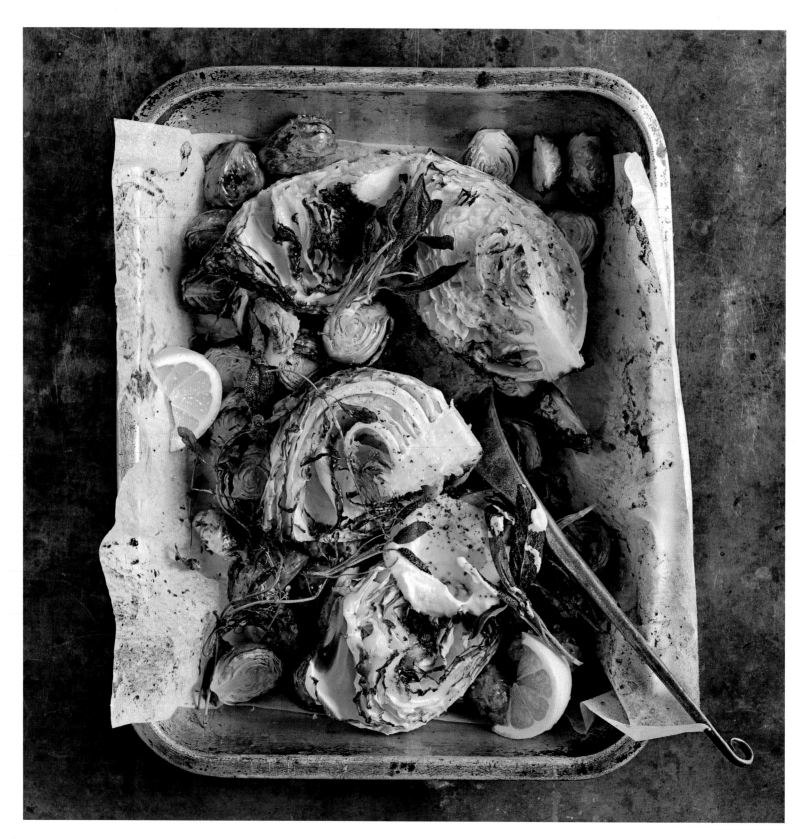

roasted cabbage and brussels sprouts with crispy herbs and tahini dressing

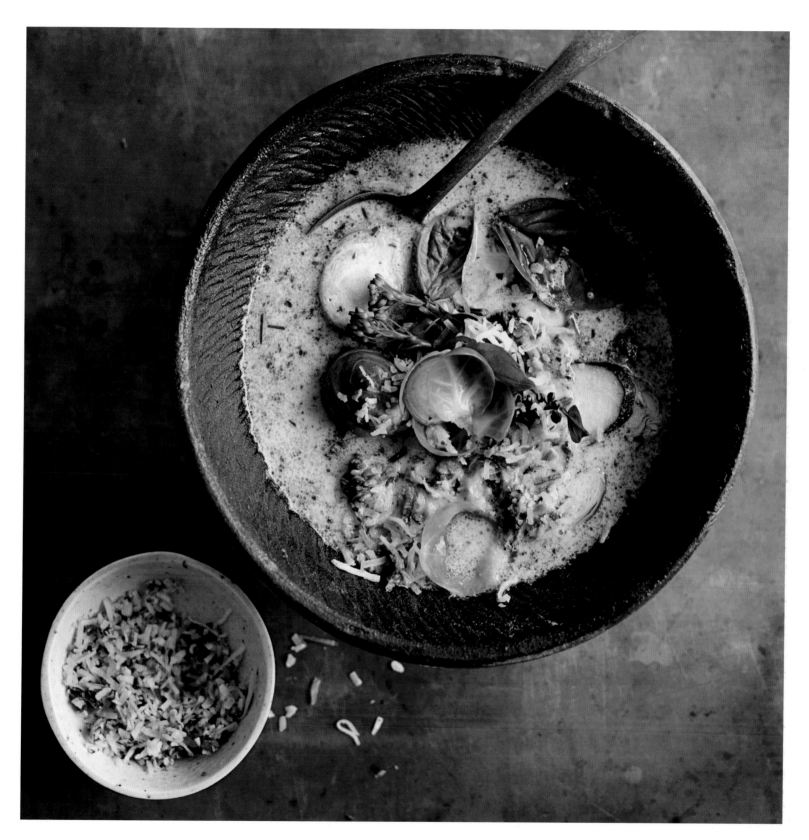

lime and coconut green vegetable curry

lime and coconut green vegetable curry

3 kaffir lime leaves*, shredded
1½ tablespoons finely grated ginger
2 cloves garlic
⅓ cup coriander (cilantro) leaves
3 long green chillies, seeded and roughly chopped
2 green onions (scallions), roughly chopped
1 teaspoon coconut sugar*
1 teaspoon finely grated lime rind
⅔ cup (50g) shredded coconut
¼ cup (60ml) vegetable oil
3 cups (750ml) coconut water
¾ cup (180ml) coconut milk
200g Brussels sprouts, trimmed and halved
2 medium zucchinis (courgettes) (260g), sliced
1 bunch broccolini (175g), trimmed and halved
2 tablespoons lime juice
Thai basil leaves, to serve

Place the kaffir lime leaf, ginger, garlic, coriander, chilli, onion, sugar and lime rind in a small food processor. Process to a coarse paste. Place 1 tablespoon of the paste in a bowl, add the coconut, mix to combine and set aside.

Add half the oil to the remaining paste in the food processor and process until smooth. Heat the remaining oil in a large deep-sided frying pan over high heat. Add the paste and cook, stirring, for 1 minute or until fragrant. Add the coconut water and coconut milk and bring to the boil. Reduce the heat to medium and simmer for 4 minutes or until thickened. Add the Brussels sprout, cover and cook for 4 minutes. Add the zucchini and broccolini, cover and cook for a further 3–4 minutes or until the vegetables are tender. Stir in the lime juice and spoon the curry into serving bowls. Sprinkle with the shredded coconut mixture and top with the basil to serve. **SERVES 4**

sage and haloumi roasted broccoli with caramelised leek

1 litre chicken or vegetable stock
1.5 litres water
4 small heads broccoli, bases trimmed
300g haloumi, sliced
12 sprigs sage
extra virgin olive oil, for drizzling
sea salt and cracked black pepper
caramelised leek
2 tablespoons extra virgin olive oil
30g unsalted butter
3 leeks, white part only, sliced
1 tablespoon thyme leaves
¼ cup (60ml) apple cider vinegar
1 tablespoon rice malt syrup*
sea salt and cracked black pepper

you can use brown sugar in place of syrup here, if you prefer

To make the caramelised leek, heat the oil and butter in a large non-stick frying pan over medium heat. Add the leek and thyme and cook, stirring occasionally, for 10 minutes or until soft. Add the vinegar, rice malt syrup, salt and pepper and cook for 5 minutes or until caramelised. Set aside.

Preheat oven to 220°C (425°F). Place the stock and water in a large saucepan over high heat. Bring to the boil, add the broccoli and cook for 4–5 minutes or until just tender. Drain and allow to cool. Place on a baking tray lined with non-stick baking paper. Make 3 incisions in each piece of broccoli at 3cm intervals. Fill each cavity with the caramelised leek, haloumi and sage. Drizzle with oil and sprinkle with salt and pepper. Roast for 10 minutes or until golden. **SERVES 4**

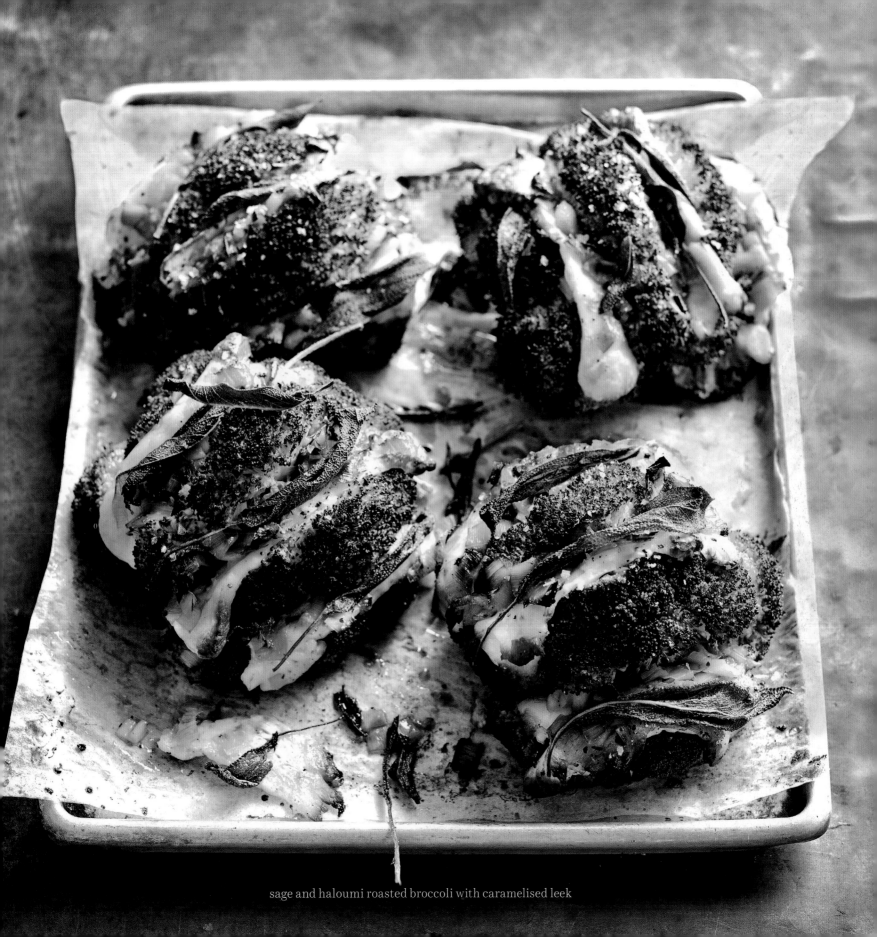

sage and haloumi roasted broccoli with caramelised leek

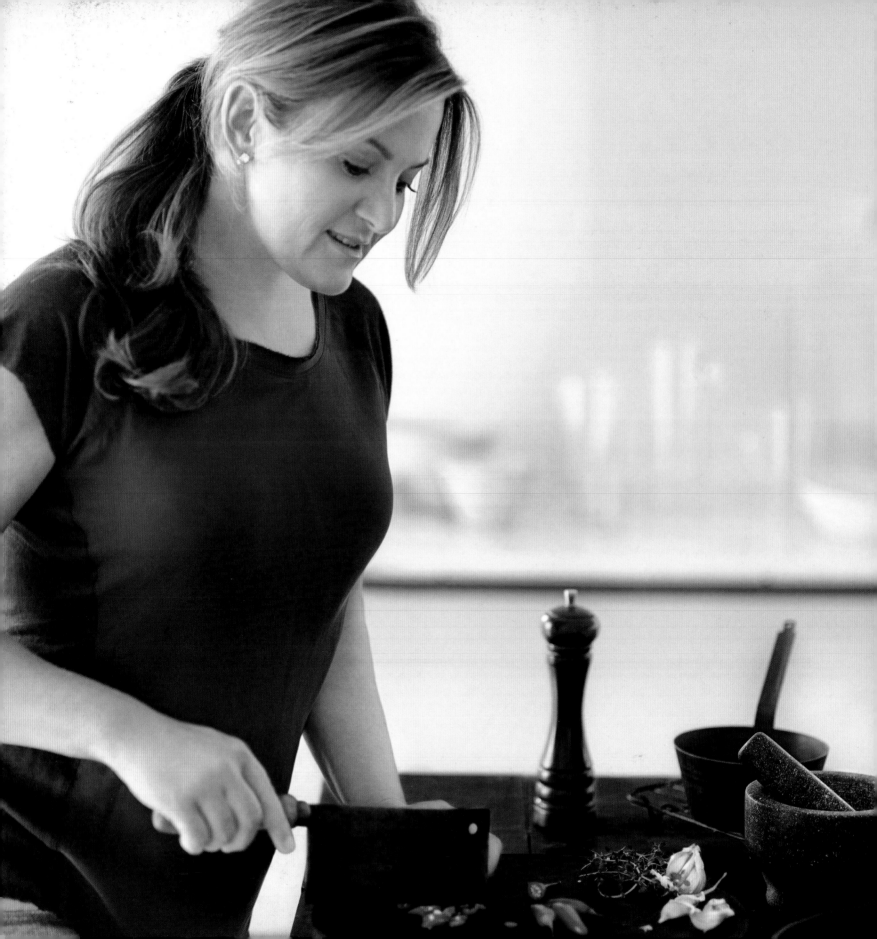

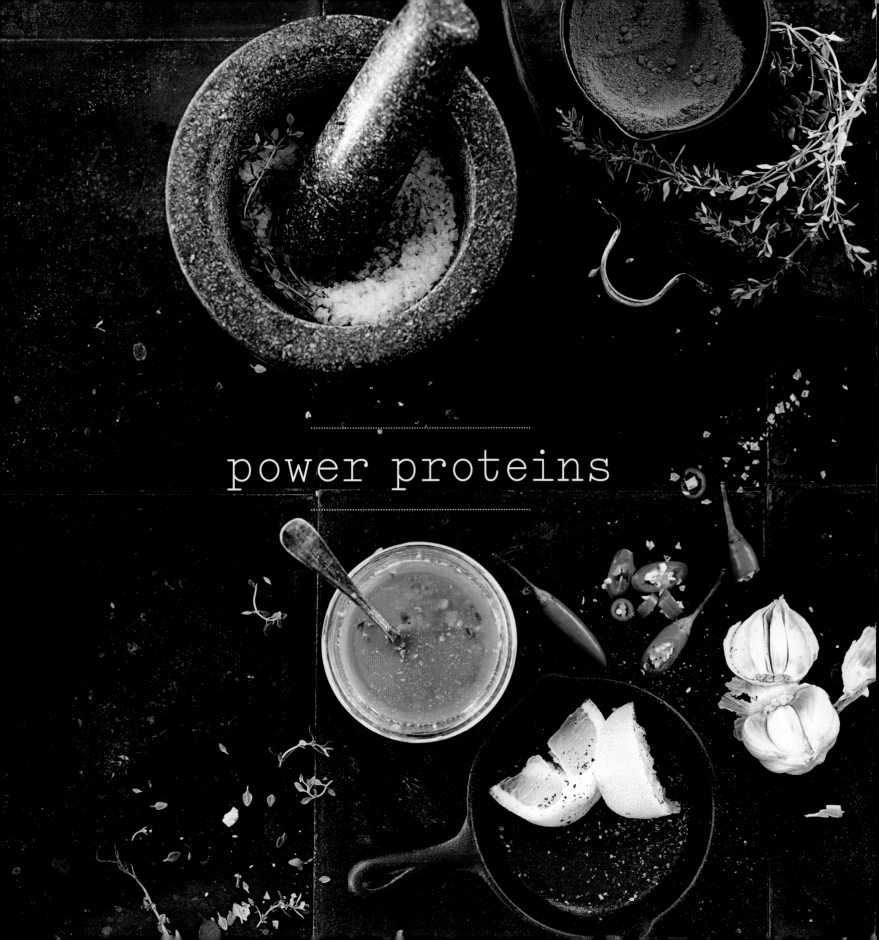

power proteins

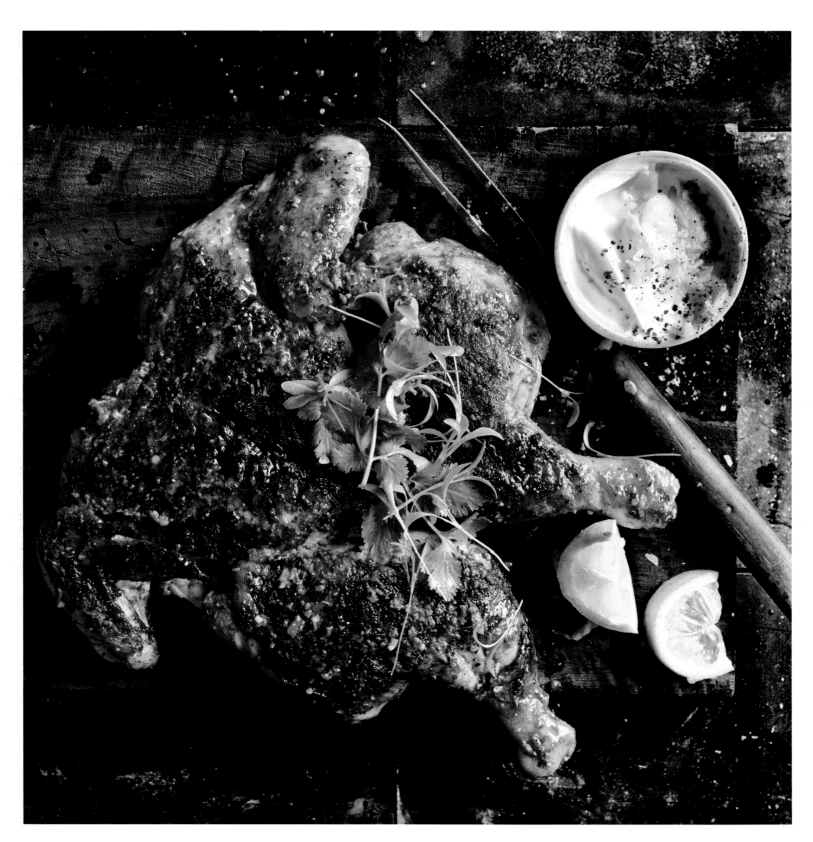

peri peri chicken

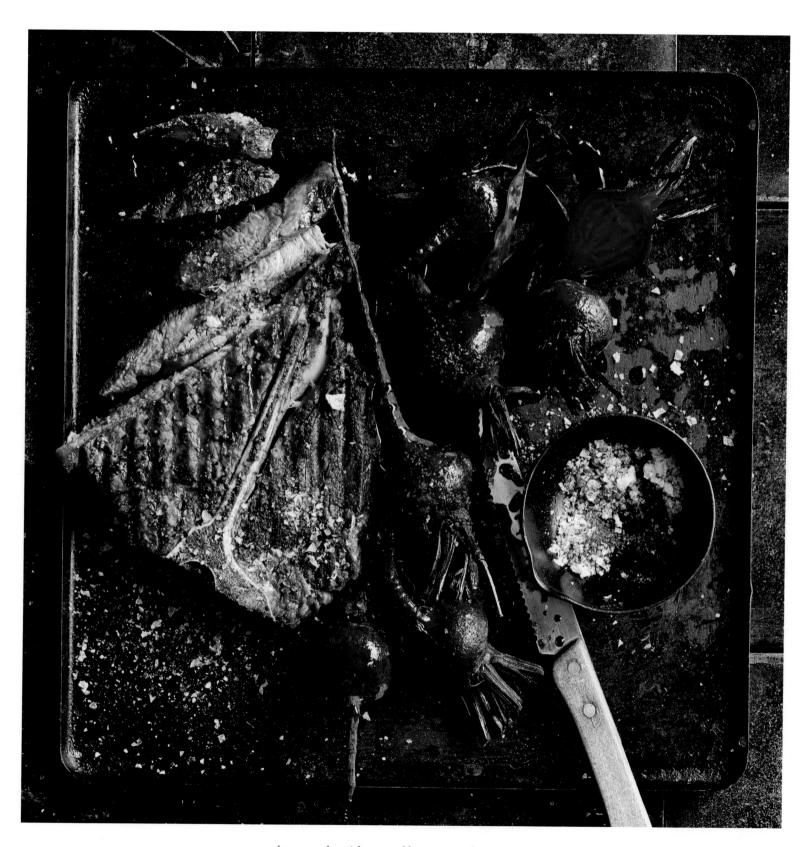

t-bone steaks with roasted beetroot and sumac salt

peri peri chicken

1 x 1.6kg whole chicken, rinsed and patted dry
1 small head garlic
1 cup (280g) plain Greek-style (thick) yoghurt
coriander (cilantro) leaves, baby (micro) coriander (cilantro)
    leaves (optional) and lemon wedges, to serve
peri peri marinade
¼ cup (60ml) extra virgin olive oil
3 cloves garlic, crushed
1 tablespoon smoked paprika
2 tablespoons chopped thyme leaves
3 small red chillies, chopped
2 tablespoons red wine vinegar
1 teaspoon sea salt flakes

To make the peri peri marinade, place the oil, crushed
garlic, paprika, thyme, chilli, vinegar and salt in a small
food processor and process until well combined. Set aside.

Place the chicken, breast-side down, on a board with
the drumsticks facing towards you. Using sharp kitchen
scissors, cut closely along either side of the backbone. Remove
and discard the bone, turn the chicken over and flatten.
Transfer to a baking tray lined with non-stick baking paper
and spoon over three-quarters of the marinade, rubbing
well to coat. Cover and refrigerate for 2–4 hours.

Preheat a char-grill pan or barbecue over high heat.
Wrap the garlic head in aluminium foil and place on the grill.
Cook, turning occasionally, for 15–20 minutes or until soft.
Place the chicken, skin-side down, on the the grill and cook
for 10 minutes. Turn and cook for a further 15 minutes or
until cooked through. Set aside and keep warm.

Remove the garlic from the foil and squeeze the cloves from
their skin into a bowl. Mash with a fork, add the yoghurt and
stir to combine. Place the chicken on a serving plate, brush
with the remaining marinade and top with the coriander.
Serve with the garlic yoghurt and lemon wedges. SERVES 4

t-bone steaks with roasted beetroot and sumac salt

2 bunches baby beetroot (600g), trimmed and cleaned
½ cup (125ml) vincotto*
¼ cup (60ml) water
2 bay leaves
4 x 450g T-bone steaks
extra virgin olive oil, for brushing
sea salt and cracked black pepper
sumac salt
2 teaspoons sea salt flakes
1 teaspoon ground sumac*

a spiced salt blend is a clever way to boost flavour, pop it on the table for sprinkling

To make the sumac salt, place the salt and sumac in a small bowl.
Mix well to combine and set aside.

Preheat oven to 180°C (350°F). Place the beetroot, vincotto, water
and bay leaves in a deep-sided roasting pan lined with non-stick
baking paper. Cover tightly with aluminium foil and roast for
30 minutes. Uncover and roast for a further 15 minutes. Preheat
a char-grill pan or barbecue over high heat. Brush the steaks with
oil and sprinkle with salt and pepper. Cook for 4–5 minutes each
side for medium rare, or until cooked to your liking. Serve the
steaks with the beetroot and sprinkle with the sumac salt. SERVES 4

ras el hanout grilled lamb

1½ cups coriander (cilantro) leaves
2 tablespoons finely chopped preserved lemon rind
3 cloves garlic, crushed
¼ cup (60ml) extra virgin olive oil, plus extra for brushing
2 teaspoons ras el hanout*
sea salt and cracked black pepper
1.6kg butterflied leg of lamb, trimmed
500g truss cherry tomatoes

Place the coriander, lemon rind, garlic, oil, ras el hanout, salt and
pepper in a small food processor and process until combined. Rub
¼ cup (125ml) over the lamb to coat. Preheat a char-grill pan or
barbecue over high heat and cook the lamb for 5 minutes each side.
Reduce heat to medium and cook for a further 5 minutes each side
for medium rare, or until cooked to your liking. Brush the tomatoes
with the extra oil and sprinkle with salt and pepper. Add to the grill
for the last 10 minutes of lamb cooking time. Slice the lamb, spoon
over the remaining marinade and serve with the tomatoes. SERVES 6

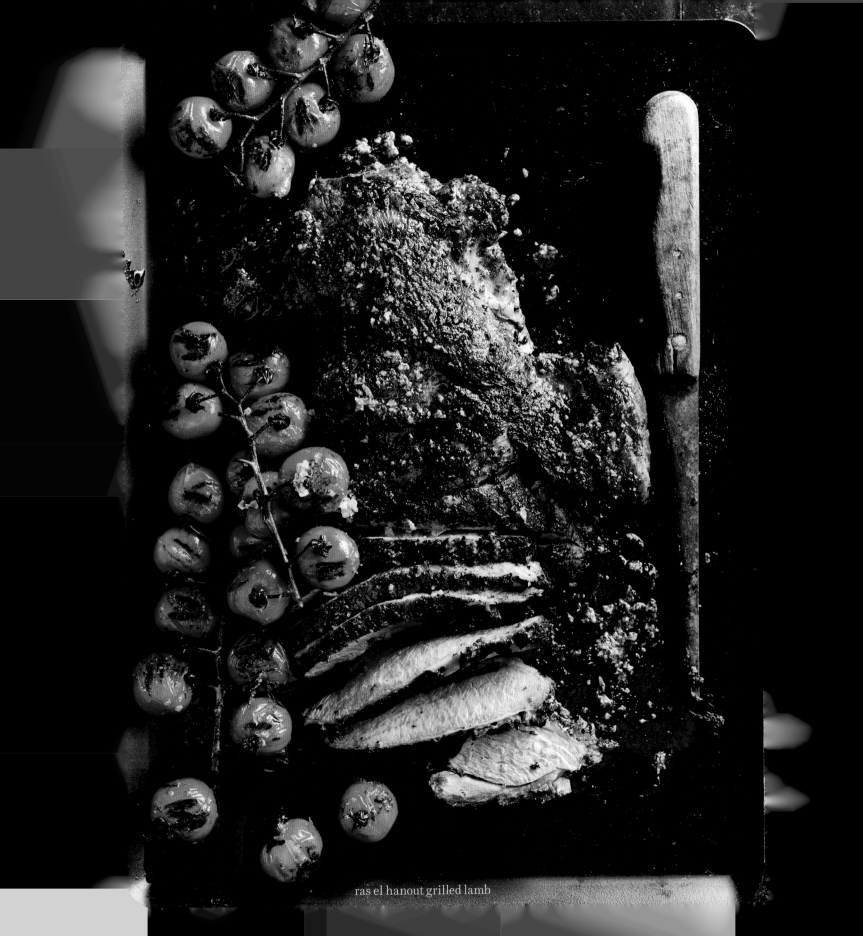

ras el hanout grilled lamb

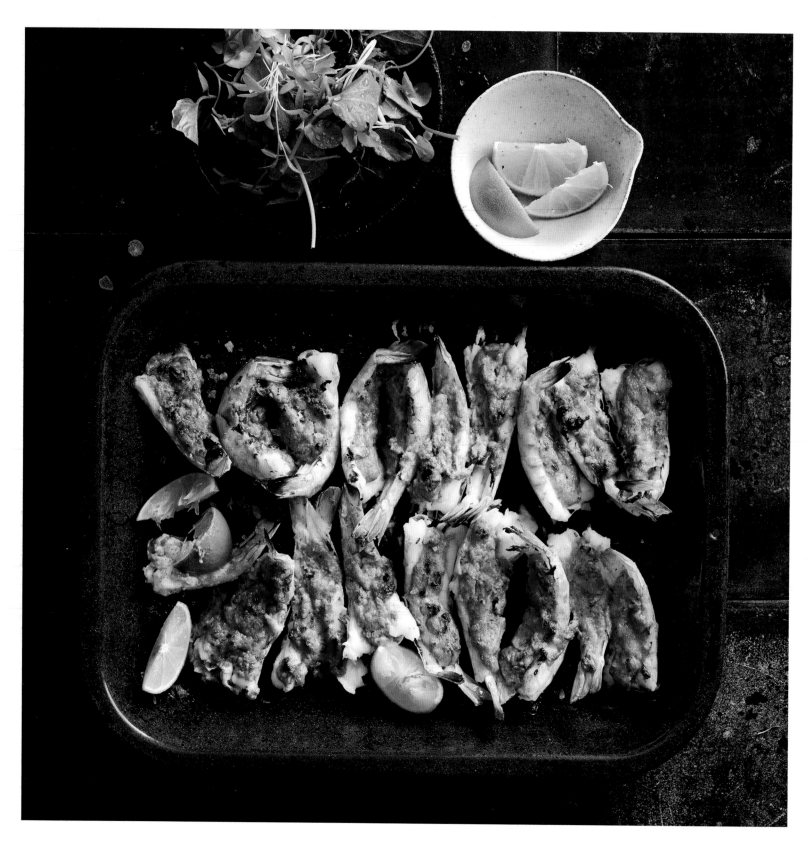

burnt almond butter prawns with chilli

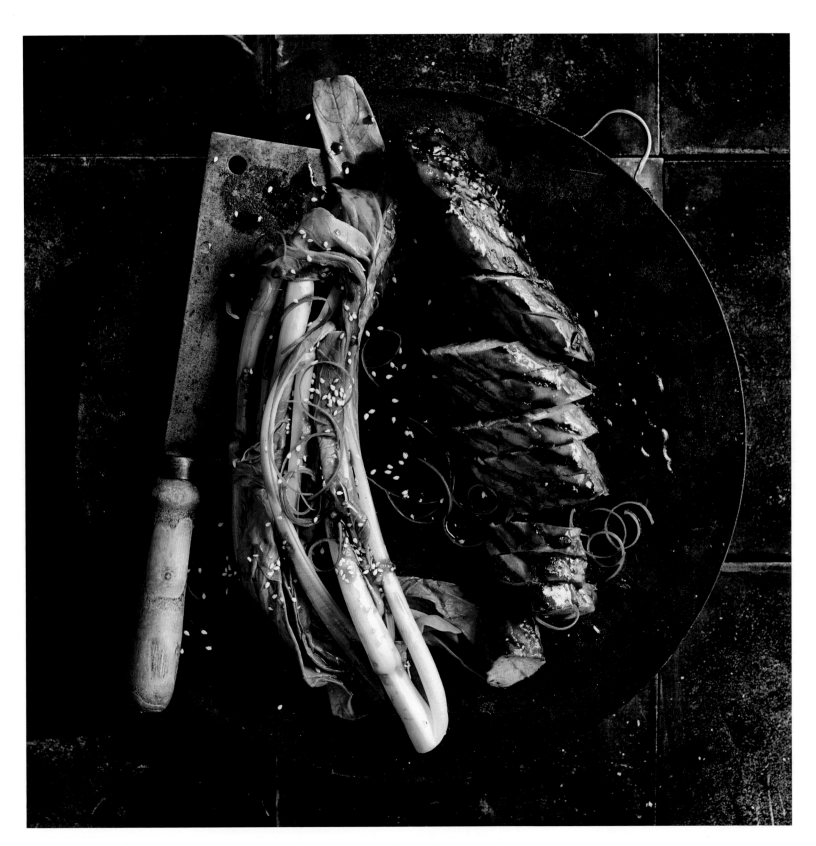

sticky barbecued pork with asian greens

burnt almond butter prawns with chilli

¼ cup (80g) almond butter*
2 small red chillies, seeded and finely chopped
2 tablespoons finely chopped coriander (cilantro)
2 cloves garlic, crushed
¼ cup (60ml) water
¼ cup (60ml) lime juice
sea salt and cracked black pepper
24 large green (uncooked) king prawns (shrimp),
    butterflied with tails intact
watercress sprigs and lime wedges, to serve

Place the almond butter, chilli, coriander, garlic, water,
lime juice, salt and pepper in a bowl and mix to combine.
    Preheat a grill (broiler) to high. Place the prawns,
flesh-side up, on a baking tray lined with non-stick baking
paper and spread with the almond butter mixture. Cook
for 5–8 minutes or until golden and cooked through. Serve
with watercress and lime wedges. SERVES 4

sticky barbecued pork with asian greens

2 tablespoons char siu or hoisin sauce
2 tablespoons spicy black bean sauce
2 x 400g pork fillets
vegetable oil, for brushing
2 bunches choy sum (640g), trimmed
2 tablespoons oyster sauce
1 tablespoon soy sauce
2 cloves garlic, crushed
3 green onions (scallions), thinly sliced
1 teaspoon sesame seeds, toasted

Place the char siu and black bean sauces in a bowl and mix to
combine. Preheat a char-grill pan or barbecue over high heat.
Brush the pork with oil and cook, turning occasionally, for
15 minutes. Brush with the sauce mixture and cook for a further
1–2 minutes or until caramelised and cooked through.
    Place the choy sum in a large saucepan of salted boiling water
and cook for 4 minutes or until tender. Drain, transfer to a bowl,
add the oyster sauce, soy sauce and garlic and toss to combine.
    Slice the pork and place on a serving plate with the choy sum.
Sprinkle with the onion and sesame seeds to serve. SERVES 4

grilled beef skewers with red chimichurri

750g rump steak, trimmed and cut into 5cm pieces
1 teaspoon each sea salt flakes and cracked black pepper
1 tablespoon extra virgin olive oil
1 tablespoon red wine vinegar
2 cloves garlic, crushed
1 lemon, halved
grilled flatbreads and store-bought hummus, to serve
coriander (cilantro) leaves, to serve
red chimichurri
½ red onion, chopped
250g cherry tomatoes
1 clove garlic, crushed
2 tablespoons chopped flat-leaf parsley leaves
2 tablespoons chopped coriander (cilantro)
½ teaspoon ground chilli
½ teaspoon smoked paprika
½ teaspoon ground cumin
¼ cup (60ml) extra virgin olive oil
1 tablespoon red wine vinegar
1 tablespoon lemon juice

To make the red chimichurri, place the onion, tomatoes,
garlic, parsley, coriander, chilli, paprika, cumin, oil,
vinegar and lemon juice in a small food processor and
process to a coarse paste. Set aside.
    Place the beef in a large bowl and add the salt, pepper,
oil, vinegar and garlic. Toss to coat and thread the beef onto
large metal skewers. Preheat a char-grill pan or barbecue
over high heat. Cook the beef skewers, turning occasionally,
for 15–18 minutes for medium rare or until cooked to your
liking. Add the lemon, cut-side down, to the grill for the
last 5 minutes of the beef cooking time. Serve the skewers
on grilled flatbreads and top with hummus, coriander,
the chimichurri and grilled lemon. SERVES 4

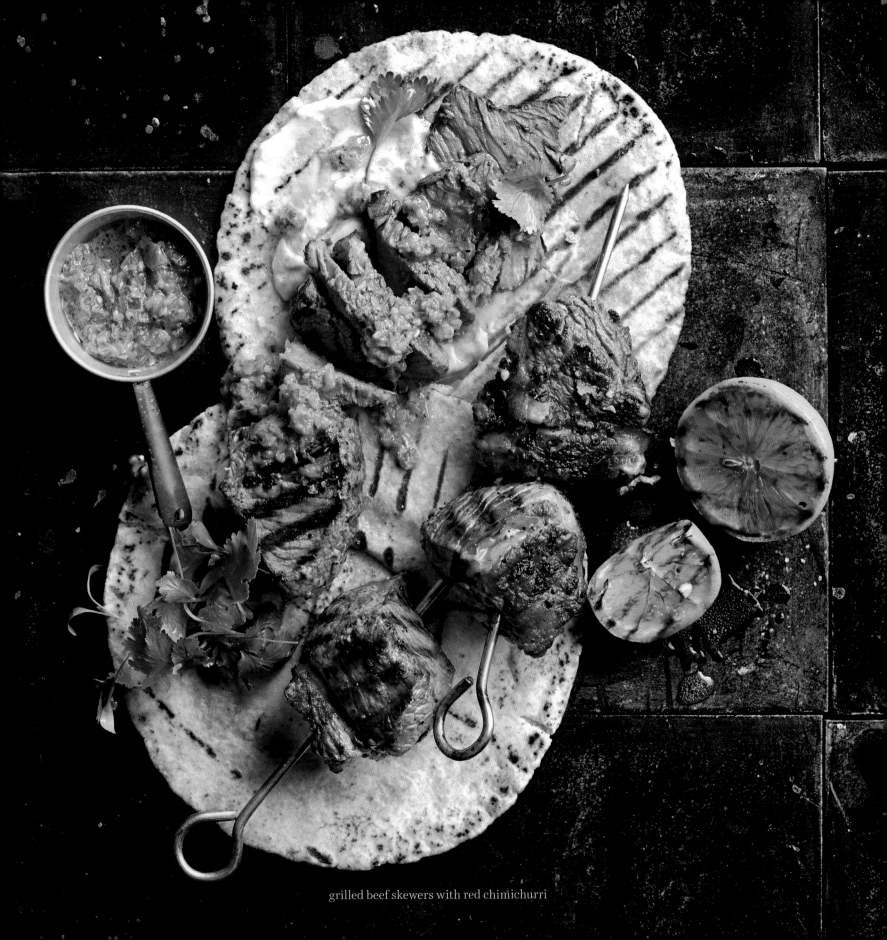

grilled beef skewers with red chimichurri

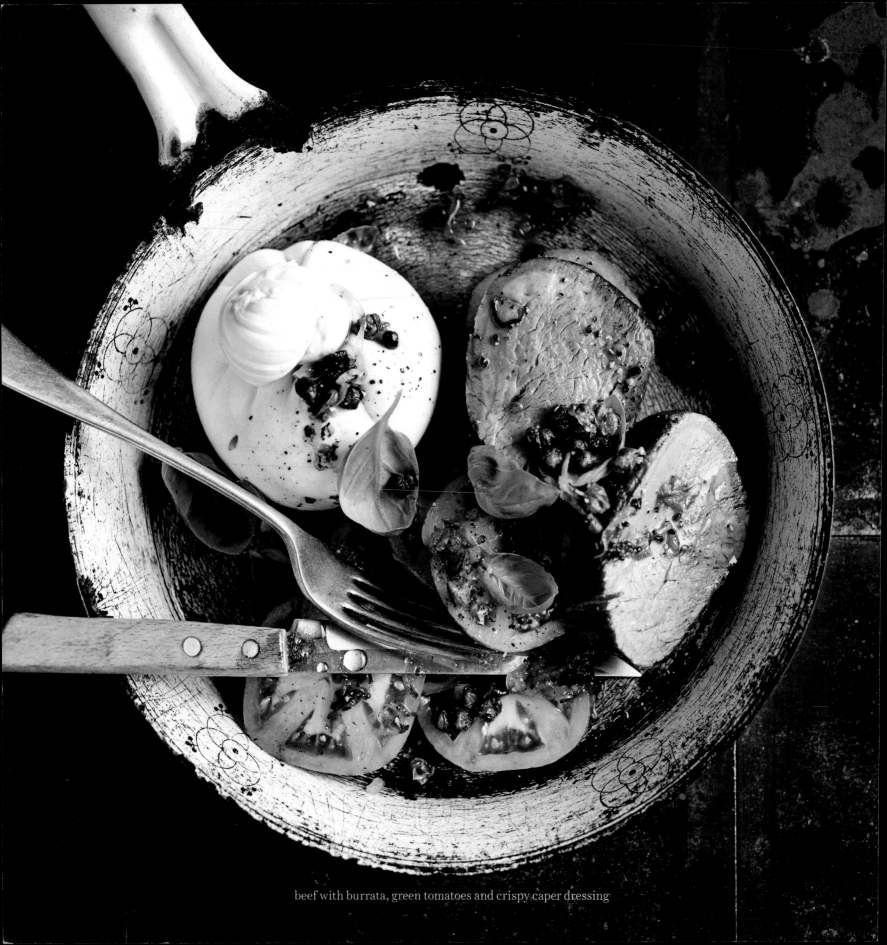

beef with burrata, green tomatoes and crispy caper dressing

beef with burrata, green tomatoes and crispy caper dressing

750g beef eye fillet
extra virgin olive oil, for brushing
sea salt and cracked black pepper
2 tablespoons extra virgin olive oil, extra
3 eschalots (French shallots), sliced
2 tablespoons salted capers, rinsed and drained
2 tablespoons white balsamic vinegar
4 green tomatoes, sliced
4 x 250g burrata or buffalo mozzarella
basil leaves, to serve

Preheat oven to 180°C (350°F). Brush the beef with oil and sprinkle with salt and pepper. Heat a large non-stick frying pan over high heat. Cook the beef, turning, for 12 minutes or until browned on all sides. Place in a roasting pan lined with non-stick baking paper. Roast for 10 minutes for rare, or until cooked to your liking.

While the beef is roasting, heat the extra oil in the pan over medium heat. Add the eschalot and capers and cook, stirring, for 3–4 minutes or until the eschalot is soft and the capers are crispy. Add the vinegar and cook for a further 1 minute or until slightly reduced.

Slice the beef and divide between serving plates with the tomato and burrata. Spoon over the caper dressing and sprinkle with basil to serve. **SERVES 4**

lamb skewers with tahini beetroot salad

500g lamb mince
1 teaspoon dried mint
2 cloves garlic, crushed
½ teaspoon ground cumin
½ teaspoon ground coriander
1 small red onion, grated
sea salt and cracked black pepper
extra virgin olive oil, for brushing
1 medium fennel bulb (300g), trimmed and thinly sliced
¼ cup fennel fronds
1 bunch baby beetroot (300g), trimmed and thinly sliced
1 bunch golden beetroot (300g), trimmed and thinly sliced
2 cups baby (micro) red-veined sorrel leaves (optional)
½ cup mint leaves
tahini dressing
¼ cup (70g) tahini*   ← *tahini is a nutty paste made from sesame seeds, sold in jars at the supermarket*
¼ cup (60ml) apple cider vinegar
2 tablespoons maple syrup
2 tablespoons lemon juice
2 tablespoons water
sea salt and cracked black pepper

To make the tahini dressing, place the tahini, vinegar, maple syrup, lemon juice, water, salt and pepper in a bowl. Whisk to combine and set aside.

Place the lamb, dried mint, garlic, cumin, coriander, onion, salt and pepper in a large bowl and mix well to combine. Preheat a char-grill pan or barbecue over medium heat. Shape tablespoons of the lamb mixture around the ends of 15cm bamboo skewers. Brush with oil and cook, turning every 2–3 minutes, for 10 minutes or until cooked through.

Place the fennel, fennel fronds, beetroot, baby sorrel, and mint leaves in a bowl and toss to combine. Top with the skewers and drizzle with the tahini dressing to serve. **SERVES 4**

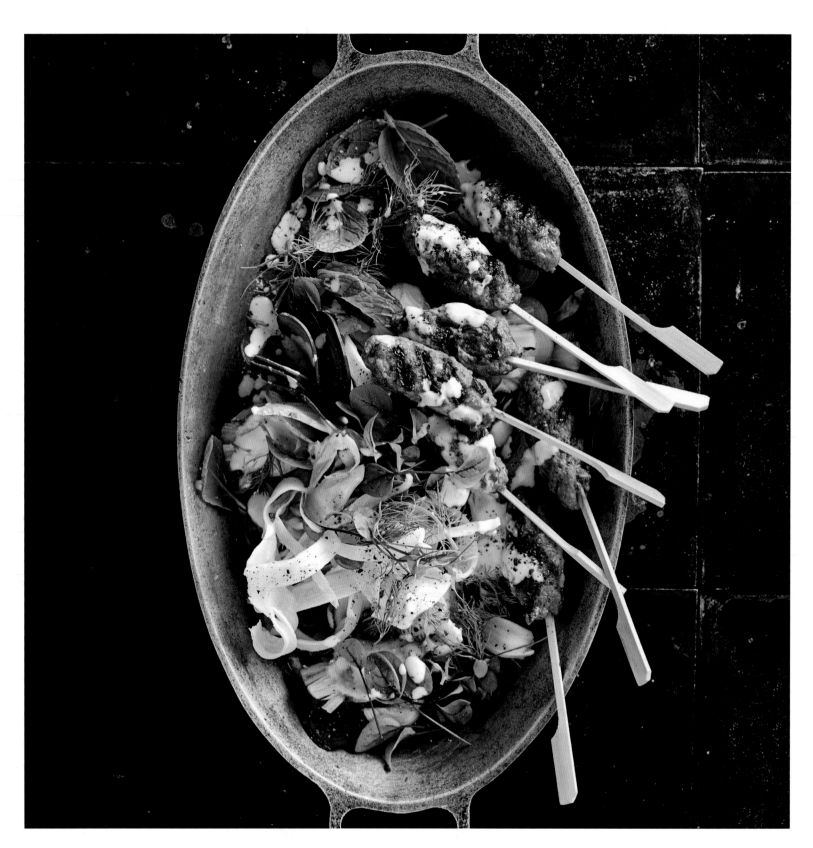

lamb skewers with tahini beetroot salad

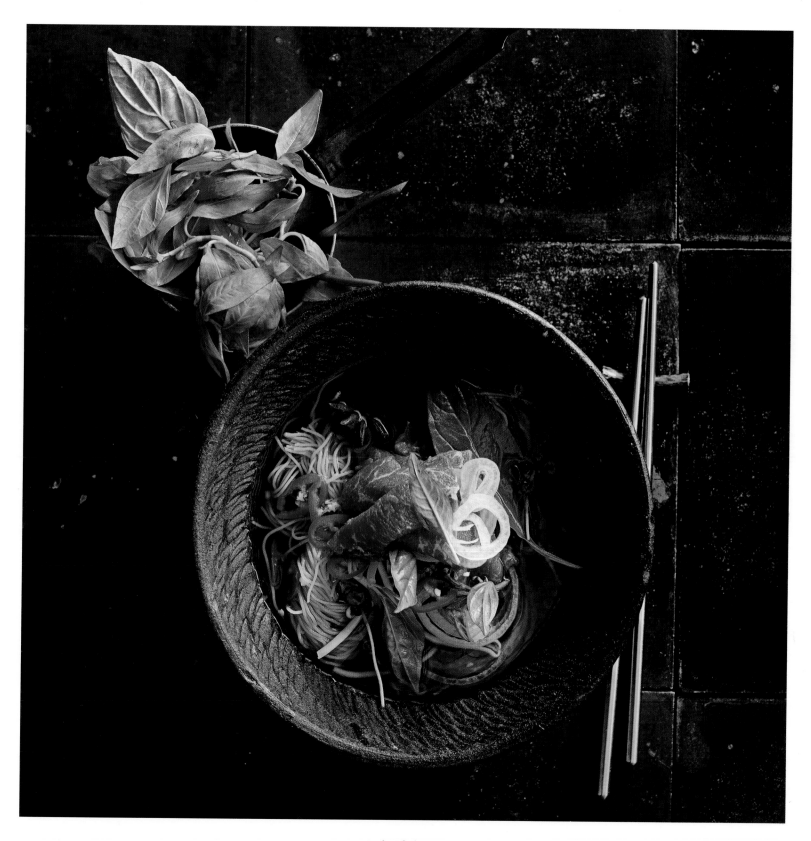

beef pho

beef pho

1 x 6cm piece ginger, peeled and halved
2 cloves garlic
1 eschalot (French shallot), halved
1.5 litres beef stock
1 star anise
1 stick cinnamon
3 teaspoons fish sauce
1 tablespoon palm sugar*
200g thin brown rice noodles, cooked and drained
1 small white onion, thinly sliced
250g beef fillet, frozen for 2 hours and thinly sliced
cracked black pepper
1 cup (100g) bean sprouts, trimmed
2 long red chillies, sliced
½ cup Thai basil leaves
½ cup Vietnamese mint leaves

Place the ginger, garlic and eschalot in a small non-stick frying pan over high heat and cook, turning, for 8–10 minutes or until charred. Transfer to a medium saucepan over high heat and add the stock, star anise and cinnamon. Bring to the boil, reduce the heat to low and simmer for 10–15 minutes or until fragrant. Add the fish sauce and sugar and stir to dissolve. Strain the stock, discarding the solids, set aside and keep warm.

Divide the noodles between serving bowls. Top with the onion and beef and ladle over the hot stock. Sprinkle with pepper and top with the sprouts, chilli, basil and mint to serve. **SERVES 4**

crispy chia tofu

¼ cup (50g) white chia seeds*
⅔ cup (70g) quinoa flakes*
⅔ cup (50g) panko (Japanese) breadcrumbs
sea salt and cracked black pepper
2 eggwhites
600g firm tofu, drained and thickly sliced
¼ cup (60ml) vegetable oil
½ teaspoon sesame oil
¼ cup (60ml) mirin (Japanese rice wine)
2 teaspoons finely grated ginger
250g baby cucumbers (cukes), sliced
1 cup mint leaves
4 cups (100g) baby (micro) watercress
    sprigs (optional), to serve
dipping sauce
2 tablespoons light soy sauce
1 small red chilli, finely chopped

chia seeds and quinoa flakes make for a delicate and crispy crumb

To make the dipping sauce, place the soy sauce and chilli in a small bowl. Mix to combine and set aside.

Place the chia seeds, quinoa flakes, breadcrumbs, salt and pepper in a bowl and mix to combine. Place the eggwhites in a bowl and whisk until fluffy. Dip the tofu in the eggwhite and press into the chia mixture to coat. Heat the vegetable oil in a large non-stick frying pan over high heat. Cook the tofu, in batches, for 1–2 minutes each side or until golden and crisp. Drain on paper towel and keep warm.

Place the sesame oil, mirin and ginger in a medium bowl and whisk to combine. Add the cucumber and mint and toss to combine. Serve the tofu with the cucumber salad, watercress and the dipping sauce. **SERVES 4**

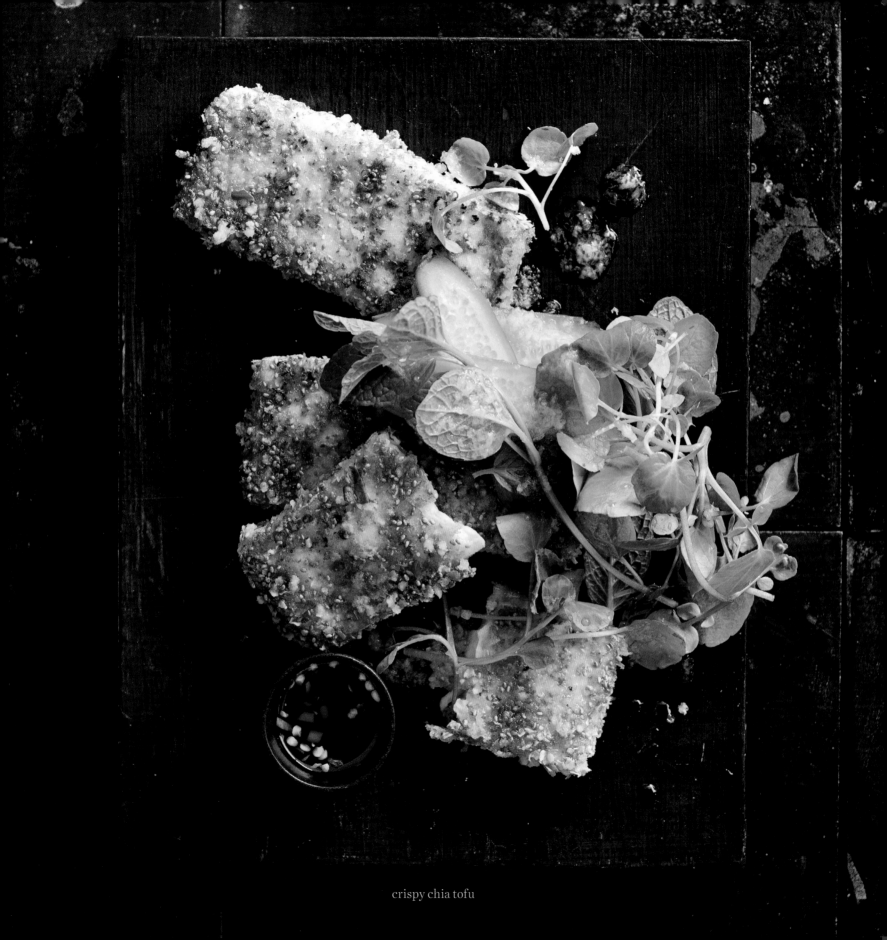

crispy chia tofu

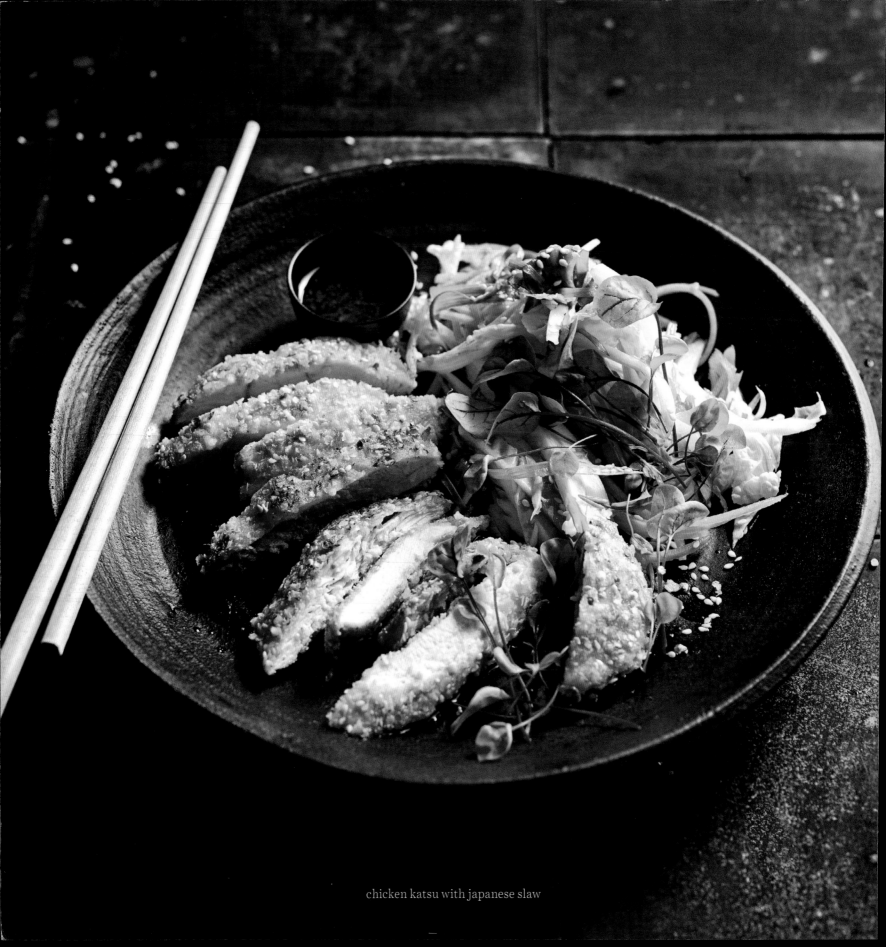

chicken katsu with japanese slaw

chicken katsu with japanese slaw

1 cup (100g) quinoa flakes*
¼ cup (20g) panko (Japanese) breadcrumbs
2 tablespoons sesame seeds, toasted, plus extra to serve
2 teaspoons coriander seeds, crushed
¼ cup (20g) finely grated parmesan
sea salt and cracked black pepper
4 x 200g chicken breast fillets, trimmed
    and halved horizontally
2 eggs, lightly beaten
2 tablespoons peanut oil
3 cups (240g) shredded Chinese cabbage (wombok)
2 carrots, peeled and shredded
2 green onions (scallions), shredded
baby (micro) red-vein sorrel leaves (optional), to serve
dressing
1 tablespoon finely grated white onion
¼ cup (60ml) soy sauce
¼ cup (60ml) rice wine vinegar
1 tablespoon maple syrup

To make the dressing, place the white onion, soy sauce, vinegar
and maple syrup in a bowl. Mix to combine and set aside.
    Place the quinoa flakes, breadcrumbs, sesame seeds, coriander
seeds, parmesan, salt and pepper in a bowl and toss to combine.
Dip the chicken pieces in the egg and press in the quinoa crumb
to coat. Heat the oil in a large non-stick frying pan over medium
heat. Cook the chicken, in batches, for 3–4 minutes each side
or until golden and cooked through. Set aside and keep warm.
    Place the cabbage, carrot and green onion in a bowl and toss
to combine. Slice the chicken and divide between serving plates
with the slaw. Sprinkle with the baby sorrel leaves and extra
sesame seeds and serve with the dressing. SERVES 4

crispy-skinned chicken
with zucchini and fennel salad

2 tablespoons extra virgin olive oil
2 tablespoons salted capers, rinsed and drained
4 x 200g chicken breast fillets, skin on
sea salt and cracked black pepper
2 medium zucchinis (courgettes) (260g), shredded
2 green (Granny smith) apples, thinly sliced
1 large fennel bulb (550g), trimmed and thinly sliced
anchovy dressing
½ cup (140g) plain Greek-style (thick) yoghurt
½ teaspoon Dijon mustard
2 tablespoons lemon juice
1 long green chilli, finely chopped
2 anchovy fillets, chopped
2 tablespoons finely shredded mint leaves
sea salt and cracked black pepper

To make the anchovy dressing, place the yoghurt, mustard,
lemon juice, chilli, anchovy, mint, salt and pepper in a bowl.
Mix to combine and set aside.
    Preheat oven to 200°C (400°F). Heat the oil in a large
non-stick frying pan over high heat. Add the capers and cook
for 2–3 minutes or until crispy. Remove with a slotted spoon
and set aside. Sprinkle the chicken with salt and pepper and
cook, skin-side down, for 3–4 minutes or until golden. Transfer
to a baking tray lined with non-stick baking paper and roast
for 12–15 minutes or until golden and cooked through.
    Place the zucchini, apple and fennel in a bowl, drizzle with
the dressing and toss to combine. Slice the chicken and divide
between serving plates with the salad. Top with the crispy
capers to serve. SERVES 4

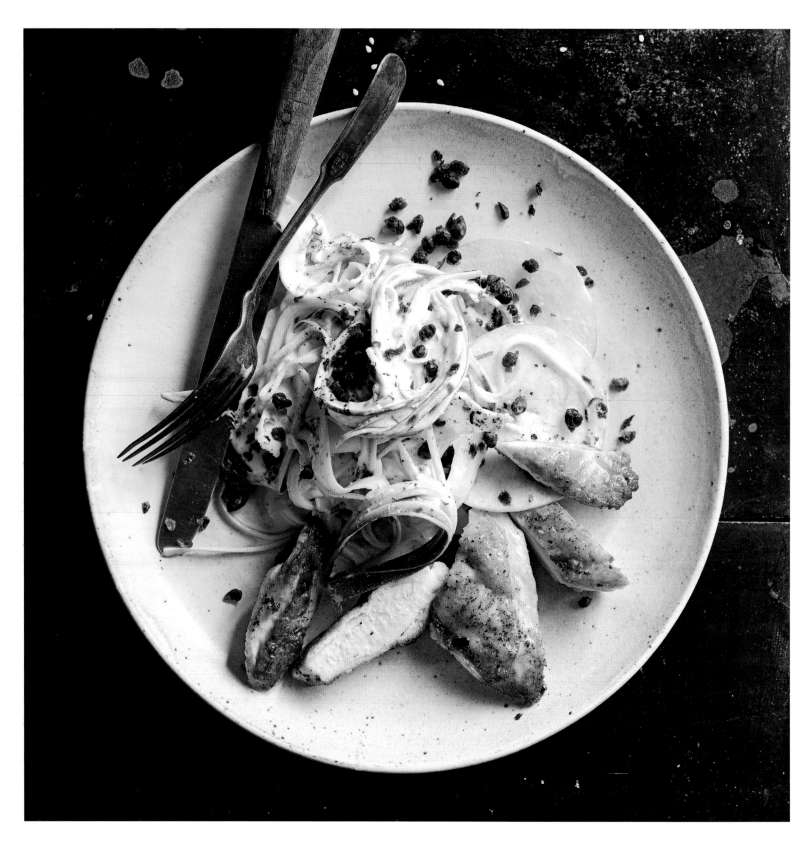

crispy-skinned chicken with zucchini and fennel salad

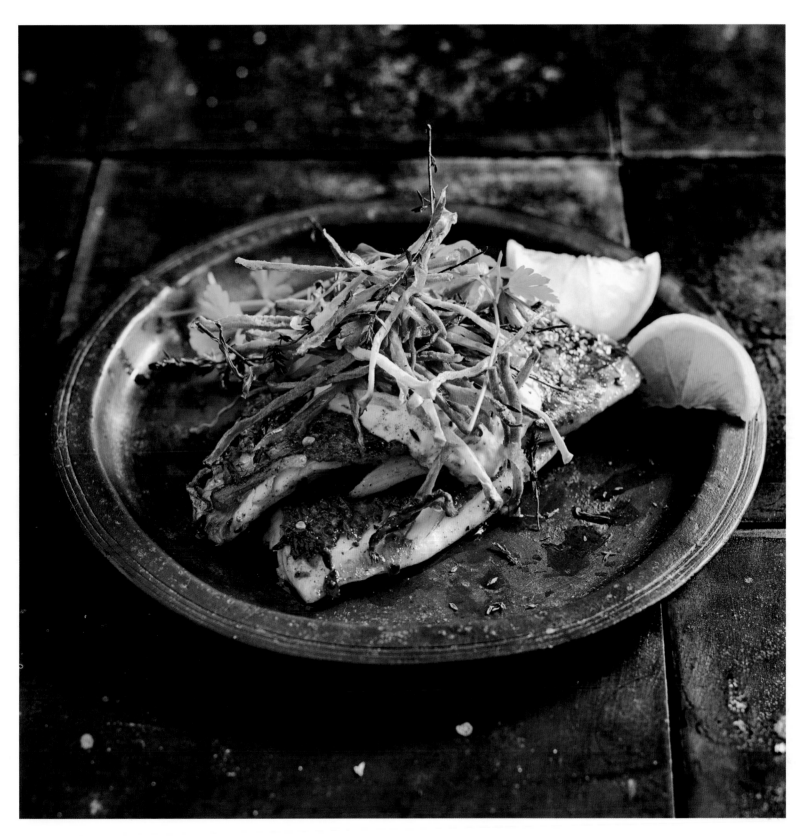

smoky chilli snapper with celeriac and sweet potato fries

smoky chilli snapper with celeriac and sweet potato fries

2 teaspoons dried chilli flakes
1 teaspoon smoked paprika
sea salt and cracked black pepper
⅓ cup (80ml) extra virgin olive oil
8 x 100g snapper fillets, skin on
store-bought tzatziki, baby (micro) parsley
   leaves (optional) and lemon wedges, to serve
celeriac and sweet potato fries
1kg sweet potato (kumara), cut into matchsticks
1kg celeriac (celery root), peeled and cut into matchsticks
2 tablespoons thyme leaves
2 tablespoons rosemary leaves
⅓ cup (80ml) extra virgin olive oil
2 teaspoons sea salt flakes

fish is an amazing source of minerals and omega-3 fats

To make the celeriac and sweet potato fries, preheat oven to
150°C (300°F). Place the sweet potato, celeriac, thyme, rosemary,
oil and salt in a large bowl and toss to coat. Place in single layers
on baking trays lined with non-stick baking paper. Roast for
35–40 minutes or until golden and crisp.

Place the chilli flakes, paprika, salt, pepper and oil in a bowl
and mix to combine. Brush over the snapper fillets. Heat a large
non-stick frying pan over high heat. Cook the fish in batches,
skin-side down, for 2 minutes. Turn and cook for a further 1 minute
or until cooked through. Divide between serving plates and top with
the tzatziki, fries and parsley and serve with lemon wedges. **SERVES 4**

spinach crepes with goat's curd and zucchini and pea salad

2 medium zucchinis (courgettes) (260g), shredded
1 cup (120g) frozen peas, thawed
2 cups (25g) snow pea tendrils
2 tablespoons extra virgin olive oil
2 tablespoons lemon juice
sea salt and cracked black pepper
200g goat's curd
lemon wedges, to serve
spinach crepes
1 cup (160g) buckwheat flour*
3 eggs
2 cups (500ml) almond milk
3 cups (75g) baby spinach leaves
1 cup flat-leaf parsley leaves
sea salt and cracked black pepper
2½ tablespoons extra virgin olive oil

smooth and creamy goat's curd lends its luscious flavour to these crepes

To make the spinach crepes, place the flour, eggs, milk, spinach,
parsley, salt and pepper in a bowl and, using a hand-held stick
blender, blend until smooth. Heat a little of the oil in a 20cm
non-stick frying pan over high heat. Add ⅓ cup (80ml) of the
batter, swirl to coat the base of the pan and cook for 1–2 minutes
or until just set. Remove from the pan, set aside and keep warm.
Repeat with the remaining oil and batter.

Place the zucchini, peas, snow pea tendrils, oil, lemon juice,
salt and pepper in a bowl and toss to combine. Divide the crepes
between serving plates and top with the goat's curd and salad.
Serve with lemon wedges. **SERVES 6**

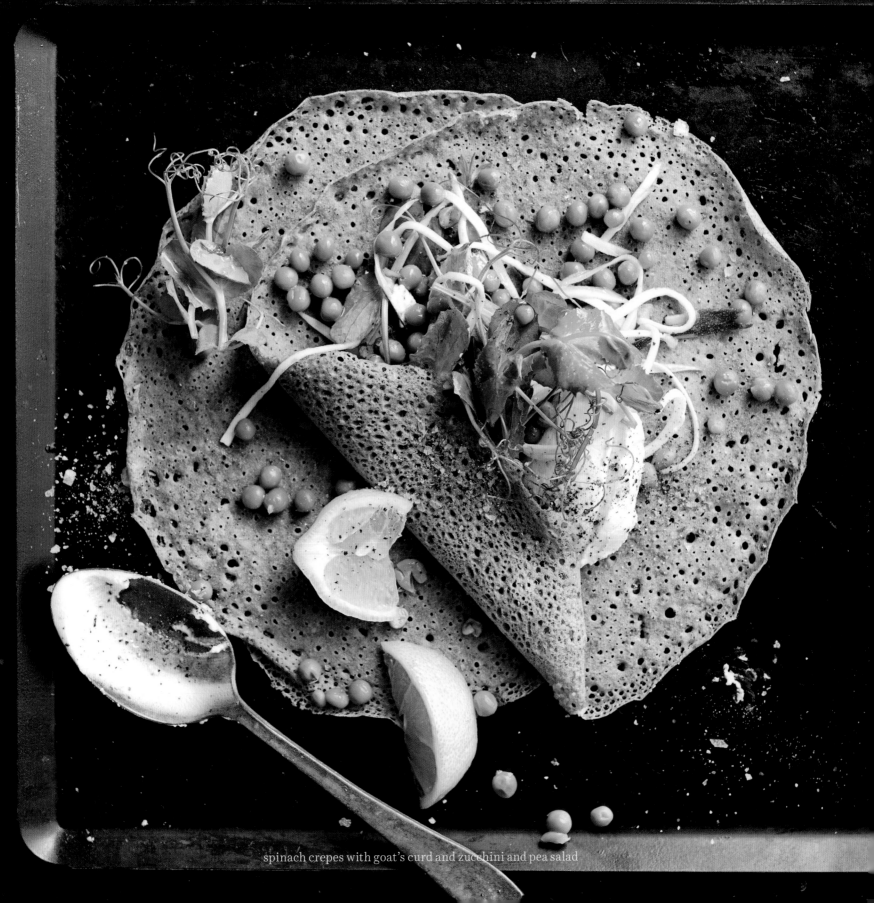

spinach crepes with goat's curd and zucchini and pea salad

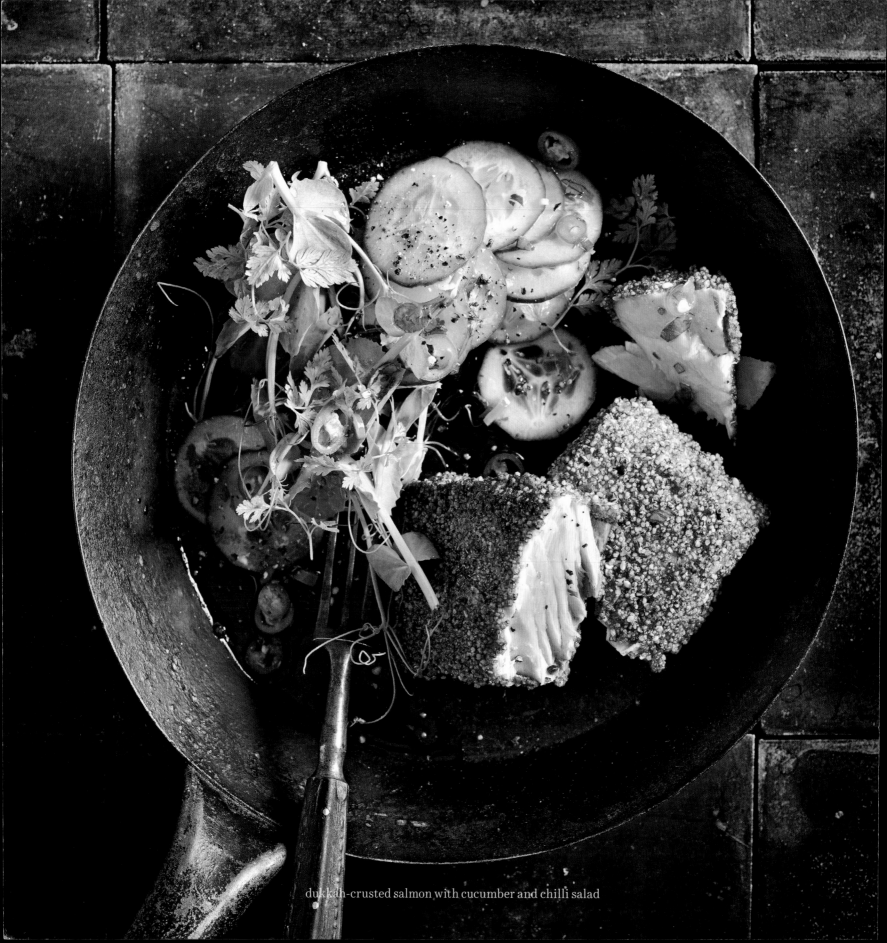

dukkah-crusted salmon with cucumber and chilli salad

dukkah-crusted salmon
with cucumber and chilli salad

1½ cups (75g) puffed amaranth*
2 tablespoons store-bought dukkah
1 teaspoon sea salt flakes
4 x 200g salmon fillets, skin removed
2 eggs, lightly beaten
2 tablespoons extra virgin olive oil
1 long green chilli, thinly sliced
¼ cup (60ml) extra virgin olive oil, extra
¼ cup (60ml) lime juice
1 clove garlic, crushed
2 tablespoons chopped coriander (cilantro)
sea salt and cracked black pepper
4 cups (50g) snow pea tendrils
2 Lebanese cucumbers (260g), thinly sliced
chervil sprigs, to serve

Place the amaranth, dukkah and salt on a small tray and toss to
combine. Dip each salmon fillet in the egg and press into the dukkah
mixture to coat. Heat the oil in a large non-stick frying pan over
medium heat. Cook the salmon, turning every 3–4 minutes, for
10–12 minutes or until just cooked through and the crumb is golden.
   Place the chilli, extra oil, lime juice, garlic, coriander, salt and
pepper in a medium bowl and whisk to combine. Add the snow pea
tendrils and cucumber and toss to coat. Divide the salmon and
salad between serving plates and top with chervil to serve. **SERVES 4**

egg and chicken soup

2 litres chicken stock
1 tablespoon finely grated ginger
1 clove garlic, thinly sliced
1 tablespoon soy sauce
2 tablespoons Shaoxing (Chinese cooking wine)
2 x 200g chicken breast fillets, trimmed
2 eggs, lightly beaten
2 bunches broccolini (350g), blanched and sliced
2 green onions (scallions), sliced
2 teaspoons sesame oil
baby (micro) Asian herbs (optional), to serve

Place the stock, ginger, garlic, soy sauce and Shaoxing in a
medium saucepan over high heat and bring to the boil. Add
the chicken, cover with a tight-fitting lid and cook for 5 minutes.
Remove from the heat and allow to stand for 10 minutes or until
the chicken is cooked through. Remove the chicken, reserving
the stock, allow to cool slightly and shred finely.
   Place the chicken stock over high heat and return to the boil.
Remove from the heat and, using a wooden spoon, stir the stock
in a circular motion to create a whirlpool effect. Gradually add
the egg in a thin, steady stream. Allow to stand for 1 minute or
until the egg is cooked. Divide the chicken and broccolini between
serving bowls. Ladle over the egg broth and top with the onion,
sesame oil and baby herbs to serve. **SERVES 4**

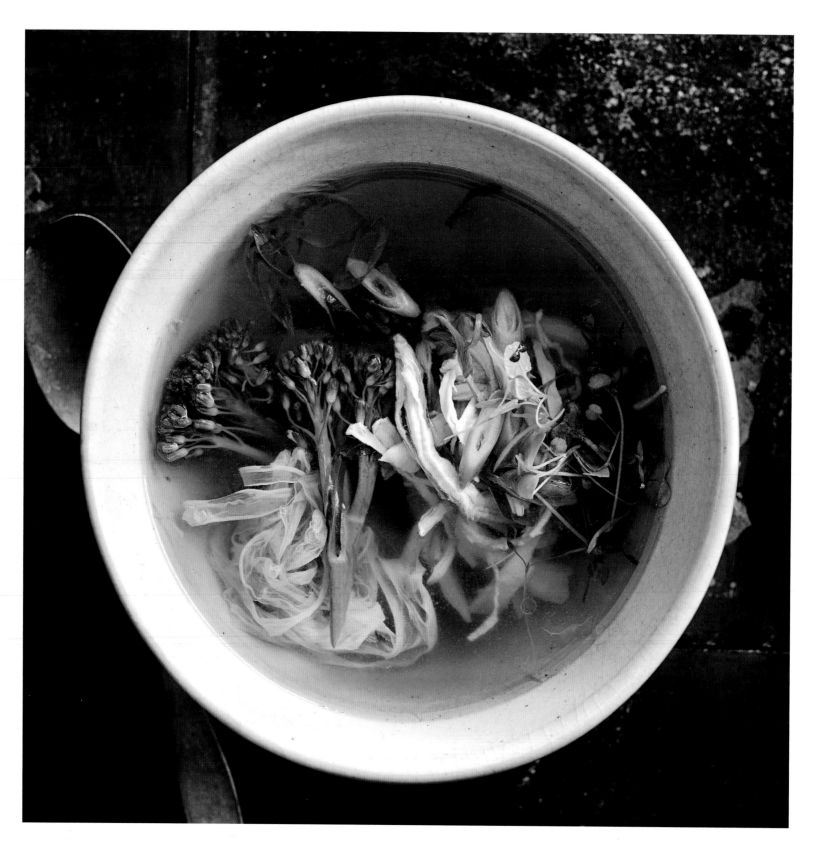

egg and chicken soup

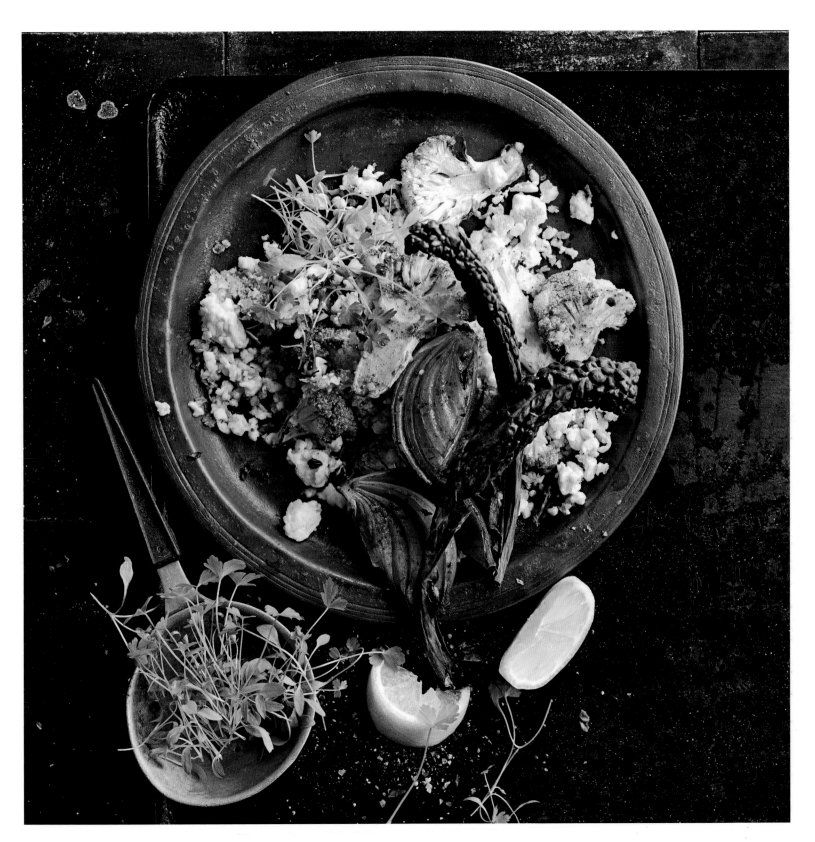

scrambled tofu with roasted cauliflower and greens

scrambled tofu with roasted cauliflower and greens

1.2kg silken tofu, drained and crumbled
1 teaspoon ras el hanout*
½ teaspoon smoked paprika
½ teaspoon dried chilli flakes
⅓ cup (80ml) extra virgin olive oil,
    plus extra for drizzling
6 cups (600g) cauliflower florets
2 red onions, quartered
1 bunch cavolo nero (Tuscan kale) (220g), trimmed
sea salt and cracked black pepper
baby (micro) parsley leaves (optional), to serve
lemon wedges, to serve

packed with protein, tofu also boasts plenty of iron and calcium

Wrap the tofu in a clean tea towel and squeeze out the moisture. Allow to drain over a sieve for 30 minutes to dry.

Preheat oven to 200°C (400°F). Place the ras el hanout, paprika, chilli and half the oil in a large bowl and whisk to combine. Add the cauliflower and onion and toss to coat. Place on 2 baking trays lined with non-stick baking paper and roast for 10 minutes. Add the cavolo nero to the trays, drizzle with extra oil and roast for a further 8 minutes or until the cauliflower and onion are golden and the cavolo nero is crisp.

Heat the remaining oil in a non-stick frying pan over high heat. Add the tofu, salt and pepper and cook, stirring occasionally, for 25–30 minutes or until golden and crisp. Divide between serving plates and top with the cauliflower, onion, cavolo nero and parsley. Serve with lemon wedges. **SERVES 4**

herb and garlic lamb with green olive salad

2 sprigs rosemary
10 sprigs thyme
6 sprigs oregano
¼ cup (60ml) extra virgin olive oil
2 cloves garlic, sliced
4 x 200g lamb backstraps
sea salt and cracked black pepper
1½ cups (260g) green (Sicilian) olives, pitted and chopped
1 Lebanese cucumber (130g), chopped
¼ cup mint leaves
1 tablespoon white balsamic vinegar
100g goat's curd

Sicilian olives are mild and fruity in flavour and have lots of beneficial fats

Tie the rosemary, thyme and oregano together with kitchen string. Heat the oil in a large non-stick frying pan over medium heat. Add the herbs and garlic and cook, stirring occasionally, for 4–5 minutes or until fragrant. Remove from the heat and set aside.

Place the lamb on a tray, sprinkle with salt and pepper and brush with some of the herb oil, using the herb bunch as a brush. Preheat a char-grill pan or barbecue over high heat. Cook the lamb for 2–3 minutes each side for medium rare, or until cooked to your liking.

Place the olive, cucumber, mint, vinegar and 1 tablespoon of the herb oil in a bowl and toss to combine. Slice the lamb and serve with the green olive salad and goat's curd. **SERVES 4**

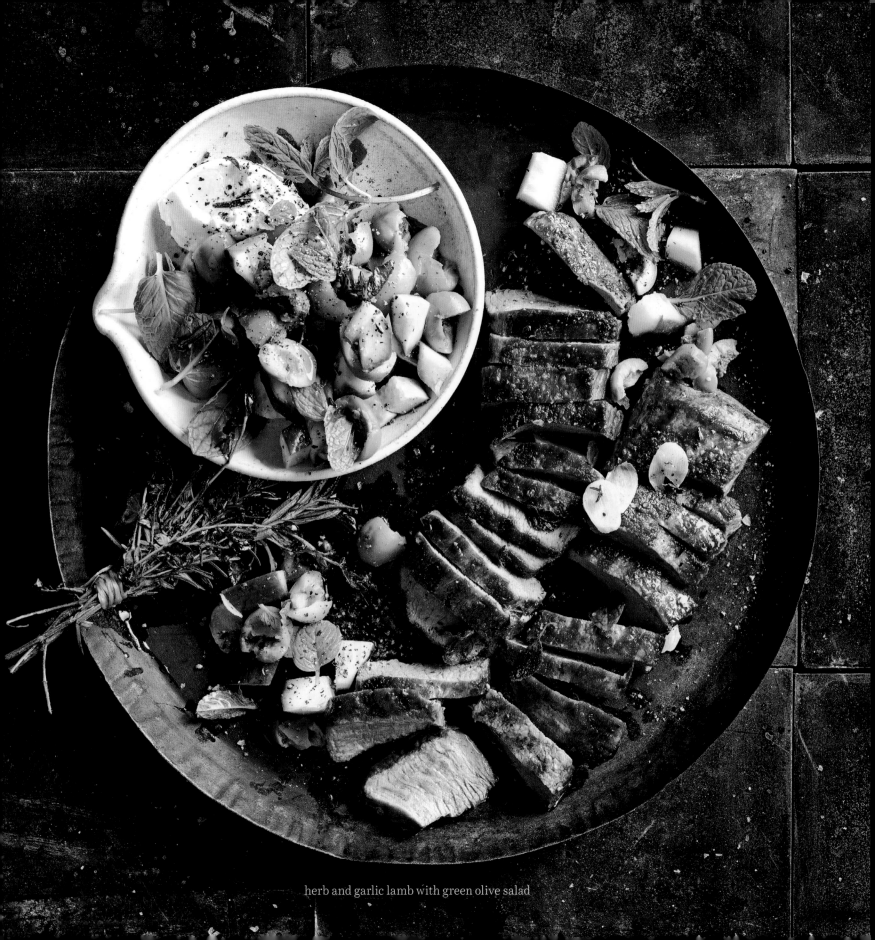

herb and garlic lamb with green olive salad

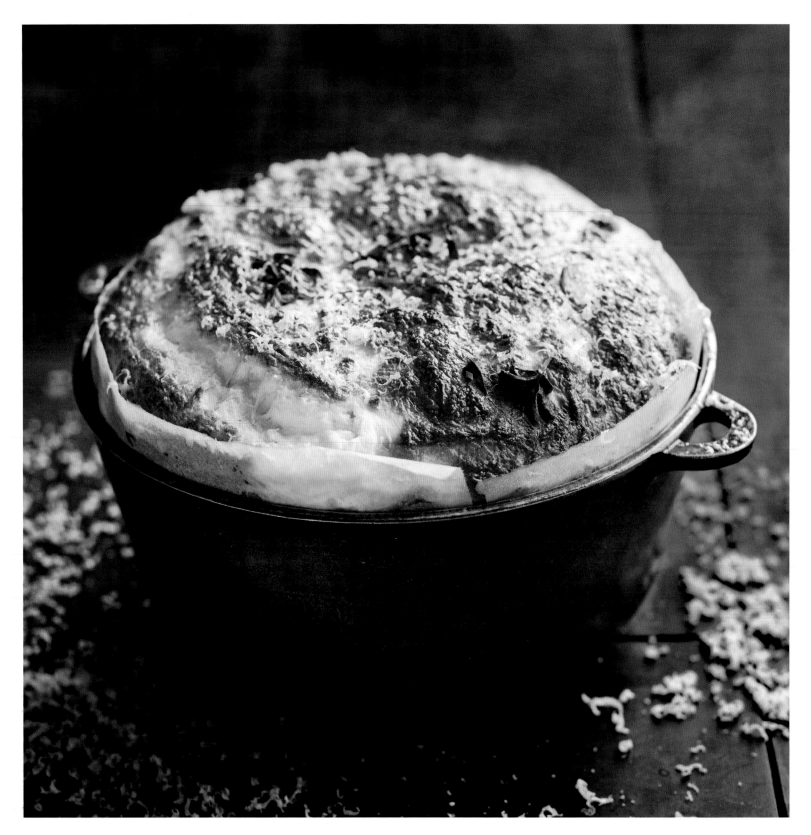

whipped ricotta soufflé

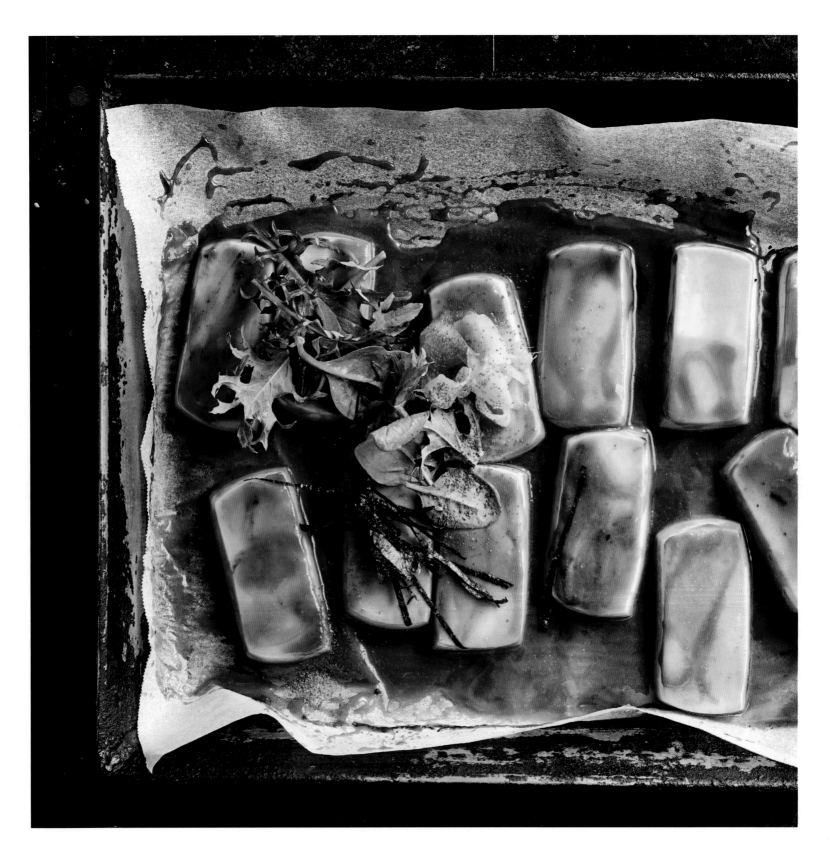

miso-glazed baked tofu

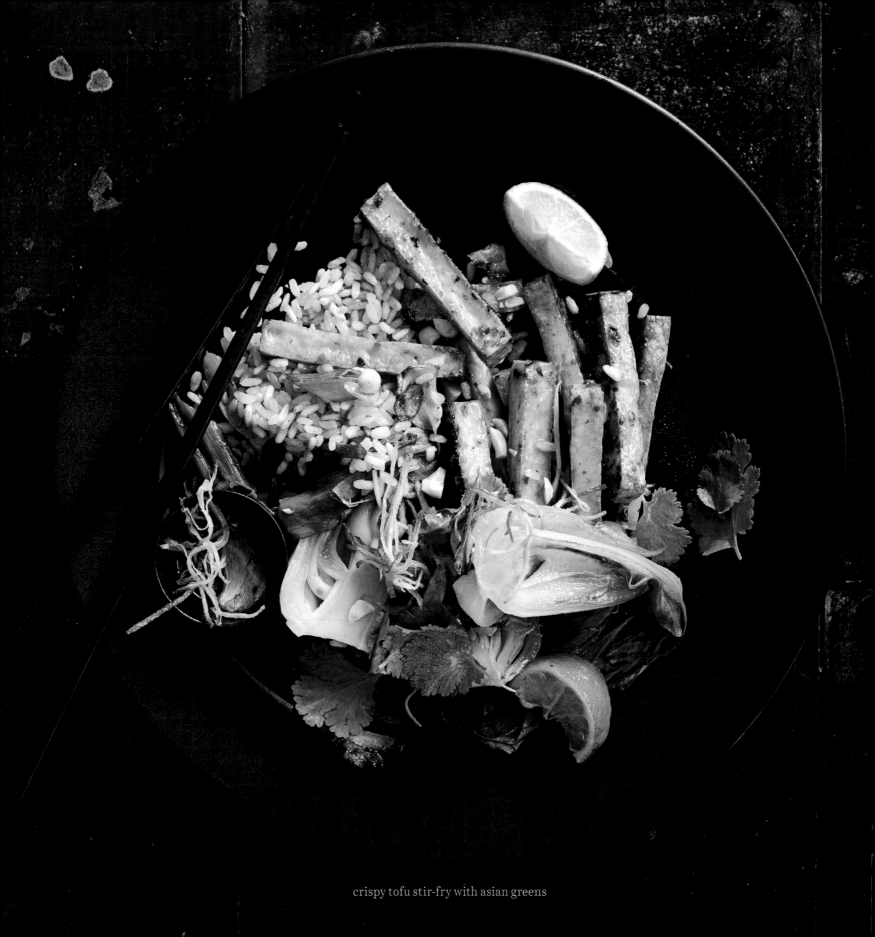

crispy tofu stir-fry with asian greens

whipped ricotta soufflé

6 egg yolks
1½ cups (120g) finely grated parmesan, plus extra to serve
3⅓ cups (800g) low-fat fresh ricotta
½ cup (125ml) milk
¼ cup oregano leaves
1 teaspoon sea salt flakes
½ teaspoon cracked black pepper
8 eggwhites
1 teaspoon white wine vinegar

Preheat oven to 180°C (350°F). Lightly grease a 20cm springform cake tin and line with non-stick baking paper. Place the egg yolks, parmesan, ricotta, milk, oregano, salt and pepper in a large bowl and mix until just combined. Place the eggwhites and vinegar in a bowl and whisk until soft peaks form. Add to the ricotta mixture and, using a large metal spoon, gently fold to combine. Spoon the mixture into the prepared tin and bake for 35–40 minutes or until golden and puffed. Sprinkle with extra parmesan to serve. **SERVES 4**

miso-glazed baked tofu

2 tablespoons each yellow miso paste*,
   rice wine vinegar, soy sauce and honey
600g firm tofu, cut into 2cm-thick slices
2 cups (50g) baby kale leaves
2 cups (50g) baby spinach leaves
1 sheet nori*, thinly sliced
pickled ginger, to serve
shichimi togarashi*, to serve
dressing
2 teaspoons yellow miso paste*
⅓ cup (80ml) orange juice
sea salt and cracked black pepper

Preheat oven to 180°C (350°F). Place the miso paste, vinegar, soy sauce and honey in a bowl and whisk until smooth. Arrange the tofu on baking trays lined with non-stick baking paper and drizzle with the miso glaze. Bake for 15–20 minutes or until caramelised.

To make the dressing, place the miso paste, orange juice, salt and pepper in a small bowl and whisk to combine.

Top the tofu with the kale, spinach, nori and ginger. Drizzle with the dressing and sprinkle with togarashi to serve. **SERVES 4**

crispy tofu stir-fry with asian greens

600g firm tofu, drained and cut into 1cm batons
1½ tablespoons peanut oil
2 cups (400g) cooked brown rice (see *glossary*, page 227)
2 cloves garlic, thinly sliced
1 tablespoon finely shredded ginger
2 green onions (scallions), sliced
4 bunches baby bok choy (600g), trimmed and halved
1 tablespoon light soy sauce
2 tablespoons store-bought Asian chilli jam
2 tablespoons lime juice
¼ cup (35g) roasted peanuts, chopped
1 cup coriander (cilantro) leaves, to serve
lime wedges, to serve

Preheat oven to 220°C (425°F). Place the tofu on a baking tray lined with non-stick baking paper and bake for 15 minutes or until golden and crisp.

Heat 1 teaspoon of the oil in a large non-stick frying pan or wok over high heat until just smoking. Add the rice and cook for 4–5 minutes or until golden and crisp. Remove from the pan, set aside and keep warm.

Heat another 1 teaspoon of the oil and add the garlic, ginger and onion to the pan. Cook, stirring, for 1 minute. Add the bok choy and soy sauce and cook for a further 1 minute or until just starting to wilt. Remove from the pan and set aside.

Place the chilli jam, lime juice and the remaining oil in a small bowl and whisk to combine. Reduce the heat to medium, add the chilli jam mixture to the pan and cook until bubbling. Add the baked tofu and cook, turning to coat, for 3–4 minutes or until golden and crisp. Return the bok choy mixture to the pan and toss to combine. Divide the rice between serving bowls and top with the stir-fry, peanuts and coriander. Serve with lime wedges. **SERVES 4**

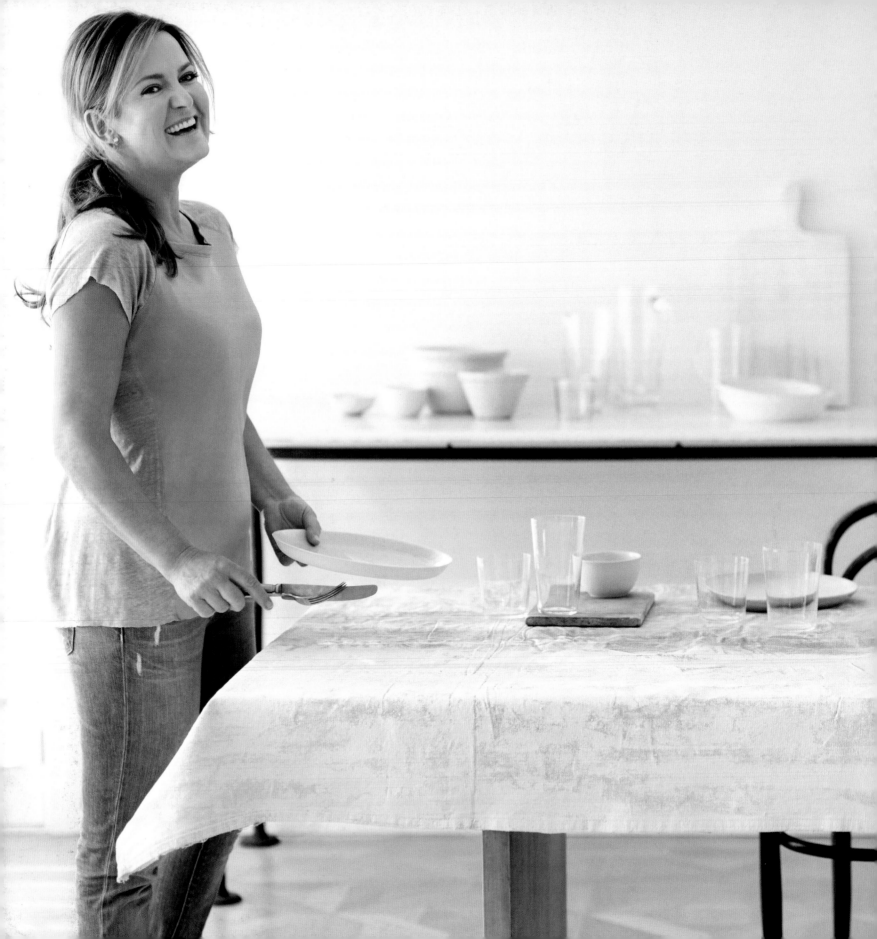

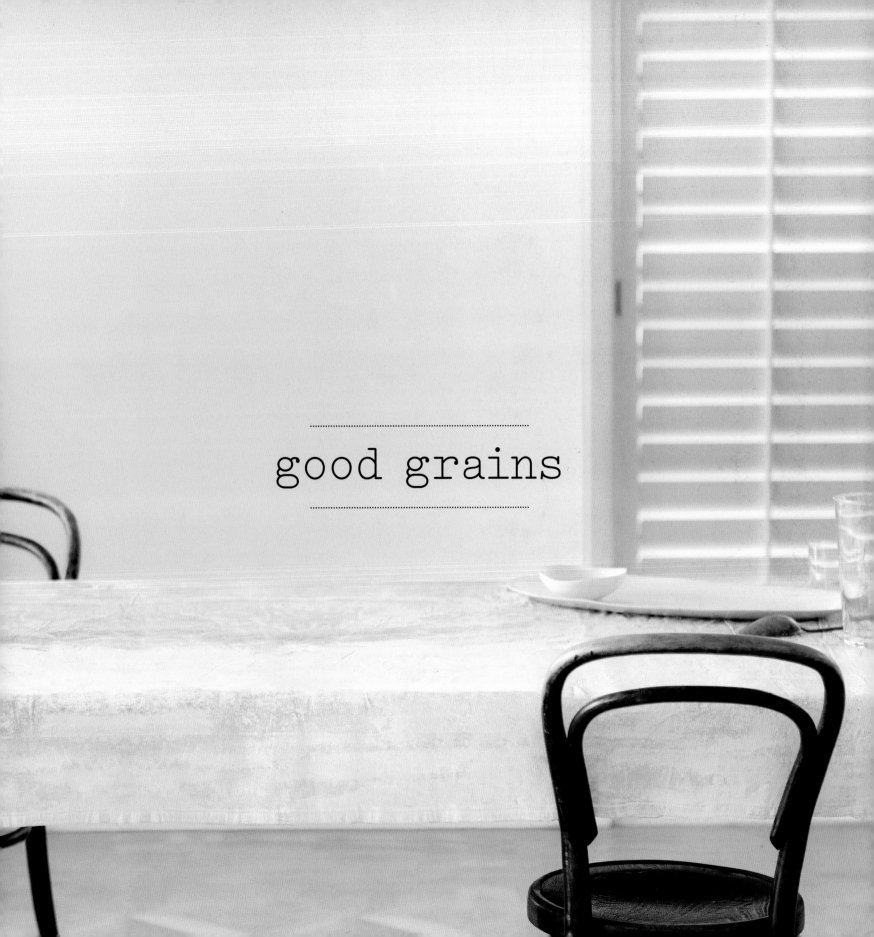

good grains

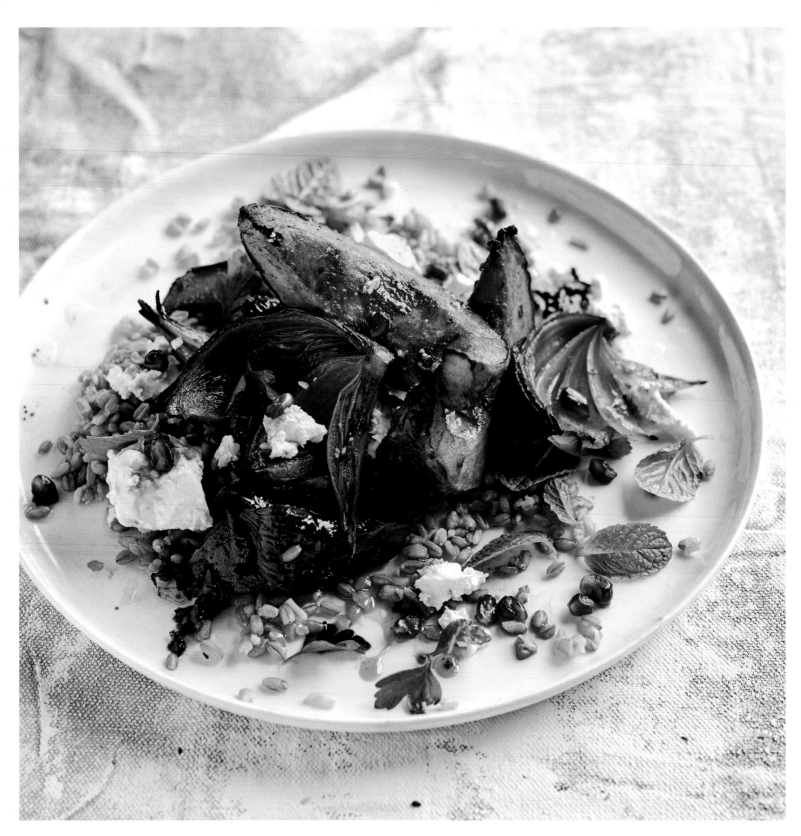

smoky pumpkin, spelt, pomegranate and feta salad

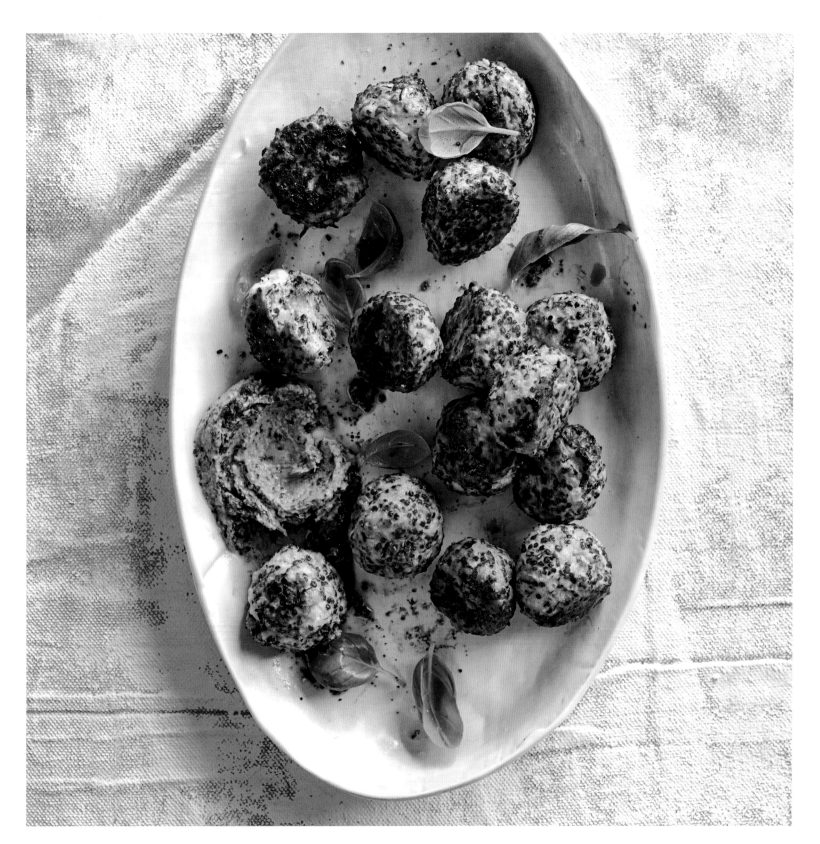

chicken, zucchini and feta meatballs

smoky pumpkin, spelt, pomegranate and feta salad

1.2kg kent pumpkin, cut into wedges
2 red onions, cut into wedges
¼ cup (60ml) extra virgin olive oil
2 tablespoons pomegranate molasses*
1 tablespoon smoked paprika
1 teaspoon dried chilli flakes
sea salt and cracked black pepper
4 cups (800g) cooked spelt* (see *glossary*, page 231)
2 cups mint leaves
1 cup flat-leaf parsley leaves
1 pomegranate, seeds removed
store-bought marinated feta, crumbled, to serve
pomegranate dressing
¼ cup (60ml) extra virgin olive oil
1 tablespoon pomegranate molasses*
1 clove garlic, crushed
sea salt and cracked black pepper

To make the pomegranate dressing, place the oil, pomegranate molasses, garlic, salt and pepper in a bowl. Whisk to combine and set aside.

Preheat oven to 200°C (400°F). Place the pumpkin, onion, oil, pomegranate molasses, paprika, chilli, salt and pepper in a large bowl and toss to combine. Transfer to a baking tray lined with non-stick baking paper and roast for 30 minutes or until golden and crisp.

Place the spelt, mint, parsley and half the pomegranate seeds in a large bowl. Add the dressing and toss to combine. Divide between serving plates and top with the pumpkin and onion. Sprinkle with feta and the remaining pomegranate seeds to serve. **SERVES 4**

chicken, zucchini and feta meatballs

2 cups (360g) coarsely grated zucchini (courgette) (about 3 zucchinis)
500g chicken mince
2 cups (340g) cooked red quinoa* (see *glossary*, page 230)
2 cloves garlic, crushed
2 tablespoons store-bought quince paste
¼ cup finely chopped flat-leaf parsley
1 tablespoon finely grated lemon rind
sea salt and cracked black pepper
150g feta, crumbled
¼ cup (20g) finely grated parmesan
extra virgin olive oil, for brushing
store-bought kale or basil pesto and basil leaves, to serve

Preheat oven to 200°C (400°F). Place the zucchini, chicken, quinoa, garlic, quince paste, parsley, lemon rind, salt and pepper in a large bowl and mix well to combine. Add the feta and parmesan and mix until just combined. Roll tablespoons of the mixture into balls and place on a baking tray lined with non-stick baking paper. Brush with oil and bake, turning halfway, for 20 minutes or until golden and cooked through. Serve meatballs with pesto and basil. **SERVES 4**

toasted grain and cauliflower tabouli

4½ cups (450g) cauliflower florets, finely chopped
1 cup (100g) cooked buckwheat* (see *glossary*, page 228)
1 cup (165g) cooked coarse burghul* (see *glossary*, page 228)
½ cup (125ml) extra virgin olive oil
2 teaspoons ras el hanout*
sea salt and cracked black pepper
3 cups flat-leaf parsley, roughly chopped
¼ cup dill, roughly chopped
½ cup (70g) pistachios, chopped
¼ cup (40g) dried currants
2 tablespoons lemon juice
fresh ricotta and lemon wedges, to serve

Preheat oven to 180°C (350°F). Place the cauliflower, buckwheat, burghul, oil, ras el hanout, salt and pepper in a large bowl and toss to combine. Spread the mixture between 2 baking trays and roast for 25–30 minutes or until golden and puffed. Allow to cool. Place in a large bowl, add the parsley, dill, pistachios, currants and lemon juice and toss to combine. Serve with ricotta and lemon wedges. **SERVES 4**

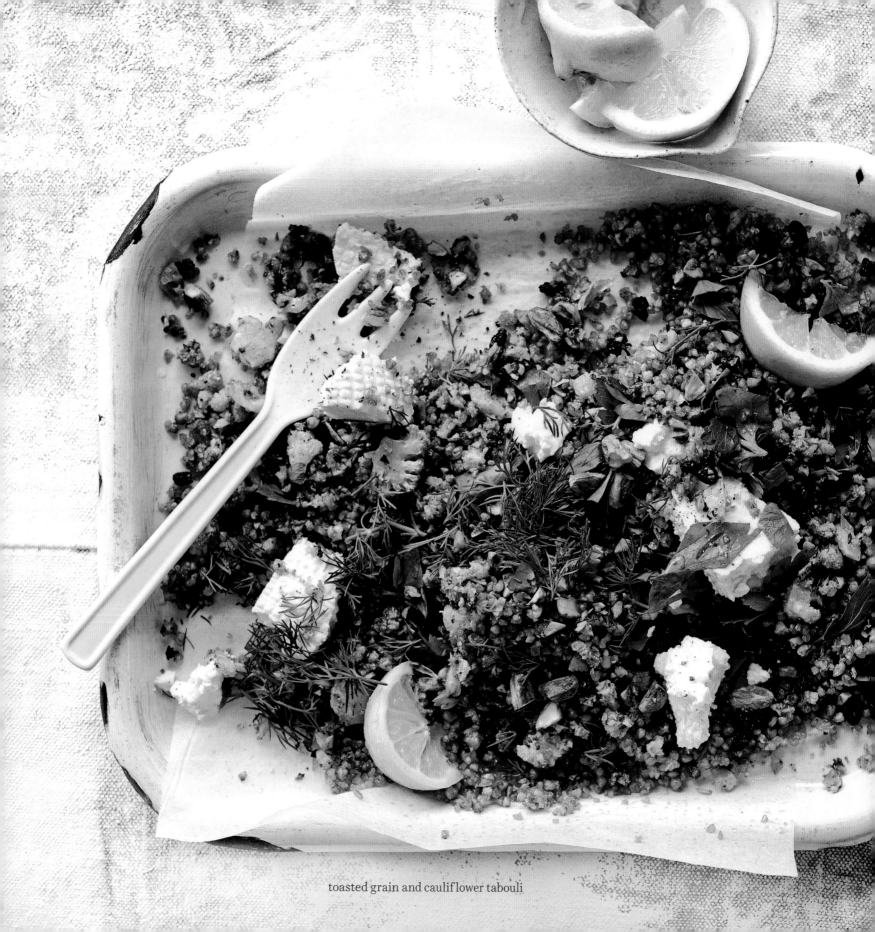

toasted grain and cauliflower tabouli

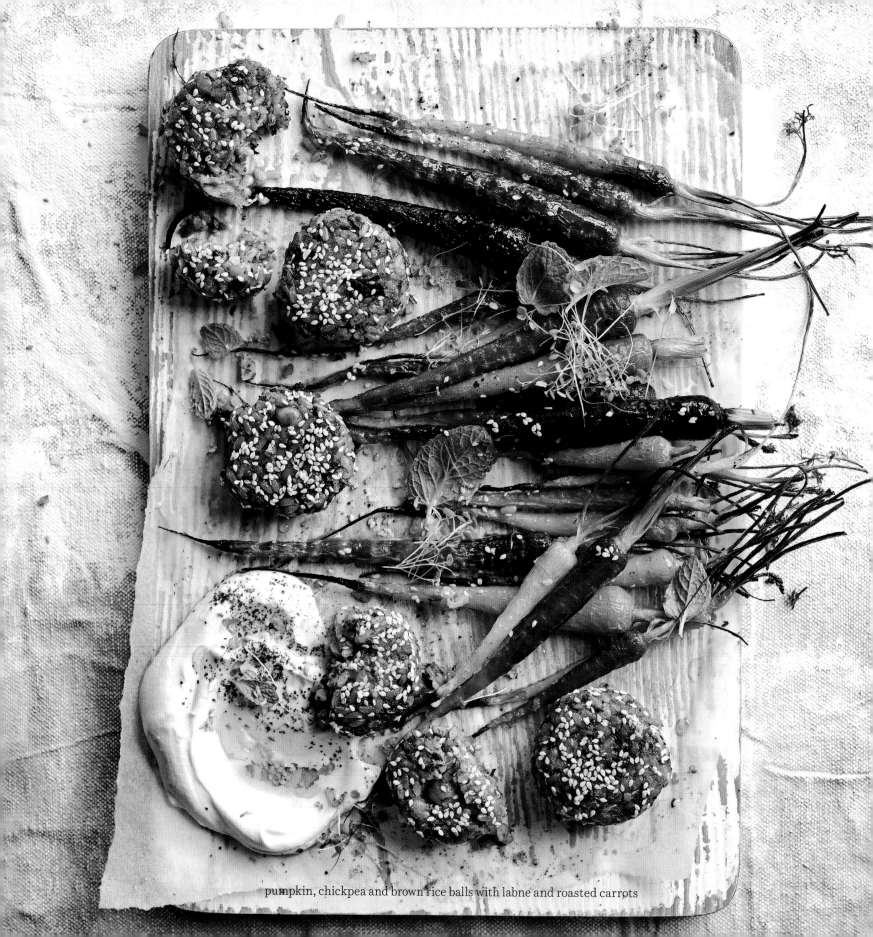

pumpkin, chickpea and brown rice balls with labne and roasted carrots

pumpkin, chickpea and brown rice balls with labne and roasted carrots

400g butternut pumpkin, peeled, seeded and chopped
24 heirloom baby carrots
2 tablespoons extra virgin olive oil, plus extra for brushing
sea salt and cracked black pepper
1 x 400g can chickpeas (garbanzo beans), rinsed and drained
2 cups (400g) cooked brown rice (see glossary, page 227)
1 tablespoon finely grated lemon rind
1 teaspoon dried chilli flakes
1 clove garlic, crushed
2 teaspoons ground sumac*, plus extra for sprinkling
1 cup coriander (cilantro) leaves, finely chopped
¼ cup (40g) sesame seeds
labne (yoghurt cheese), to serve
mint leaves and baby (micro) watercress (optional), to serve

Preheat oven to 200°C (400°F). Place the pumpkin and carrots on a large baking tray. Drizzle with the oil, sprinkle with salt and pepper and toss to coat. Roast for 20 minutes or until golden and tender.

Place the chickpeas in a large bowl and roughly mash with a fork. Add the pumpkin, rice, lemon rind, chilli, garlic, sumac, coriander, salt and pepper and mix well to combine. Divide and shape the mixture into 2-tablespoon balls and flatten slightly. Press into the sesame seeds to coat and brush with extra oil. Place on a baking tray lined with non-stick baking paper and roast, turning halfway, for 20 minutes or until golden. Sprinkle with extra sumac and serve with the carrots, labne, mint and baby watercress. **SERVES 4**

pumpernickel bagels

1¼ cups (310ml) water, at room temperature
14g dry yeast
2½ cups (375g) whole-wheat flour*
1 cup (120g) rye flour*
2 tablespoons raw cacao powder*
1 tablespoon brown sugar
1 tablespoon instant coffee granules
2 teaspoons sea salt flakes
¼ cup (95g) molasses*   ← *find molasses in supermarkets – it's usually near the honey*
¼ cup (60ml) vegetable oil
4 litres water, extra
2 tablespoons molasses*, extra
1 tablespoon black sesame seeds
2 teaspoons caraway seeds
1 eggwhite, lightly beaten
cream cheese, gravlax and sliced dill pickles, to serve

Place the water, yeast and 1 cup (150g) of the whole-wheat flour in a large bowl and stir to combine. Allow to stand in a warm place for 5–10 minutes or until bubbly. Add the remaining whole-wheat flour, the rye flour, cacao, sugar, coffee, salt, molasses and oil and mix until well combined. Turn out the dough onto a lightly floured surface and knead for 8–10 minutes or until smooth and elastic. Place in a lightly oiled bowl, cover with a clean tea towel and set aside in a warm place for 1 hour or until doubled in size.

Divide and shape the dough into 8 equal rounds and, using your thumb, make a small hole in the centre of each. Cover with the tea towel and set aside for 10 minutes.

Preheat oven to 200°C (400°F). Place the extra water and extra molasses in a large saucepan over high heat and bring to the boil. Reduce the heat to medium and bring to a gentle simmer. Working in batches, add the bagels and cook for 1 minute. Turn, using a slotted spoon, and cook for a further 1 minute. Remove the bagels from the water and place on a baking tray lined with non-stick baking paper. Place the sesame and caraway seeds in a bowl and mix to combine. Brush the bagels with the eggwhite and sprinkle with the seed mix. Bake for 20–25 minutes or until the bagels are crisp on the outside. Slice, spread with cream cheese and top with gravlax and pickles to serve. **MAKES 8**

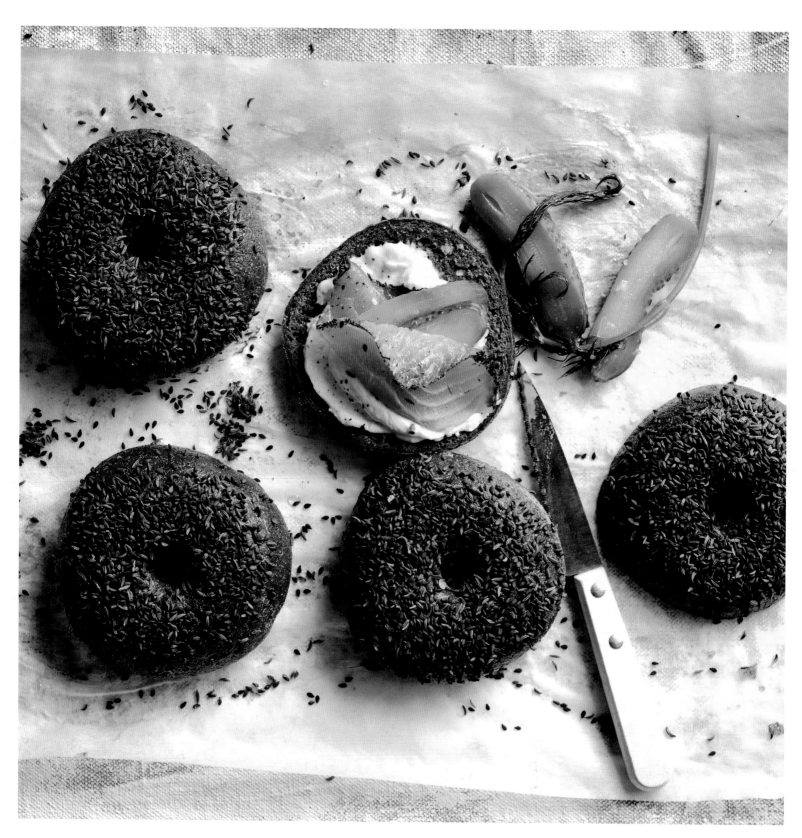

pumpernickel bagels

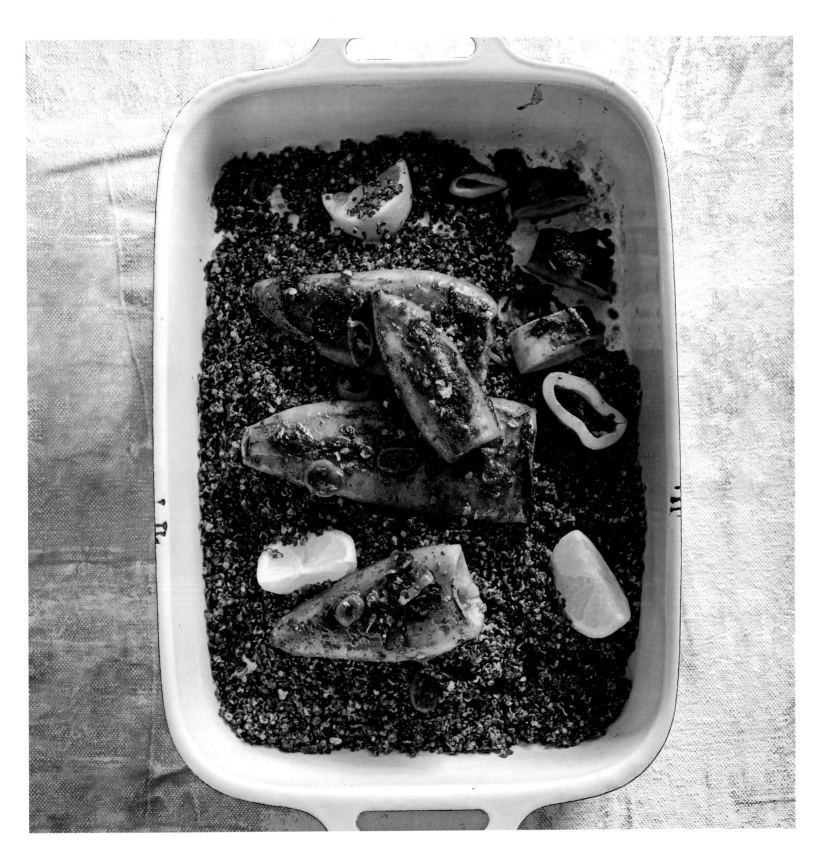

sticky wok-fried calamari with black quinoa

sticky wok-fried calamari with black quinoa

⅓ cup (80ml) peanut oil
650g cleaned squid hoods
2 tablespoons finely grated ginger
3 cloves garlic, crushed
2 tablespoons kecap manis (sweet Indonesian soy sauce)
3 tablespoons Chinese black vinegar
1 tablespoon finely grated orange rind
2 long red chillies, thinly sliced
3 cups (510g) cooked black quinoa* (see *glossary*, page 230)
sea salt and cracked Sichuan pepper (optional)
lemon wedges, to serve

Place 2 tablespoons of the oil, the squid, ginger, garlic, kecap manis, vinegar, orange rind and chilli in a bowl and toss to coat. Cover and set aside in the refrigerator for 1 hour to marinate.

Heat the remaining oil in a large non-stick frying pan or wok over high heat. Working in batches add the squid, reserving the marinade, and cook for 3 minutes each side or until cooked through. Set aside and keep warm. Add the reserved marinade to the pan and cook for 3–4 minutes or until thickened.

Place the quinoa on a serving plate, top with the squid and pour over the sticky sauce. Sprinkle with salt and Sichuan pepper and serve with lemon wedges. **SERVES 4**

beef skewers with crispy amaranth and brown rice noodle pancakes

800g beef rump, trimmed and thinly sliced
¼ cup (60ml) store-bought Asian chilli jam
¼ cup (60ml) oyster sauce
¼ cup (60ml) brown rice vinegar
2 cloves garlic, crushed
1 tablespoon finely grated ginger
2 Lebanese cucumbers (260g), peeled and thinly sliced
2 tablespoons rice wine vinegar
sea salt and cracked black pepper
baby (micro) coriander (cilantro) (optional), to serve
lime wedges, to serve
crispy amaranth and noodle pancakes
150g thin brown rice noodles, cooked and drained
1 cup (285g) cooked amaranth* (see *glossary*, page 228)
3 long red chillies, seeded and finely chopped
3 green onions (scallions), sliced
5 kaffir lime leaves*, thinly sliced
1 teaspoon sesame oil
1 teaspoon sea salt flakes
2 eggwhites, lightly beaten
2 tablespoons vegetable oil

Place the beef, chilli jam, oyster sauce, brown rice vinegar, garlic and ginger in a bowl and toss to coat. Cover and refrigerate for 30 minutes to marinate.

To make the crispy amaranth and noodle pancakes, place the noodles, amaranth, chilli, onion, lime leaf, sesame oil, salt and eggwhite in a bowl and mix to combine. Heat a little of the vegetable oil in a large non-stick frying pan over high heat. Cook the pancakes, in ½-cup (60ml) batches, for 4–5 minutes each side or until golden and crisp. Set aside and keep warm.

Preheat a char-grill pan or barbecue over high heat. Thread the beef onto bamboo skewers and cook for 2–3 minutes each side or until charred and just cooked. Place the cucumber and rice wine vinegar in a bowl and toss to combine. Divide the crispy pancakes between serving plates and top with cucumber and the beef skewers. Sprinkle with salt, pepper and coriander and serve with lime wedges. **SERVES 4**

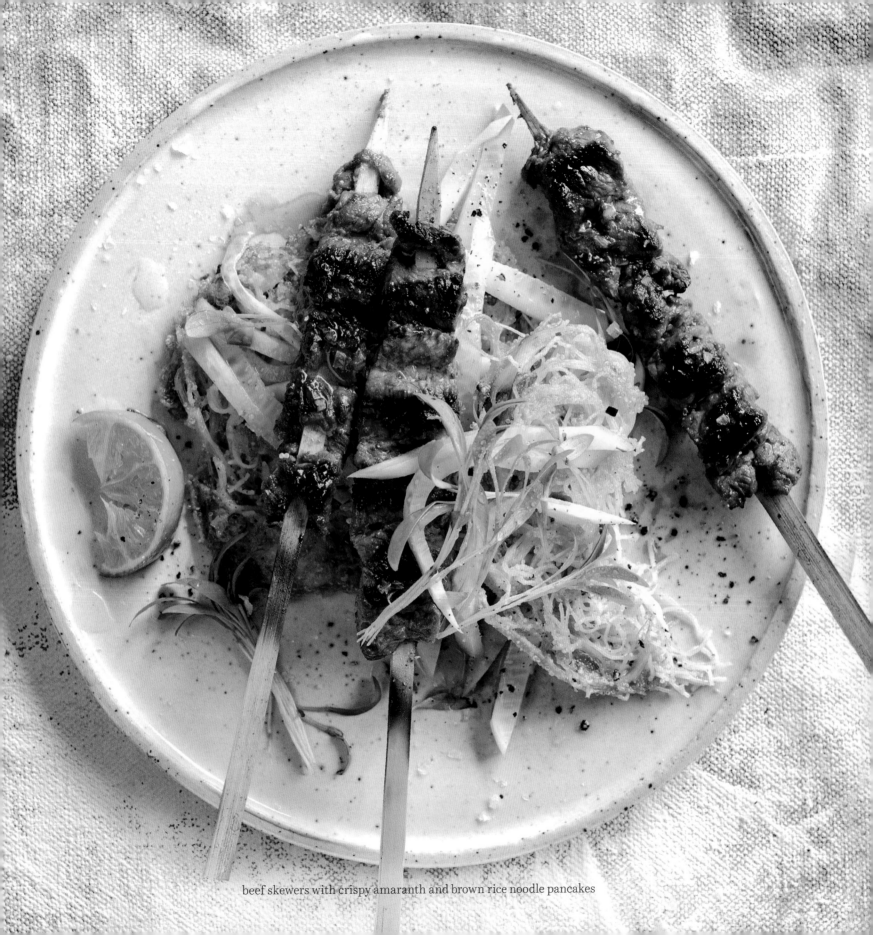

beef skewers with crispy amaranth and brown rice noodle pancakes

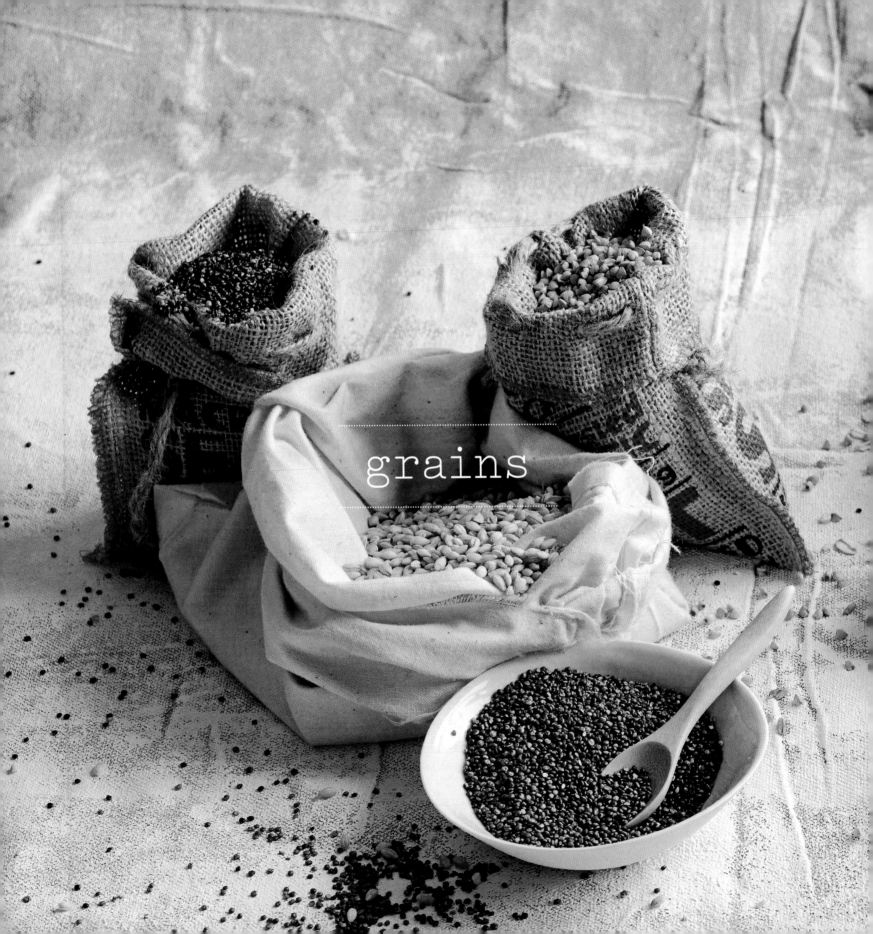

grains

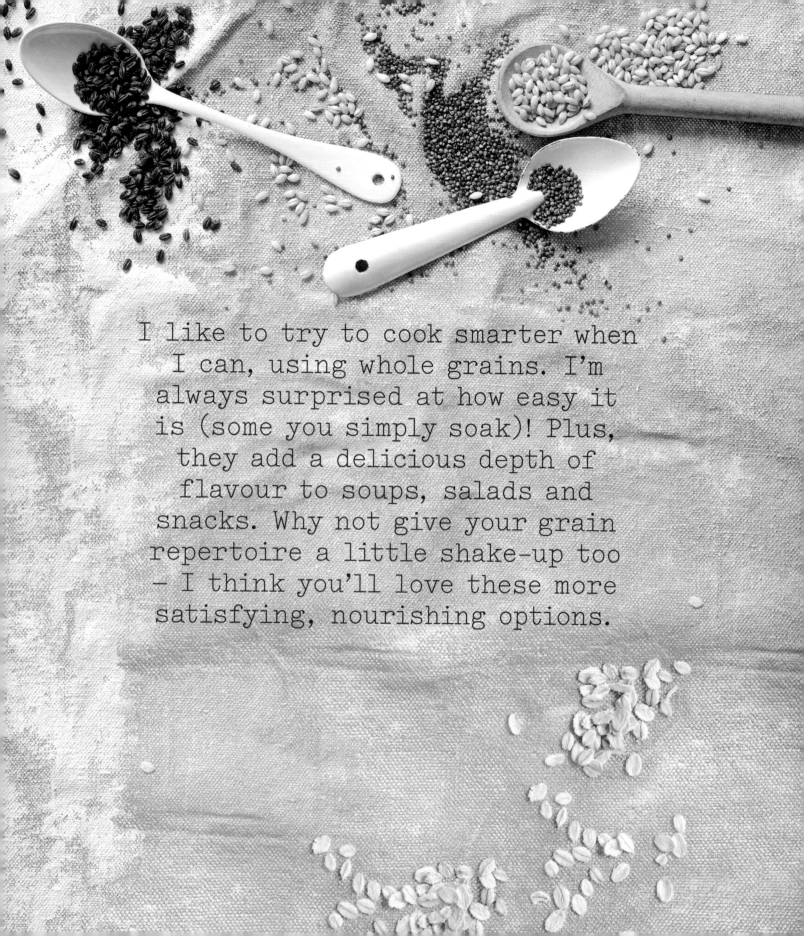

I like to try to cook smarter when I can, using whole grains. I'm always surprised at how easy it is (some you simply soak)! Plus, they add a delicious depth of flavour to soups, salads and snacks. Why not give your grain repertoire a little shake-up too — I think you'll love these more satisfying, nourishing options.

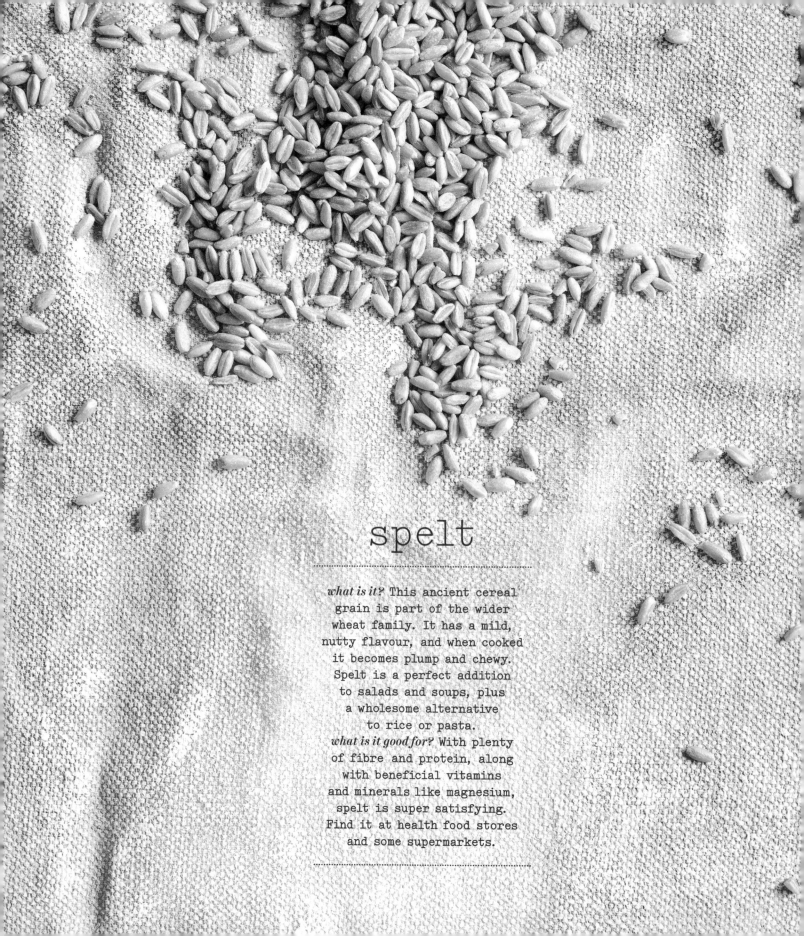

spelt

what is it? This ancient cereal
grain is part of the wider
wheat family. It has a mild,
nutty flavour, and when cooked
it becomes plump and chewy.
Spelt is a perfect addition
to salads and soups, plus
a wholesome alternative
to rice or pasta.
what is it good for? With plenty
of fibre and protein, along
with beneficial vitamins
and minerals like magnesium,
spelt is super satisfying.
Find it at health food stores
and some supermarkets.

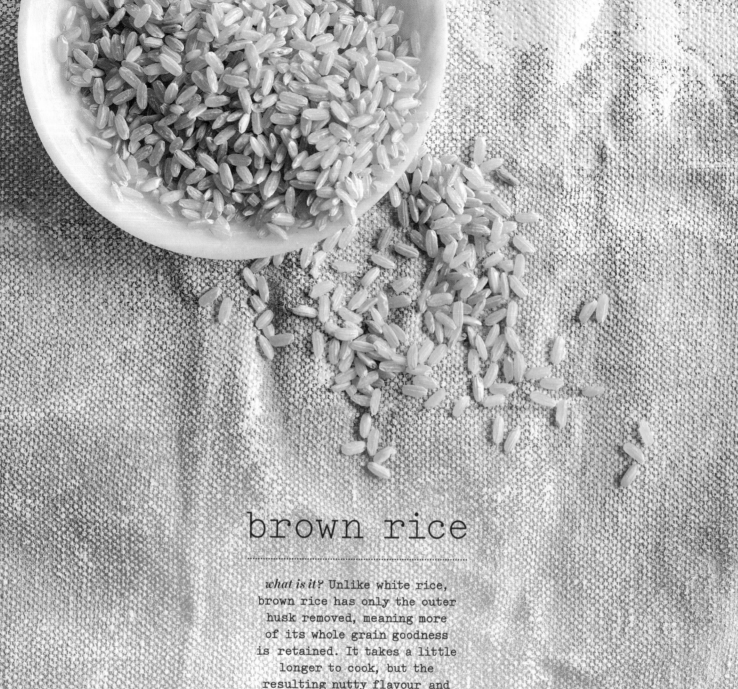

brown rice

what is it? Unlike white rice,
brown rice has only the outer
husk removed, meaning more
of its whole grain goodness
is retained. It takes a little
longer to cook, but the
resulting nutty flavour and
firm but fluffy texture
are worth it.
what is it good for? High in
minerals such as manganese
and selenium, and with
beneficial B-group vitamins,
brown rice is a great grain
choice. It's gluten-free, too
— a perfect pantry staple!

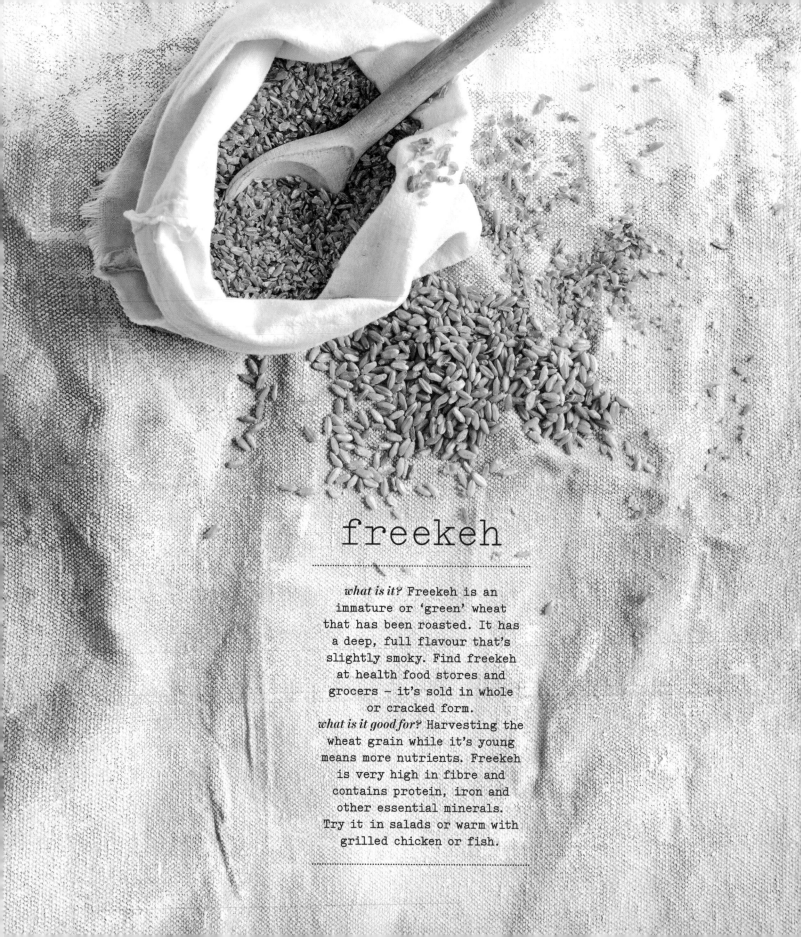

freekeh

what is it? Freekeh is an immature or 'green' wheat that has been roasted. It has a deep, full flavour that's slightly smoky. Find freekeh at health food stores and grocers – it's sold in whole or cracked form.

what is it good for? Harvesting the wheat grain while it's young means more nutrients. Freekeh is very high in fibre and contains protein, iron and other essential minerals. Try it in salads or warm with grilled chicken or fish.

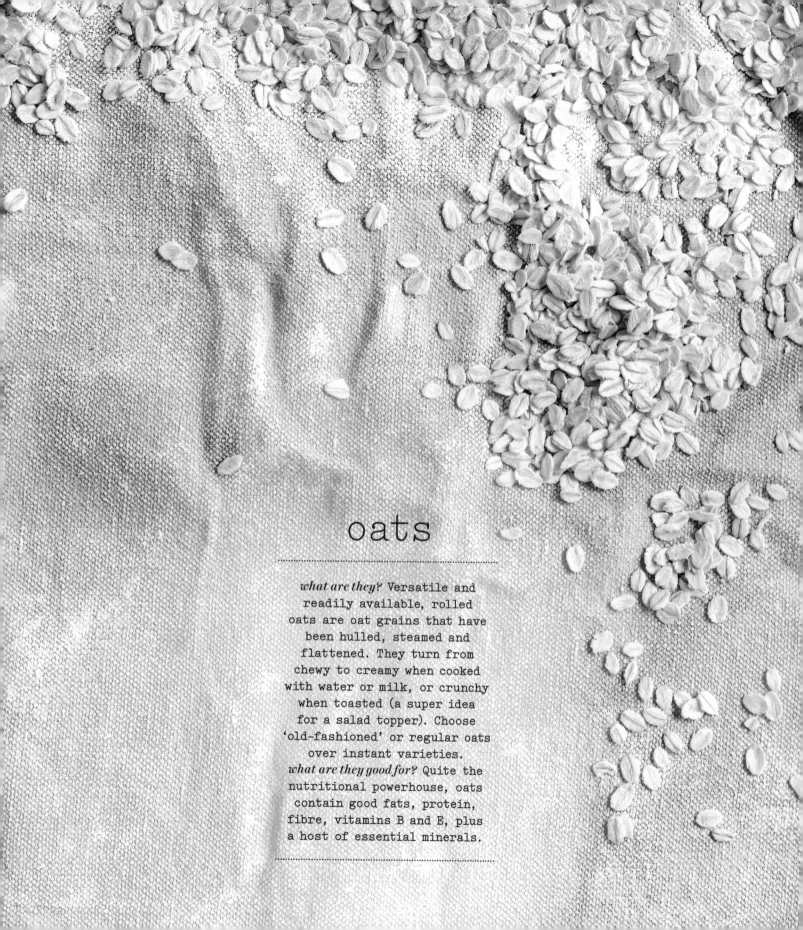

oats

what are they? Versatile and readily available, rolled oats are oat grains that have been hulled, steamed and flattened. They turn from chewy to creamy when cooked with water or milk, or crunchy when toasted (a super idea for a salad topper). Choose 'old-fashioned' or regular oats over instant varieties.

what are they good for? Quite the nutritional powerhouse, oats contain good fats, protein, fibre, vitamins B and E, plus a host of essential minerals.

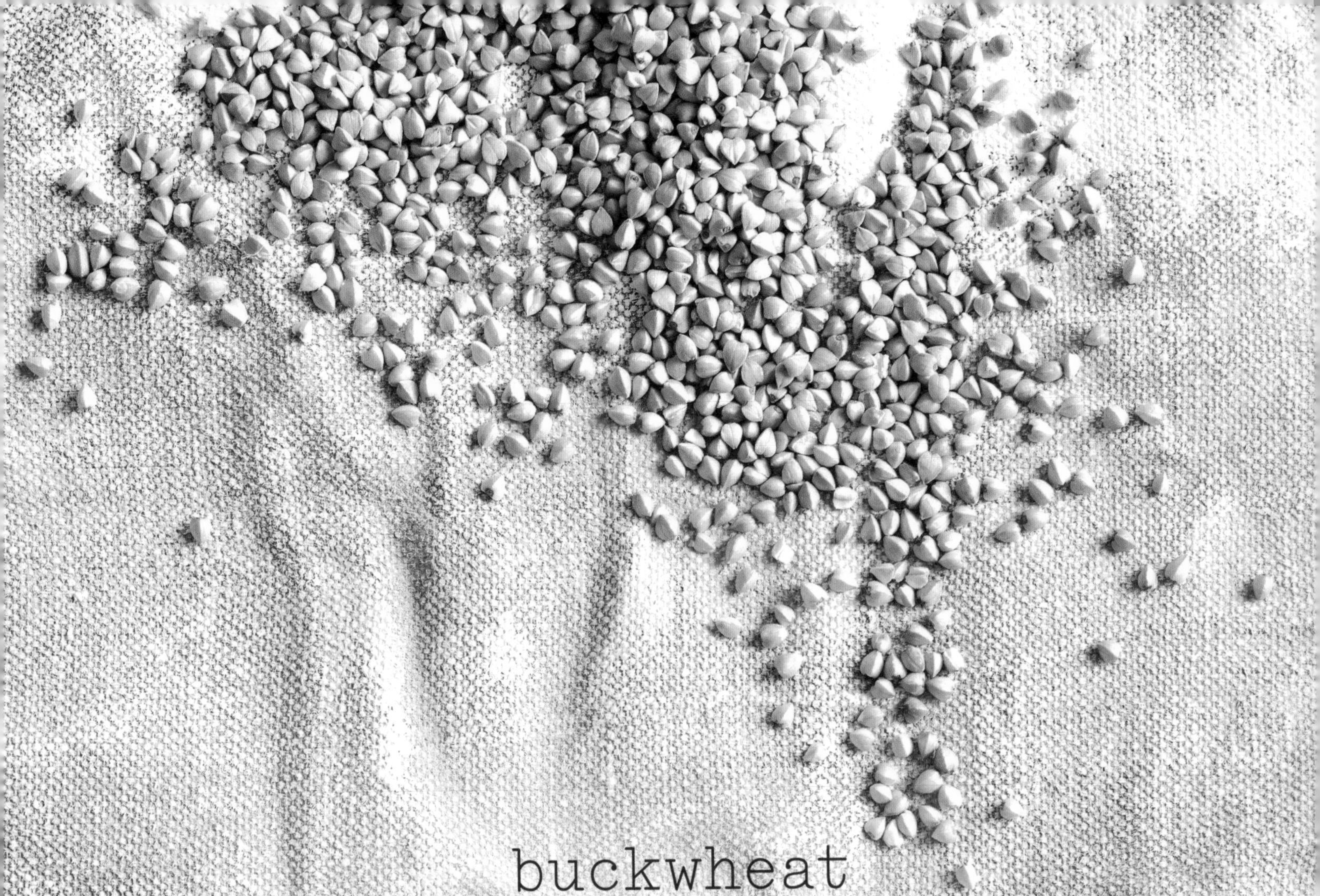

buckwheat

what is it? Buckwheat is in
fact not a wheat at all, but
the seeds of a plant related
to rhubarb. These little
pyramid-shaped kernels
are light brown or green in
colour and, once cooked, can
be used just like rice or
pasta. Buy raw buckwheat
at health food stores and
some supermarkets.
what is it good for? Gluten-free,
fibre-rich and full of
minerals, raw buckwheat is
a clever way to add substance
to breakfast bowls or salads.

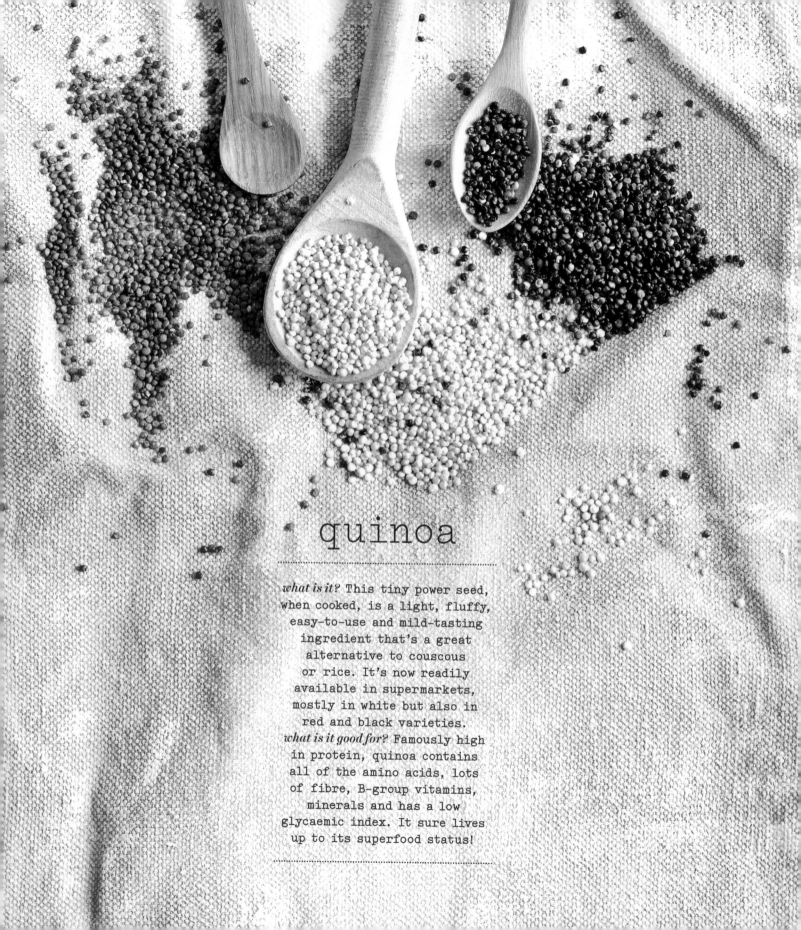

quinoa

what is it? This tiny power seed, when cooked, is a light, fluffy, easy-to-use and mild-tasting ingredient that's a great alternative to couscous or rice. It's now readily available in supermarkets, mostly in white but also in red and black varieties.

what is it good for? Famously high in protein, quinoa contains all of the amino acids, lots of fibre, B-group vitamins, minerals and has a low glycaemic index. It sure lives up to its superfood status!

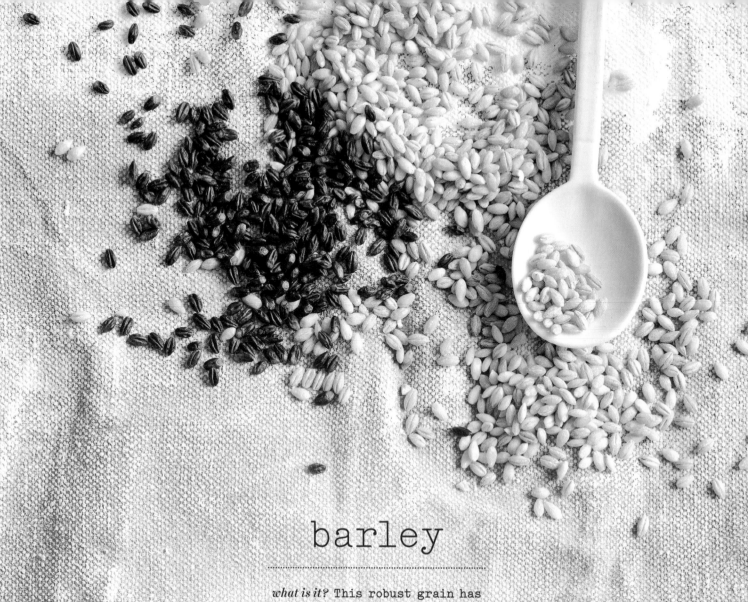

barley

what is it? This robust grain has been used for centuries. To make pearl barley, the barley husk and bran are removed and the grains are steamed and polished until smooth. Black barley is an heirloom variety and can be found at health food stores. Both are creamy and satisfying in soups, stews and wintry salads.

what is it good for? Barley is high in fibre and has a good amount of protein. With B-group vitamins, iron and selenium, too, it's a smart carbohydrate.

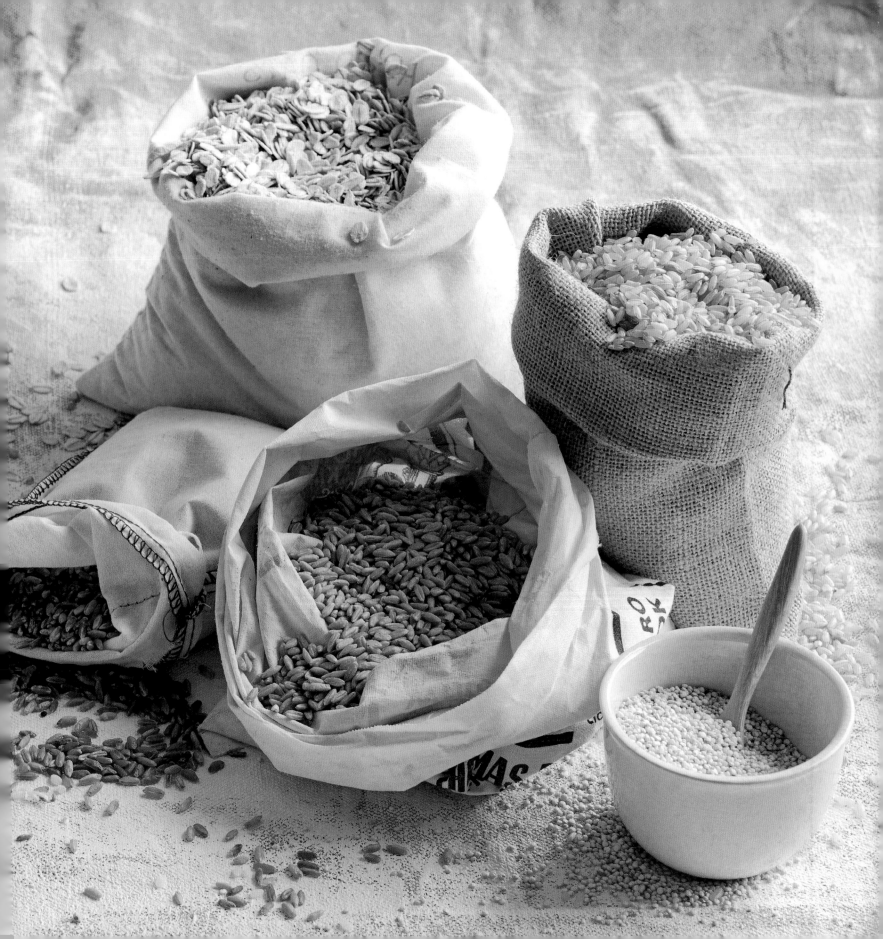

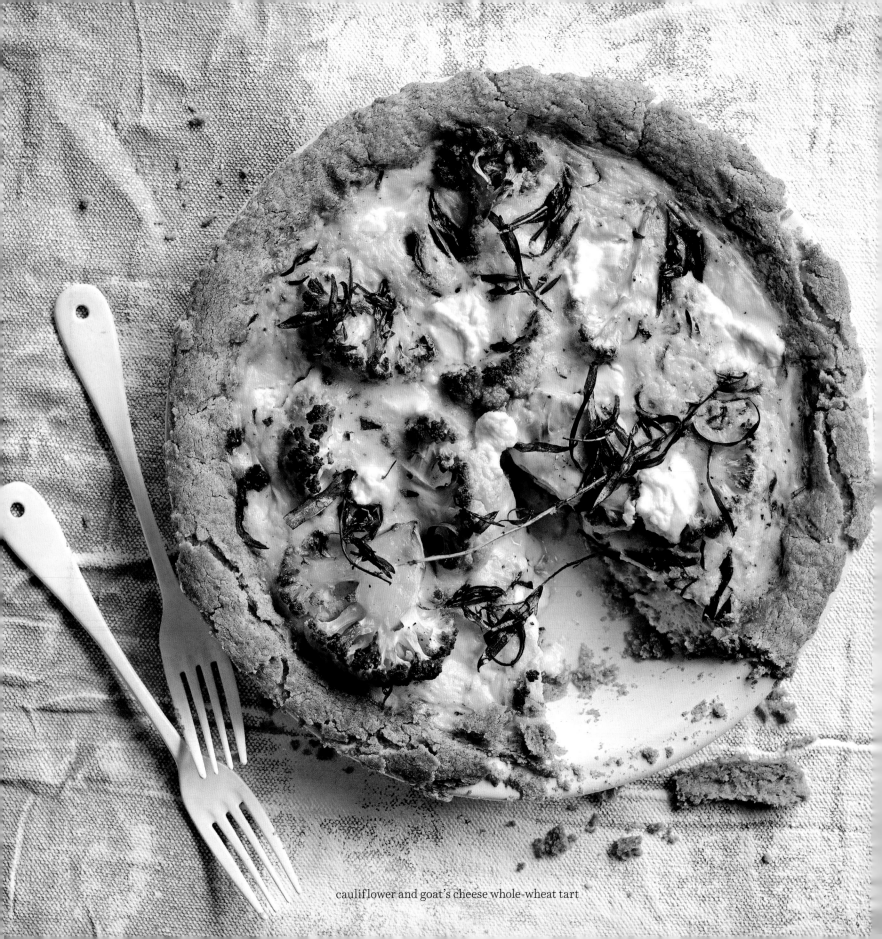

cauliflower and goat's cheese whole-wheat tart

barley lends this zesty slaw its nourishing fibre and essential minerals

cauliflower and goat's cheese whole-wheat tart

3½ cups (350g) cauliflower florets
½ cup tarragon leaves
¼ cup (60ml) extra virgin olive oil
sea salt and cracked black pepper
4 eggs
¾ cup (180ml) milk
¼ cup (20g) finely grated parmesan
100g goat's curd
whole-wheat pastry
½ cup (70g) wholemeal spelt flour*
¾ cup (120g) brown rice flour*
1 teaspoon psyllium husk powder*
1 teaspoon sea salt flakes
150g cold unsalted butter, chopped
1 tablespoon iced water

Preheat oven to 180°C (350°F). To make the whole-wheat pastry, place both the flours, the psyllium husk powder, salt and butter in a food processor and process until the mixture resembles coarse breadcrumbs. Add the water, a little at a time, until a soft dough forms. Turn out onto a lightly floured surface and bring together to form a flat disc. Wrap in plastic wrap and refrigerate for 30 minutes.

Place the cauliflower and tarragon on a baking tray lined with non-stick baking paper. Drizzle with the oil, sprinkle with salt and pepper and toss to coat. Roast for 20 minutes or until golden.

Roll out the dough between 2 sheets of non-stick baking paper to a 5mm-thick round. Line a 23cm pie tin with the pastry, trimming any excess. Line the pastry case with non-stick baking paper and fill with baking beans or uncooked rice. Bake for 25 minutes, remove the paper and beans and bake for a further 10 minutes or until crisp. Remove from the oven and reduce the temperature to 160°C (320°F).

Place the eggs, milk, parmesan, salt, pepper and half the goat's curd in a bowl and whisk to combine. Place the roasted cauliflower mixture in the pastry case and pour over the egg mixture. Spoon over the remaining goat's curd and bake for 30–35 minutes or until just set. Slice and serve warm. **SERVES 4–6**

asian barley slaw

2 cups (370g) cooked pearl barley (see *glossary*, page 226)
2 cups (160g) shredded Chinese cabbage (wombok)
2 cups (240g) shredded green mango
1 eschalot (French shallot), thinly sliced
1 cup (140g) podded edamame*, cooked
1 cup coriander (cilantro) leaves
1 cup Thai basil leaves
½ cup (80g) roasted cashews, chopped
sesame omelette
4 eggs
1 teaspoon fish sauce
2 teaspoons sesame oil
2 teaspoons black sesame seeds
2 tablespoons vegetable oil
dressing
¼ cup (60ml) rice wine vinegar
¼ cup (60ml) mirin (Japanese rice wine)
2 tablespoons fish sauce
2 tablespoons lime juice
1 clove garlic, crushed
1 long red chilli, seeded and finely chopped

To make the dressing, place the vinegar, mirin, fish sauce, lime juice, garlic and chilli in a bowl. Whisk to combine and set aside.

To make the sesame omelette, place the eggs, fish sauce, sesame oil and sesame seeds in a bowl and whisk to combine. Heat 2 teaspoons of the vegetable oil in a small non-stick frying pan over medium heat. Add one-quarter of the egg mixture and cook, stirring a little at first, for 2 minutes or until just set. Set aside and keep warm. Repeat with the remaining vegetable oil and egg mixture.

Place the barley, cabbage, mango, eschalot, edamame, coriander, basil and cashews in a large bowl. Pour over the dressing and toss to combine. Divide the slaw between serving plates and top with the warm sesame omelettes. **SERVES 4**

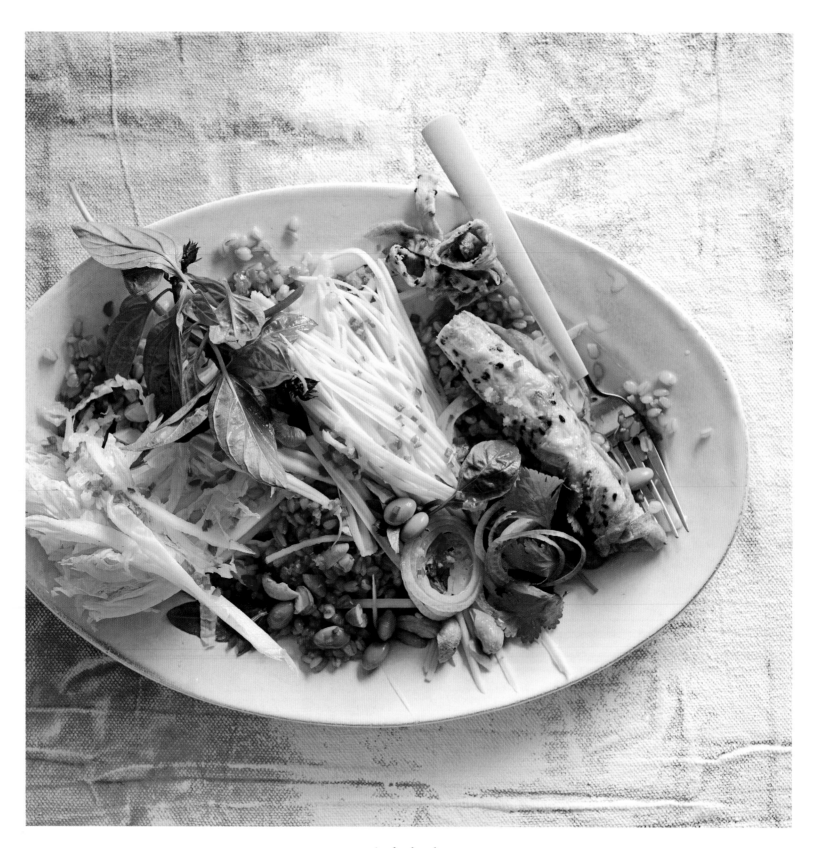

asian barley slaw

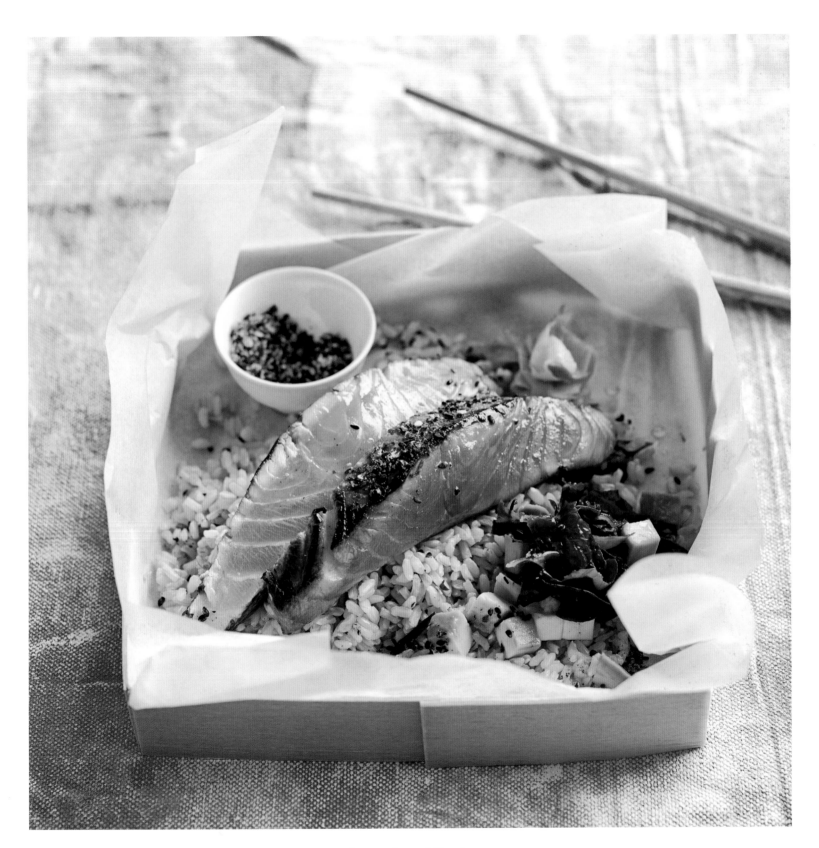

brown rice sushi bowls

brown rice sushi bowls

1½ cups (300g) brown rice
2¼ cups (560ml) cold water
¼ cup dried wakame* pieces
1 cup (250ml) cold water, extra
2 tablespoons peanut oil
4 x 250g skinless salmon fillets
1 tablespoon kecap manis (sweet Indonesian soy sauce)
1 avocado, chopped
½ cup (140g) pickled ginger, drained, liquid reserved
chilli sesame salt
1 tablespoon black sesame seeds
½ teaspoon dried chilli flakes
½ teaspoon sea salt flakes

To make the chilli sesame salt, place the sesame seeds, chilli
and salt in a mortar and lightly crush with a pestle. Set aside.

Place the rice and water in a medium saucepan over high
heat and bring to the boil. Reduce the heat to low, cover with
a tight-fitting lid and cook for 30 minutes or until tender.
Set aside and keep warm.

Place the wakame and the extra water in a bowl. Allow to
stand for 10 minutes or until softened. Drain and set aside.

Heat the oil in a large non-stick frying pan over medium heat.
Brush the salmon with the kecap manis and cook, in batches,
for 1–2 minutes each side or until seared. Remove from the pan,
cover and allow to rest for 5 minutes before slicing each fillet
into 3 pieces. Spoon the rice into serving bowls and top with the
salmon, avocado, wakame, ginger and a little of the reserved
pickling liquid. Sprinkle with the sesame salt to serve. **SERVES 4**

freekeh, avocado and cucumber rice paper rolls with coriander dressing

2 cups (340g) cooked cracked freekeh* (see *glossary*, page 229)
12 x 20cm rice paper rounds
4 radishes, trimmed and thinly sliced
½ cup mint leaves
12 butter lettuce leaves
1 Lebanese cucumber (130g), cut into batons
1 avocado, sliced
½ cup (70g) salted roasted peanuts, chopped
coriander dressing
1 cup coriander (cilantro) leaves
2 green onions (scallions), chopped
1 teaspoon finely grated ginger
¼ cup (60ml) mirin (Japanese rice wine)
¼ cup (60ml) rice wine vinegar
2 tablespoons lime juice

To make the coriander dressing, place the coriander, green
onion, ginger, mirin, vinegar and lime juice in a small food
processor and process until finely chopped.

Place the freekeh in a bowl, add half the coriander dressing
and toss to combine. Dip 1 rice paper round in a bowl of cold
water for 10 seconds or until slightly softened. Place on a clean
surface and line the centre by alternating slices of radish with
mint leaves. Top with a lettuce leaf and a little of the freekeh,
cucumber, avocado and peanuts. Fold in three of the edges and
roll to enclose. Set aside under a clean damp tea towel and repeat
with the remaining rice paper rounds and ingredients. Serve
immediately with the remaining coriander dressing. **MAKES 12**

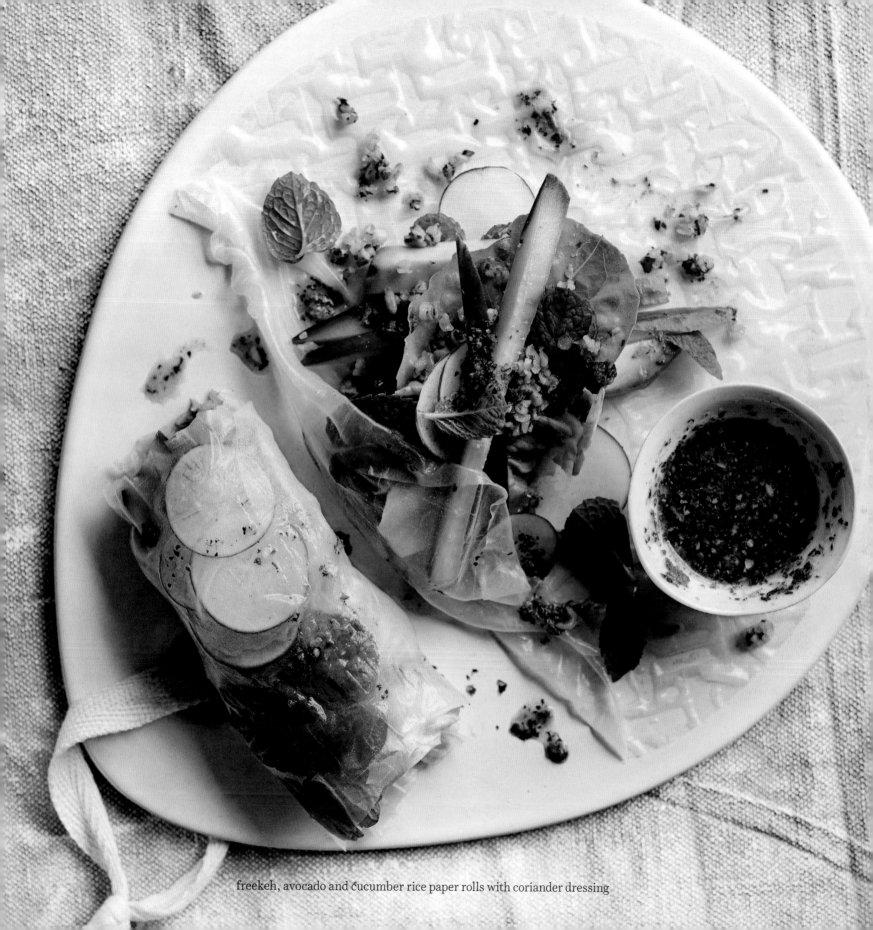

freekeh, avocado and cucumber rice paper rolls with coriander dressing

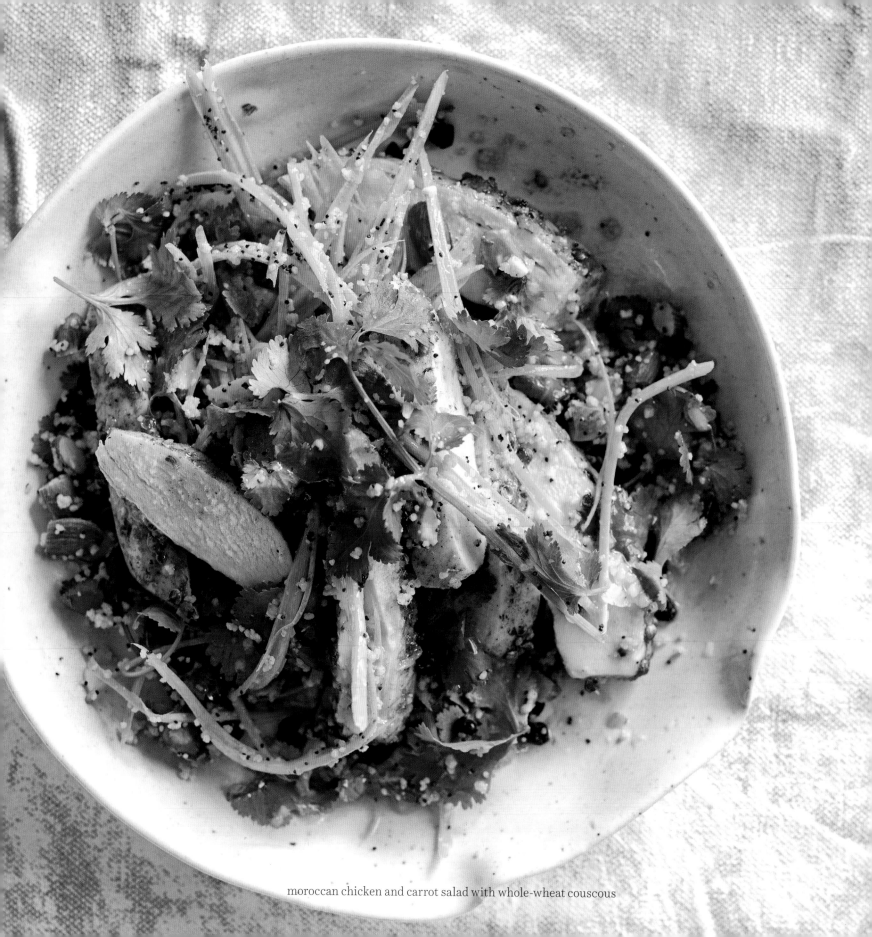

moroccan chicken and carrot salad with whole-wheat couscous

moroccan chicken and carrot salad with whole-wheat couscous

2 tablespoons extra virgin olive oil
1 teaspoon ras el hanout*
1 tablespoon chopped preserved lemon rind
1 teaspoon coriander seeds, crushed
3 x 200g chicken breast fillets, trimmed
1½ cups (240g) dried whole-wheat couscous*
1½ cups (375ml) boiling water
sea salt flakes
3 carrots, peeled and shredded
1 cup (160g) smoked almonds, chopped
½ cup (80g) dried currants
2 tablespoons poppyseeds
3 cups coriander (cilantro) leaves
orange dressing
2 tablespoons extra virgin olive oil
¼ cup (60ml) orange juice
2 tablespoons white wine vinegar
1 clove garlic, crushed
1 teaspoon Dijon mustard

almonds give this salad a hint of smokiness and a delicious crunch

To make the orange dressing, place the oil, orange juice, vinegar, garlic and mustard in a bowl. Whisk to combine and set aside.

Preheat oven to 220°C (425°F). Place the oil, ras el hanout, lemon rind and coriander seeds in a small bowl and mix to combine. Place the chicken on a baking tray lined with non-stick baking paper and brush with the ras el hanout mixture. Roast for 12–15 minutes or until golden and cooked through. Allow to cool slightly before slicing into strips.

While the chicken is roasting, place the couscous, water and a pinch of salt in a large bowl and cover with plastic wrap. Set aside for 5 minutes or until the water is absorbed. Fluff the couscous with a fork and add the carrot, almonds, currants, poppyseeds, coriander and the chicken. Top with the orange dressing, toss to combine and divide between bowls to serve. **SERVES 4**

quinoa and sweet potato bakes

2 sweet potatoes (kumara) (800g), peeled and chopped
    into 2cm cubes
2 tablespoons extra virgin olive oil, plus extra for drizzling
1 teaspoon sea salt flakes
2 cups (340g) cooked blacked quinoa* (see *glossary*, page 230),
    plus extra for sprinkling
2 tablespoons linseeds (flaxseeds)*
2 tablespoons store-bought caramelised onion
1¾ cups (420g) fresh ricotta
1½ cups (120g) finely grated parmesan
2 tablespoons thyme leaves
2 eggs
cracked black pepper
150g goat's cheese, sliced
6 sprigs thyme, extra

this is a cheat's trick to instant sweet flavour – keep a jar in your pantry

Preheat oven to 200°C (400°F). Lightly grease 6 x ¾-cup-capacity (180ml) Texas muffin tins, line with non-stick baking paper and set aside.

Place the sweet potato, oil and salt on a baking tray lined with baking paper and toss to combine. Roast for 20–25 minutes or until golden brown. Allow to cool slightly and transfer to a large bowl. Add the quinoa, linseeds, onion, ricotta, parmesan, thyme, eggs and pepper and mix until just combined.

Spoon into the prepared tins and top with the goat's cheese and extra thyme. Sprinkle with the extra quinoa, drizzle with extra oil and bake for 30–35 minutes or until golden. Serve warm. **MAKES 6**

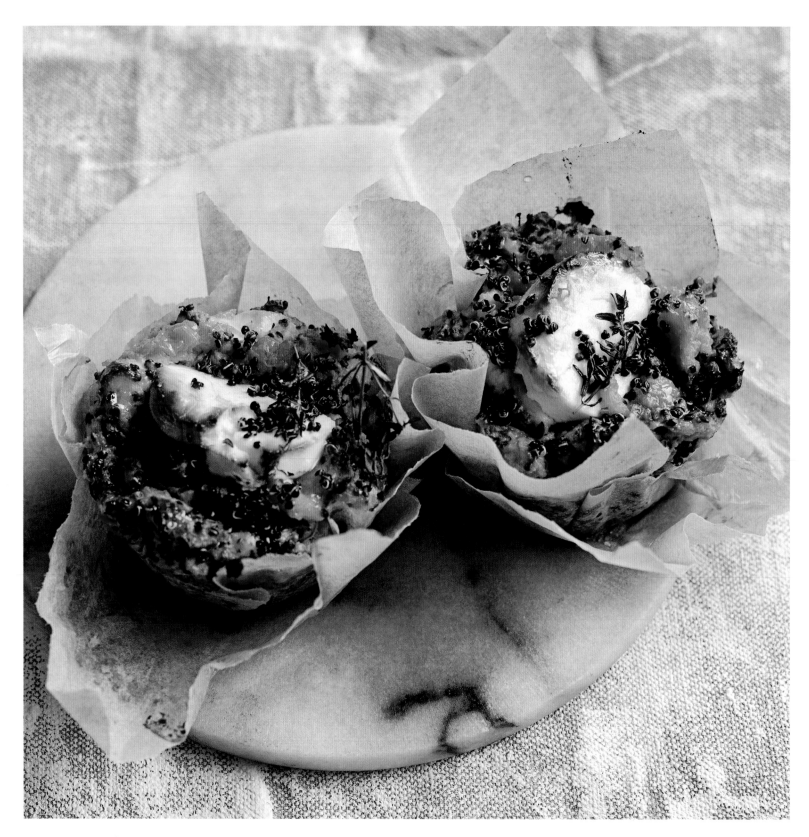

quinoa and sweet potato bakes

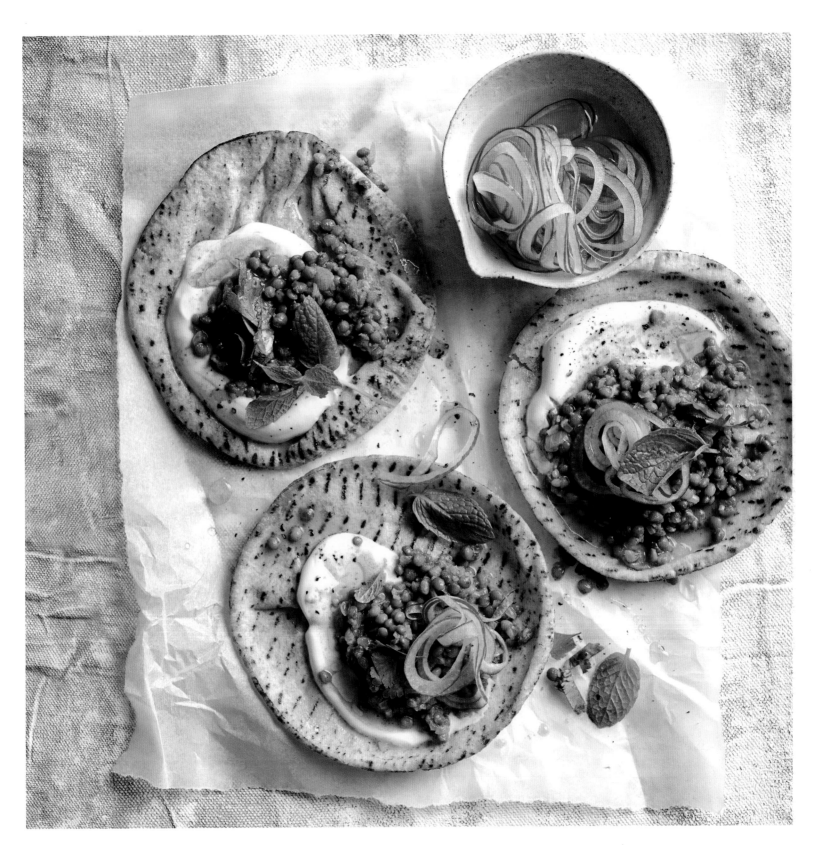

harissa lentils with pickled onion

harissa lentils with pickled onion

¼ cup (60ml) extra virgin olive oil
1 brown onion, finely chopped
2 cloves garlic, crushed
1½ tablespoons harissa*
½ teaspoon ground cumin
2 x 400g cans lentils, rinsed and drained
2 cups (500ml) chicken stock
2 cups coriander (cilantro) leaves, chopped
¼ cup (60ml) lemon juice
4 wholemeal pita breads, baked until crisp
plain Greek-style (thick) yoghurt and mint leaves, to serve
pickled onion
1 red onion, thinly sliced
½ cup (125ml) white wine vinegar
sea salt and cracked black pepper

To make the pickled onion, place the red onion, vinegar, salt
and pepper in a bowl and allow to stand for 10 minutes or until
softened. Drain and set aside.

Heat the oil in a large non-stick frying pan over medium
heat. Add the brown onion and cook for 6–7 minutes or until
softened. Add the garlic, harissa and cumin and cook for a further
1 minute. Add the lentils and stock and cook for 10 minutes or until
thickened. Add the coriander and lemon juice and stir to combine.

Divide the pita breads between serving plates, top with yoghurt,
the lentil mixture, pickled onion and mint to serve. **SERVES 4**

harissa roasted eggplant
with black lentil and herb salad

3 eggplants (aubergines) (840g), halved lengthways
    and flesh scored
1 tablespoon harissa*
2 cloves garlic, crushed
2 tablespoons pomegranate molasses*
2 tablespoons finely grated lemon rind
extra virgin olive oil, for drizzling
1 cup (210g) black lentils
2 cups (500ml) water
1 cup flat-leaf parsley leaves, roughly chopped
1 cup coriander (cilantro) leaves, roughly chopped
1 cup mint leaves, roughly chopped
¼ cup (50g) chia seeds*
plain Greek-style (thick) yoghurt, to serve
dressing
¼ cup (60ml) extra virgin olive oil
2 tablespoons balsamic vinegar
1 tablespoon pomegranate molasses*   ← *middle-eastern and specialty food shops stock pomegranate molasses*
¼ cup (60ml) lemon juice

To make the dressing, place the oil, vinegar, pomegranate molasses
and lemon juice in a bowl, whisk to combine and set aside.

Preheat oven to 170°C (340°F). Place the eggplant, cut-side up,
on a baking tray lined with non-stick baking paper. Place the
harissa, garlic, pomegranate molasses and lemon rind in a bowl
and mix to combine. Spoon over the eggplant, drizzle with oil
and roast for 1 hour or until tender.

Place the lentils and water in a small saucepan over high heat
and bring to the boil. Reduce the heat to medium, cover with a
tight-fitting lid and simmer for 20 minutes or until just tender.
Drain and refresh under cold running water.

Place the lentils, parsley, coriander, mint and chia seeds in
a large bowl. Top with the dressing and toss to combine. Divide
the eggplant between serving plates and spoon over the salad.
Top with yoghurt to serve. **SERVES 6**

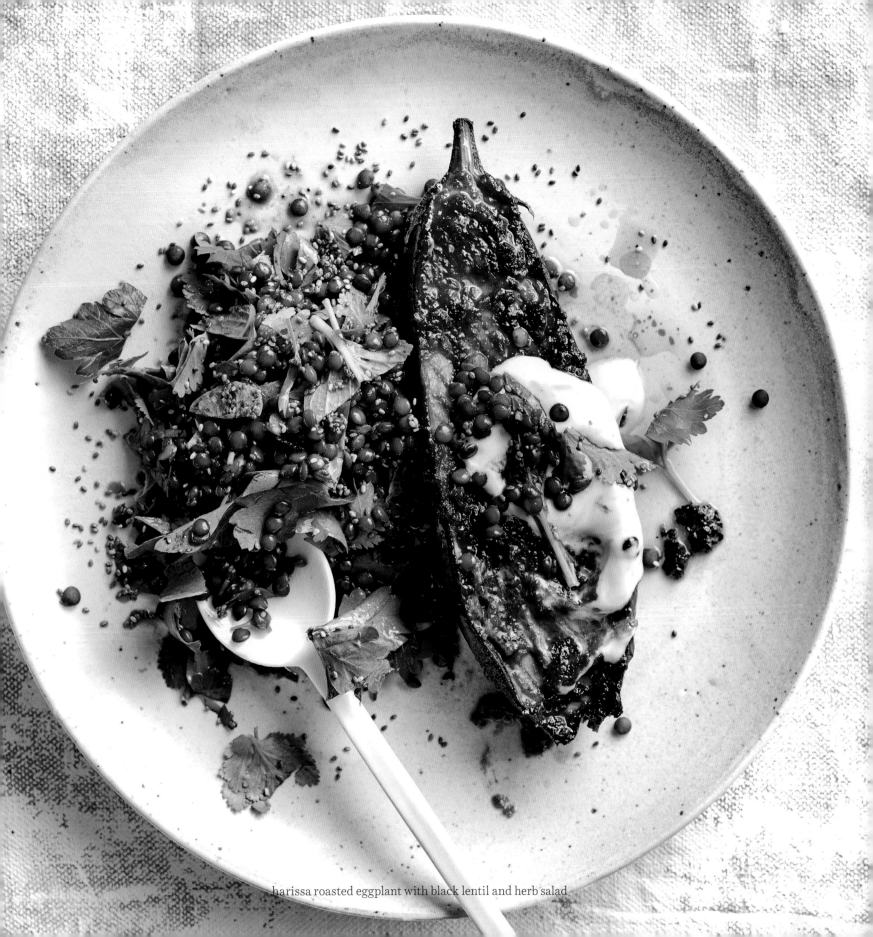

harissa roasted eggplant with black lentil and herb salad

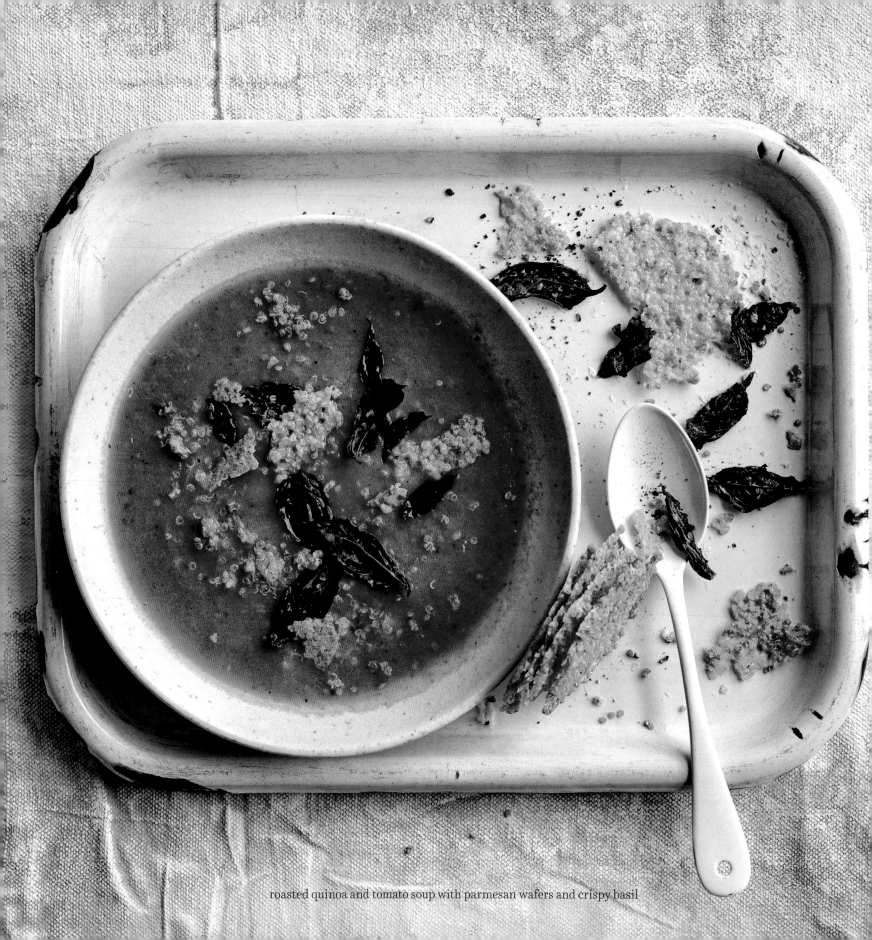

roasted quinoa and tomato soup with parmesan wafers and crispy basil

roasted quinoa and tomato soup with parmesan wafers and crispy basil

2kg tomatoes, halved
1 cup basil leaves
1 head garlic
extra virgin olive oil, for drizzling
2 cups (320g) cooked quinoa* (see *glossary*, page 230)
1.5 litres chicken stock
sea salt and cracked black pepper
parmesan wafers
½ cup (80g) cooked quinoa* (see *glossary*, page 230)
½ cup (40g) finely grated parmesan
cracked black pepper

Preheat oven to 200°C (400°F). To make the parmesan wafers, place the quinoa, parmesan and pepper in a bowl and toss to combine. Place tablespoons of the mixture on a baking tray lined with non-stick baking paper and bake for 5–7 minutes or until golden. Allow to cool on the tray and set aside.

Place the tomatoes, basil and garlic on a baking tray lined with non-stick baking paper and drizzle with oil. Roast for 45 minutes or until the tomatoes are soft and the basil is crisp. Spread the quinoa on a separate baking tray lined with non-stick baking paper, drizzle with oil and toss to coat. Roast for the last 15 minutes of the tomato cooking time.

Reserve and set aside the crispy basil leaves. Squeeze the roasted garlic from its skin into a large saucepan. Add the tomatoes and stock and bring to the boil over high heat. Reduce the heat to medium and simmer for 10 minutes or until thickened. Using a hand-held stick blender, blend until smooth. Add the roasted quinoa, salt and pepper and stir to combine. Divide the soup between serving bowls and top with the reserved basil. Serve with the parmesan wafers. SERVES 4

fried brown rice with lettuce cups

1 teaspoon dried chilli flakes
2 tablespoons sesame seeds, toasted
2 tablespoons chia seeds*
¼ cup (40g) pepitas (pumpkin seeds)*, toasted
¼ cup store-bought crispy fried shallots (eschalots)*
2 tablespoons vegetable oil
¼ cup (30g) finely shredded ginger
4 cloves garlic, thinly sliced
2 tablespoons store-bought Asian chilli jam
1 tablespoon soy sauce
4 green onions (scallions), thinly sliced
4 cups (800g) cooked brown rice (see *glossary*, page 227)
4 eggs
4 iceberg lettuce leaves
bean sprouts, coriander (cilantro) leaves, Thai basil leaves
    and Chinese black vinegar, to serve

Place the chilli, sesame seeds, chia seeds, pepitas and crispy shallots in a bowl, stir to combine and set aside.

Heat 1 tablespoon of the oil in a large non-stick frying pan or wok over high heat. Add the ginger and garlic and cook for 2–3 minutes or until golden. Remove from the pan with a slotted spoon and set aside. Add the chilli jam, soy sauce, onion and rice to the pan and cook, stirring, for 10 minutes or until the rice is crispy. Remove from the pan, set aside and keep warm. Add the remaining oil to the pan and reduce the heat to medium. Fry the eggs for 2–3 minutes or until just set.

Divide the fried rice, lettuce leaves and eggs between serving plates. Top with the bean sprouts, coriander, basil, ginger and garlic. Sprinkle with the seed mixture and serve with black vinegar. SERVES 4

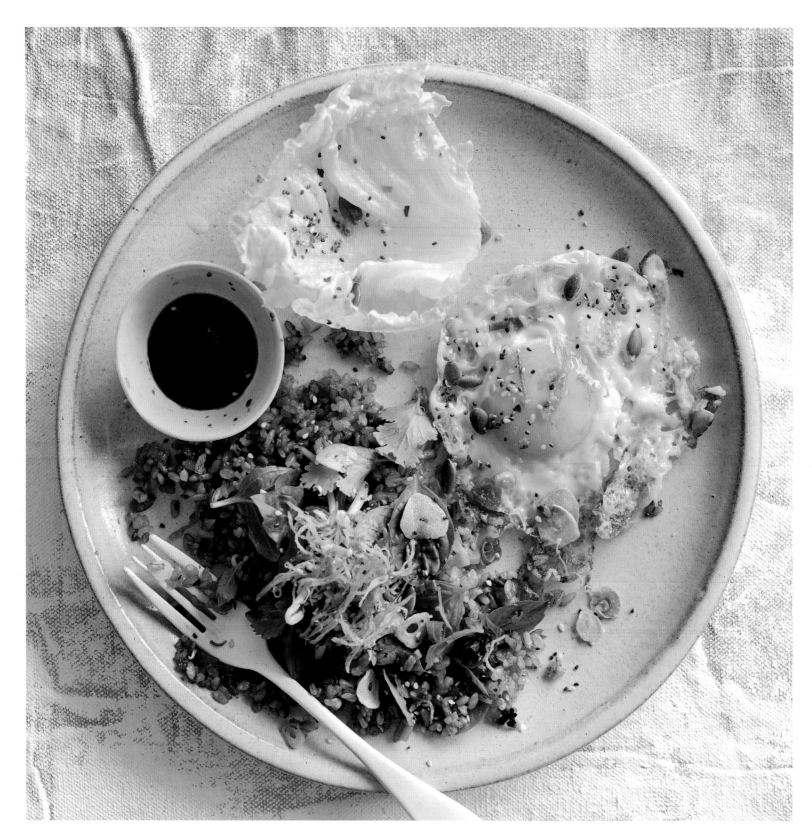

fried brown rice with lettuce cups

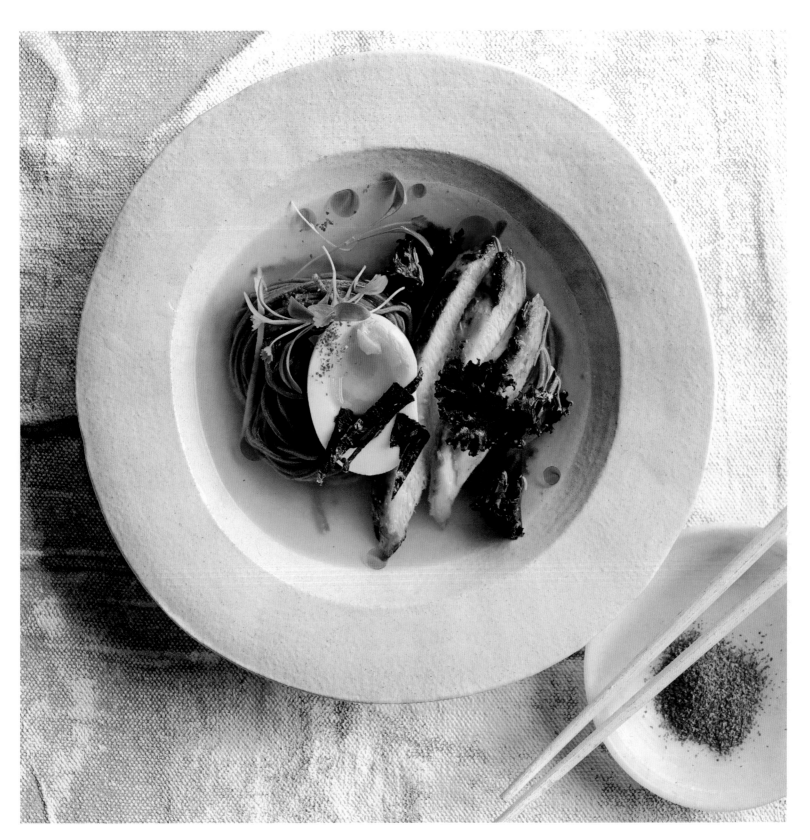

whole-wheat ramen with miso-glazed chicken and kale

whole-wheat ramen with miso-glazed chicken and kale

3 x 200g chicken breast fillets, trimmed
1 tablespoon vegetable oil
2 tablespoons finely grated ginger
2 tablespoons white miso paste*
1.5 litres chicken stock
250g whole-wheat Japanese noodles
2 cups (60g) torn kale leaves
2 soft-boiled eggs, halved
4 strips toasted nori*
baby (micro) coriander (cilantro) (optional), to serve
shichimi togarashi* and chilli oil, to serve
miso glaze
2 tablespoons vegetable oil
2 tablespoons white miso paste*
2 tablespoons mirin (Japanese rice wine)

To make the miso glaze, place the oil, miso and mirin in a bowl and whisk until well combined.

Brush the miso glaze over the chicken. Heat the oil in a large non-stick frying pan over medium heat. Cook the chicken for 5 minutes each side or until golden and cooked through. Set aside and keep warm.

Place the ginger, miso paste and stock in a medium saucepan over medium heat. Stir to combine and bring to the boil. Reduce the heat to low and simmer for 5 minutes.

Cook the noodles in a large saucepan of salted boiling water for 4–6 minutes or until just tender. Drain and divide between serving bowls. Slice the chicken and place on top of the noodles. Top with the kale and ladle over the miso broth. Top each bowl with half an egg, a strip of nori and baby coriander. Serve with togarashi and chilli oil. **SERVES 4**

creamy quinoa risotto with sage and almond brussels sprouts

3 cups (750ml) chicken stock
1 tablespoon extra virgin olive oil
½ onion, finely chopped
1 clove garlic, crushed
1 cup (180g) quinoa*
¼ cup (20g) finely grated parmesan, plus extra to serve
¼ cup (60g) crème fraîche
sea salt and cracked black pepper
sage and almond brussels sprouts
60g unsalted butter
500g Brussels sprouts, trimmed and leaves separated
½ cup (80g) chopped almonds
2 cups sage leaves
1 tablespoon finely grated lemon rind

Place the stock in a saucepan over medium heat and bring to a simmer. Heat the oil in a large deep-sided frying pan over medium heat. Add the onion and cook, stirring, for 5–6 minutes or until softened. Add the garlic and cook for a further 1 minute. Add the quinoa and cook, stirring, for 1 minute or until slightly toasted. Gradually add the warm stock to the pan, 1 cup (250ml) at a time, stirring occasionally for 10–15 minutes or until most of the stock is absorbed and the quinoa has softened. Add the parmesan and crème fraîche and stir to combine. Set aside and keep warm.

To make the sage and almond Brussels sprouts, melt the butter in a large non-stick frying pan over medium heat. Add the sprout leaves and cook, tossing, for 3 minutes. Add the almonds, sage and lemon rind and cook for a further 3 minutes or until golden and crisp.

Divide the risotto between serving bowls and top with the sage and almond Brussels sprouts. Sprinkle with salt, pepper and extra parmesan to serve. **SERVES 4**

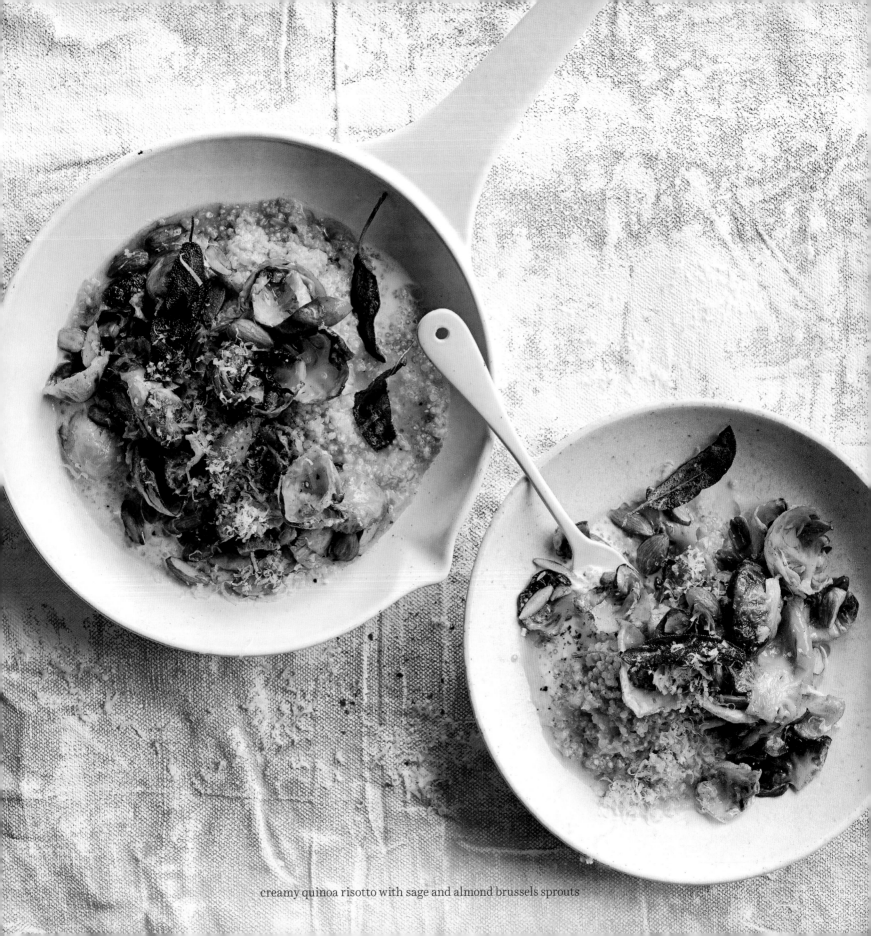

creamy quinoa risotto with sage and almond brussels sprouts

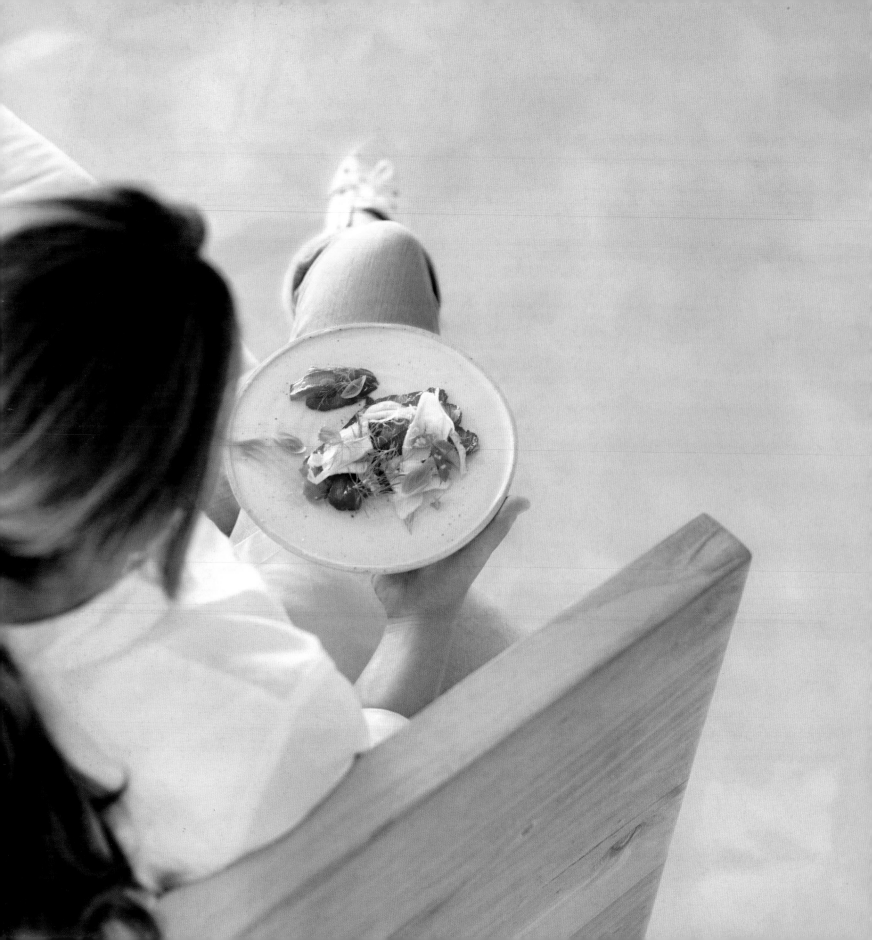

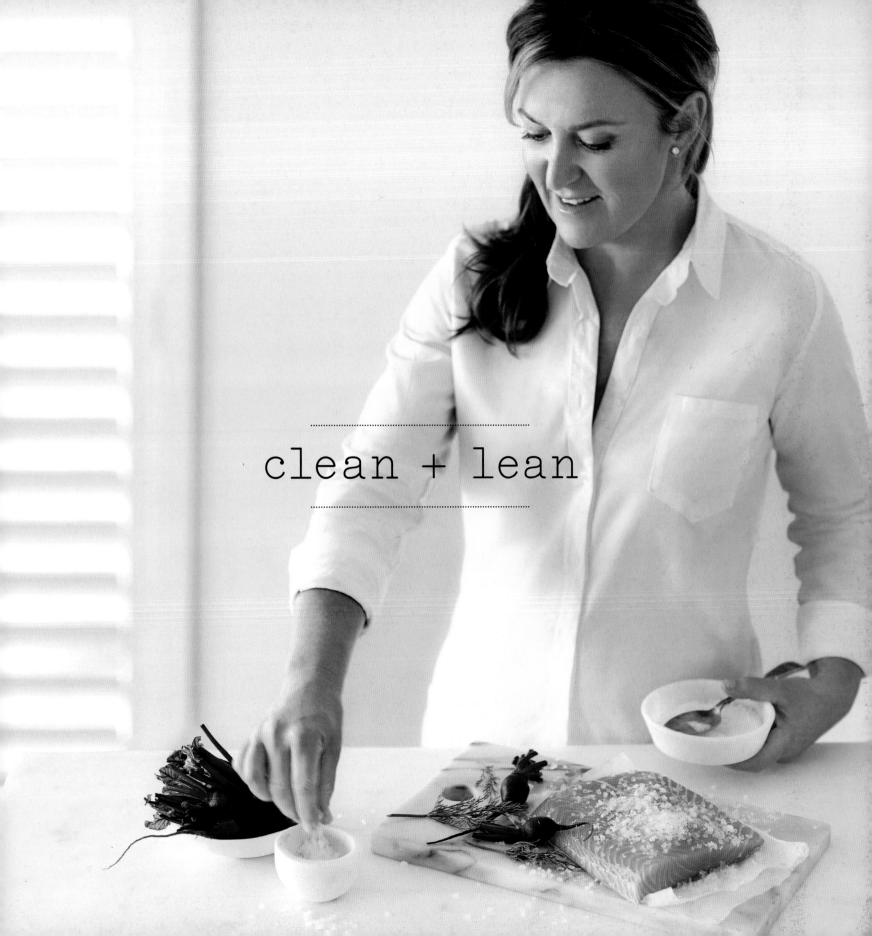

clean + lean

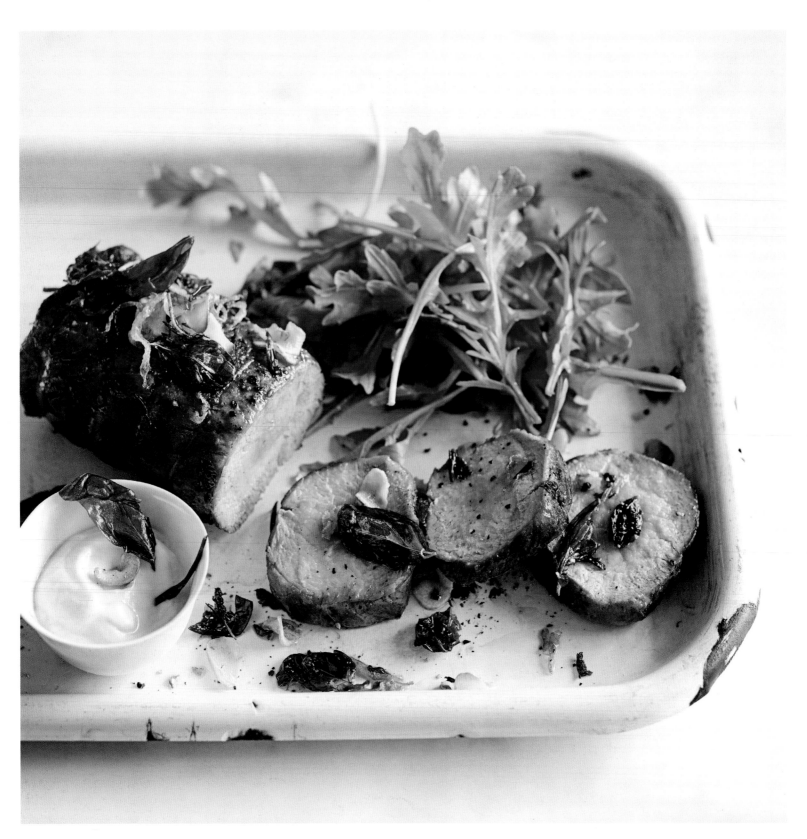

vitello tonnato with crispy garlic and herbs

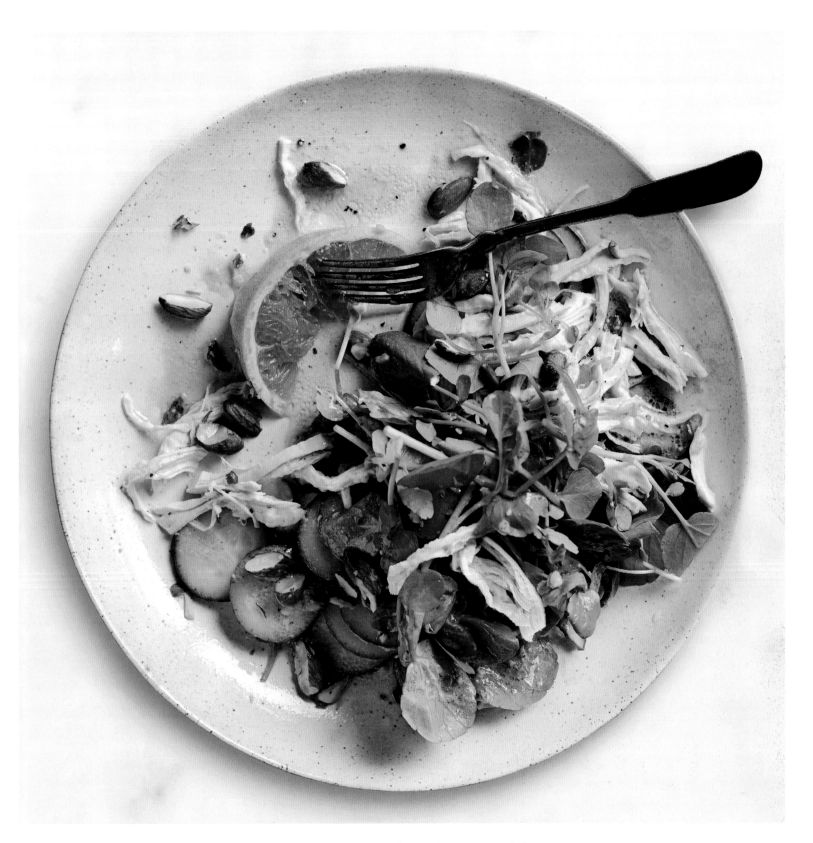

tarragon poached chicken and watercress salad

vitello tonnato with crispy garlic and herbs

750g veal fillet
extra virgin olive oil, for brushing
sea salt and cracked black pepper
¼ cup (60ml) extra virgin olive oil, extra
3 cloves garlic, thinly sliced
2 cups basil leaves
1 cup tarragon leaves
rocket (arugula) leaves, to serve
anchovy mayonnaise
300g silken tofu
1 clove garlic, crushed
2 anchovy fillets
¼ cup (60ml) lemon juice
⅓ cup (25g) finely grated parmesan

To make the anchovy mayonnaise, place the tofu, garlic, anchovies, lemon juice and parmesan in a food processor and process until smooth. Refrigerate until ready to use.

Preheat oven to 180°C (350°F). Brush the veal with oil and sprinkle with salt and pepper. Heat a large non-stick frying pan over medium heat and cook the veal, turning, for 12 minutes or until browned on all sides. Transfer to a baking tray lined with non-stick baking paper and roast for 10 minutes. Allow to cool to room temperature.

Heat the extra oil in a clean large non-stick frying pan over medium heat. Add the garlic and cook for 1 minute. Add the basil and tarragon and cook for 2–3 minutes or until the garlic is golden and the herbs are crisp. Remove with a slotted spoon and set aside on paper towel to drain.

Slice the veal and top with the crispy garlic and herbs. Serve with the anchovy mayonnaise and rocket. **SERVES 4**

tarragon poached chicken and watercress salad

1 litre chicken stock
1 lemon, sliced
4 sprigs tarragon
3 x 200g chicken breast fillets, trimmed
4 cups (60g) watercress sprigs
2 Lebanese cucumbers (260g), sliced
½ cup (80g) smoked almonds, chopped
baby (micro) mint (optional) and pink grapefruit wedges, to serve
dressing
¼ cup (60ml) pink grapefruit juice
2 tablespoons extra virgin olive oil
1 tablespoon Dijon mustard
sea salt and cracked black pepper

To make the dressing, place the grapefruit juice, oil, mustard, salt and pepper in a bowl and whisk to combine. Set aside.

Place the stock, lemon and tarragon in a deep-sided frying pan over high heat and bring to the boil. Add the chicken and cook for 4 minutes. Remove the pan from the heat and allow to stand, covered, for 10 minutes or until the chicken is cooked through. Drain and shred the chicken.

Place the watercress, cucumber, almond, chicken and the dressing in a bowl and toss to combine. Sprinkle with mint and serve with grapefruit wedges. **SERVES 4**

kingfish ceviche

400g sashimi-grade kingfish, cut into 1cm cubes
2 tablespoons lime juice
2 teaspoons finely grated lime rind
½ teaspoon sea salt flakes
4 jalapeño chillies, seeded and finely chopped
2 Lebanese cucumbers (260g), peeled and sliced
⅓ cup (45g) roasted unsalted peanuts, roughly chopped
¼ cup baby (micro) coriander (cilantro) leaves (optional)
baby cos (romaine) lettuce leaves and lime wedges, to serve

Place the fish, lime juice, lime rind, salt and chilli in a bowl and toss to coat. Allow to stand for 5–10 minutes. Place the cucumber in a large bowl and top with the ceviche mixture, peanut and coriander. Spoon onto lettuce leaves and serve with lime wedges. **SERVES 4**

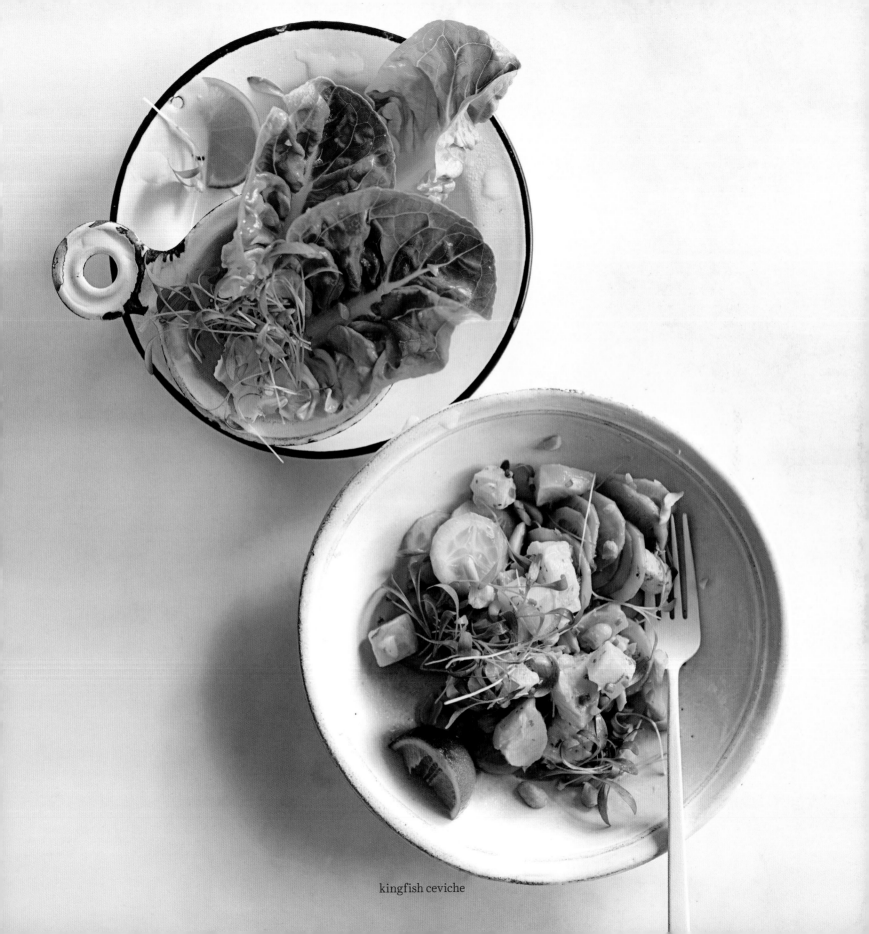

kingfish ceviche

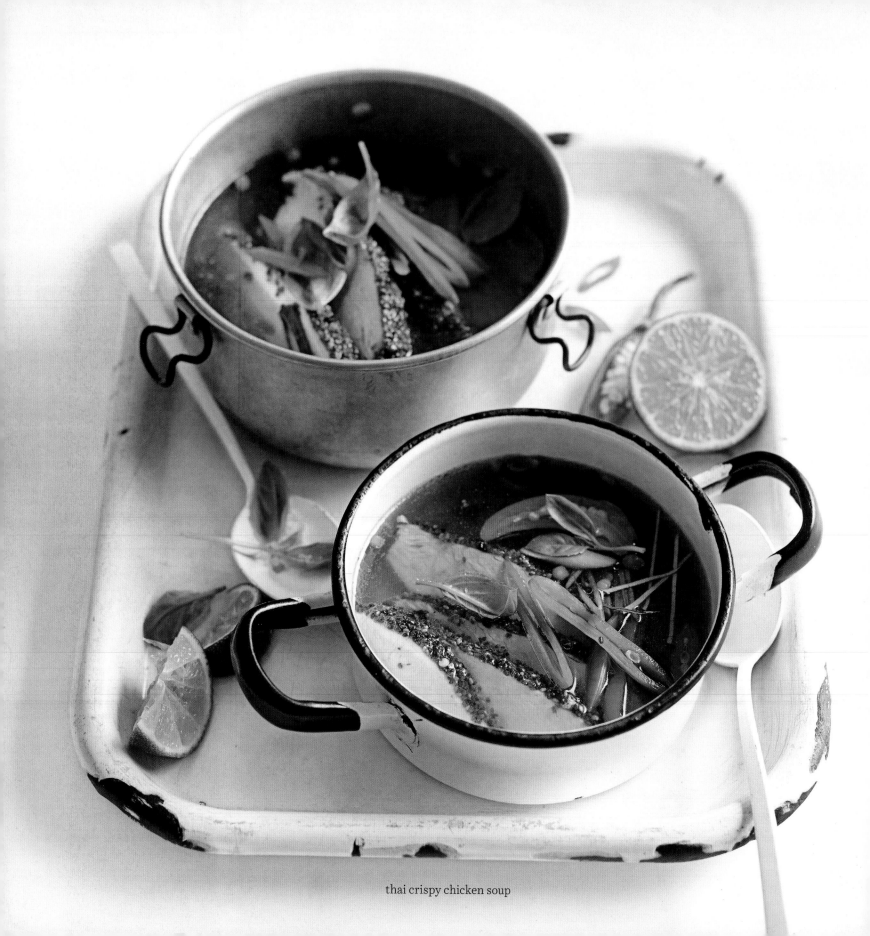

thai crispy chicken soup

thai crispy chicken soup

2 litres chicken stock
1 x 5cm piece ginger, peeled and sliced
1 teaspoon soy sauce
2 tablespoons fish sauce
1 stalk lemongrass, white part only, bruised
4 kaffir lime leaves*
2 small red chillies, halved lengthways
½ cup (100g) black chia seeds*
1 teaspoon dried chilli flakes
sea salt flakes
3 x 200g chicken breast fillets, trimmed
1 eggwhite, lightly beaten
2 tablespoons vegetable oil
200g sugar snap peas, trimmed and shredded
2 green onions (scallions), thinly sliced
basil leaves and lime wedges, to serve

Place the stock, ginger, soy sauce, fish sauce, lemongrass, lime leaves and chilli halves in a large saucepan over high heat. Bring to the boil, reduce the heat to medium and simmer for 10 minutes or until fragrant.

While the broth is simmering, place the chia seeds, chilli flakes and salt in a bowl and mix to combine. Brush the chicken fillets with the eggwhite and sprinkle both sides with the seed mix to coat. Heat the oil in a large non-stick frying pan over medium heat. Cook the chicken for 5–6 minutes each side or until golden and cooked through. Set aside and keep warm.

Add the peas to the broth and cook for a further 1 minute. Remove and discard the ginger, lemongrass and lime leaves.

Slice the chicken and divide between serving bowls. Ladle over the hot broth and peas and top with the onion and basil. Serve with lime wedges. **SERVES 4**

chicken, fennel and edamame salad

1 cup (160g) pepitas (pumpkin seeds)*, roughly chopped
⅓ cup (55g) sesame seeds
sea salt and cracked black pepper
2 x 200g chicken breast fillets, trimmed
    and halved horizontally
2 eggs, lightly beaten
1 tablespoon extra virgin olive oil
2 stalks celery, shaved
1 medium fennel bulb (400g),
    trimmed and thinly sliced
1 cup (140g) podded edamame*, blanched
100g ricotta salata*, shaved
baby (micro) mint (optional), to serve
dressing
2 tablespoons extra virgin olive oil
2 tablespoons lemon juice
1 clove garlic, crushed
1 teaspoon hot English mustard

← *ricotta salata is a salted, pressed ricotta – it's perfect in salads*

To make the dressing, place the oil, lemon juice, garlic and mustard in a bowl and whisk to combine. Set aside.

Place the pepitas, sesame seeds, salt and pepper in a bowl and toss to combine. Dip the chicken pieces in the egg and press into the seed mixture to coat. Heat the oil in a large non-stick frying pan over medium heat. Cook the chicken, in batches, for 3–4 minutes each side or until golden and cooked through. Slice the chicken and divide between serving plates with the celery, fennel and edamame. Drizzle with the dressing and top with the ricotta salata and mint to serve. **SERVES 4**

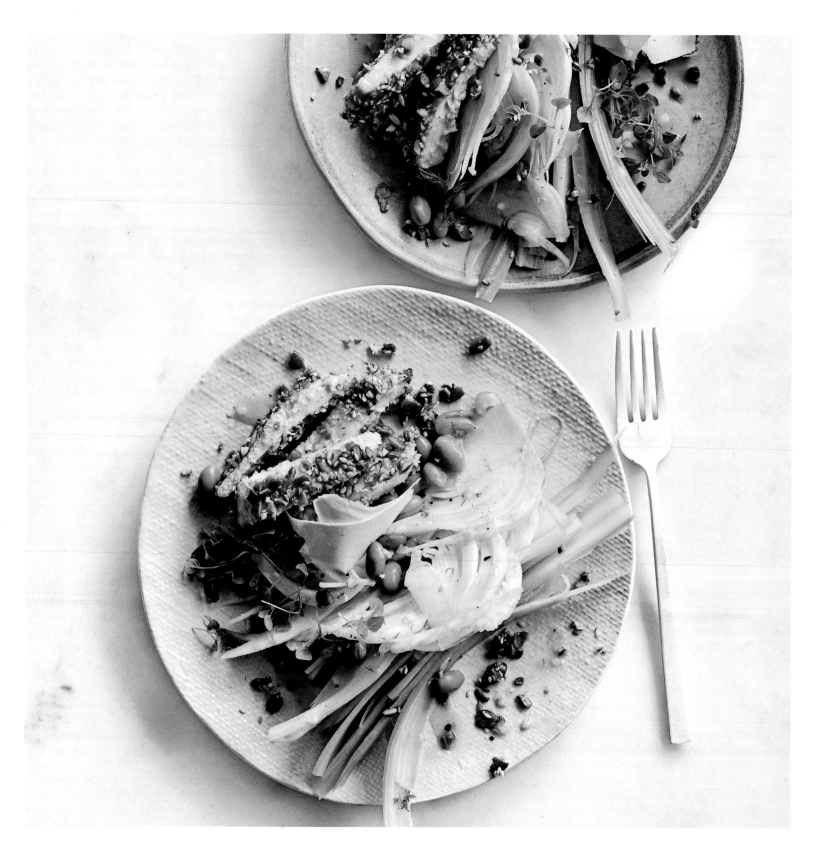

chicken, fennel and edamame salad

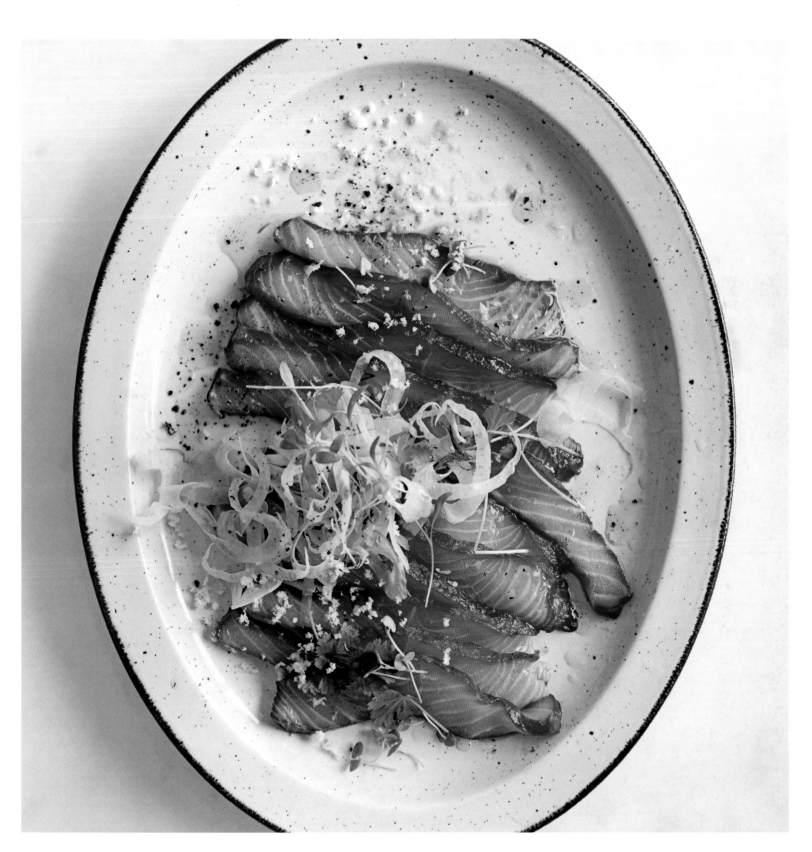

beetroot and horseradish cured salmon

beetroot and horseradish cured salmon

⅓ cup (100g) coarse rock salt
2 tablespoons caster (superfine) sugar
2 tablespoons finely chopped dill
1 x 500g salmon fillet, skin and bones removed
1 tablespoon finely grated fresh horseradish*
1 large beetroot (200g), coarsely grated
¼ cup each baby (micro) parsley
    and basil leaves (optional), to serve
fennel salad
2 teaspoons finely grated fresh horseradish*
¼ teaspoon rice wine vinegar
2 tablespoons extra virgin olive oil
sea salt and cracked black pepper
4 small fennel bulbs (800g), trimmed and thinly sliced

Place the salt, sugar and dill in a bowl and stir to combine.
Sprinkle both sides of the salmon with the horseradish. Place
half the salt mixture in the base of a glass or ceramic dish
large enough to snugly fit the salmon. Top with half the
beetroot and the salmon. Layer with the remaining beetroot
and salt mixture. Cover with plastic wrap, weigh down with
cans of beans or tomatoes and refrigerate for 3 hours.

While the salmon is curing, make the fennel salad. Place
the horseradish, vinegar, oil, salt and pepper in a large bowl
and whisk to combine. Add the fennel and toss to combine.

Remove the salmon from the salt and beetroot and slice
thinly. Divide between serving plates and top with the salad
and baby herbs to serve. SERVES 4

cauliflower and tofu soup with salsa verde

2 tablespoons extra virgin olive oil
1 leek, white part only, sliced
1 white onion, finely chopped
3 cloves garlic, sliced
1 medium cauliflower (1.5kg), chopped
2 litres chicken stock
600g silken tofu
sea salt and cracked black pepper
salsa verde
1 cup flat-leaf parsley leaves
1 cup oregano leaves
¼ cup chopped chives
1 tablespoon finely grated lemon rind
2 tablespoons lemon juice
1 tablespoon water
¼ cup (60ml) extra virgin olive oil
sea salt and cracked black pepper

← full of green goodness, this zesty dressing is also great spooned over grilled chicken or fish

To make the salsa verde, place the parsley, oregano, chives,
lemon rind, lemon juice, water, oil, salt and pepper in a small
food processor and process until finely chopped. Set aside.

Heat the oil in a large saucepan over high heat. Add the leek,
onion and garlic and cook, stirring, for 5–7 minutes or until
soft. Add the cauliflower and stock and bring to the boil. Reduce
the heat to medium and simmer for 10 minutes or until the
cauliflower is tender. Add the tofu, salt and pepper and, using
a hand-held stick blender, blend until smooth. Divide the soup
between serving bowls and top with salsa verde to serve. SERVES 4

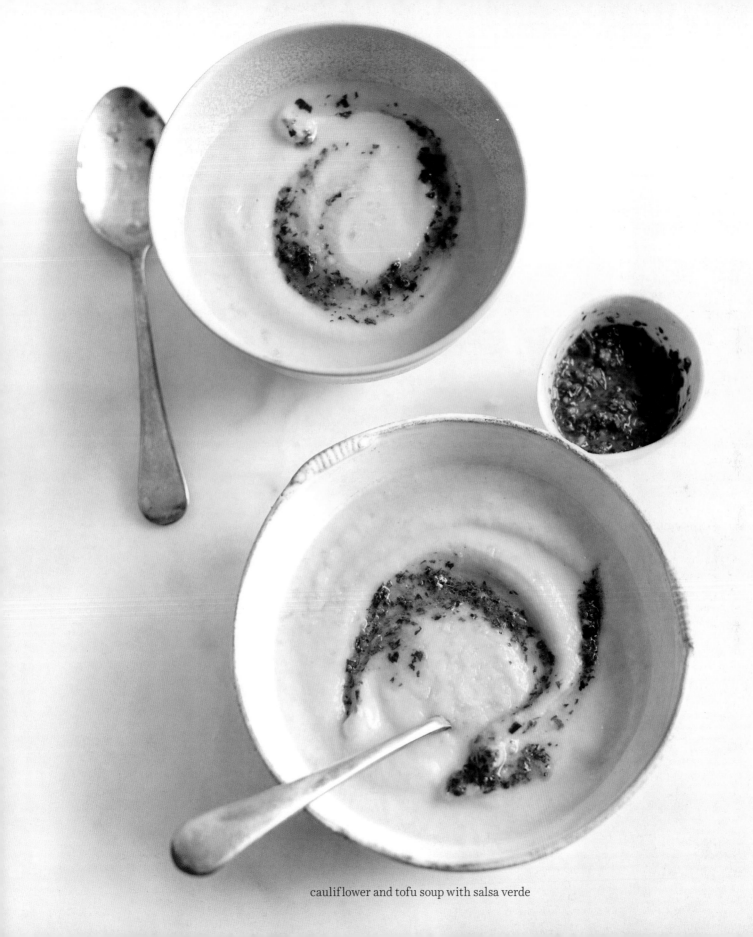

cauliflower and tofu soup with salsa verde

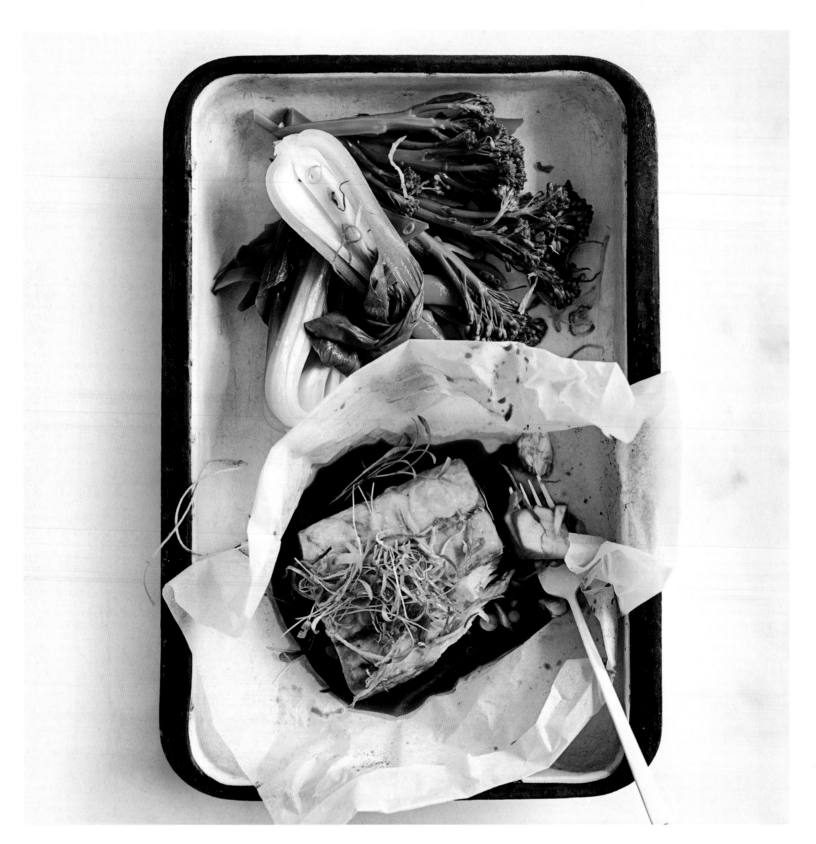

steamed barramundi parcels with crispy ginger

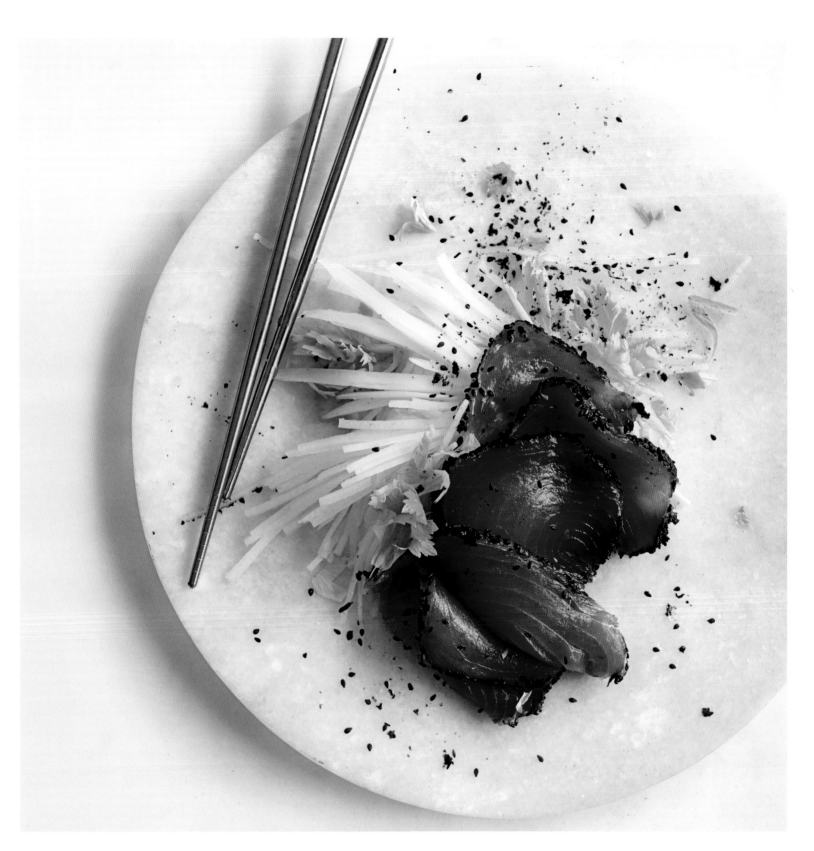

nori and sesame crusted tuna

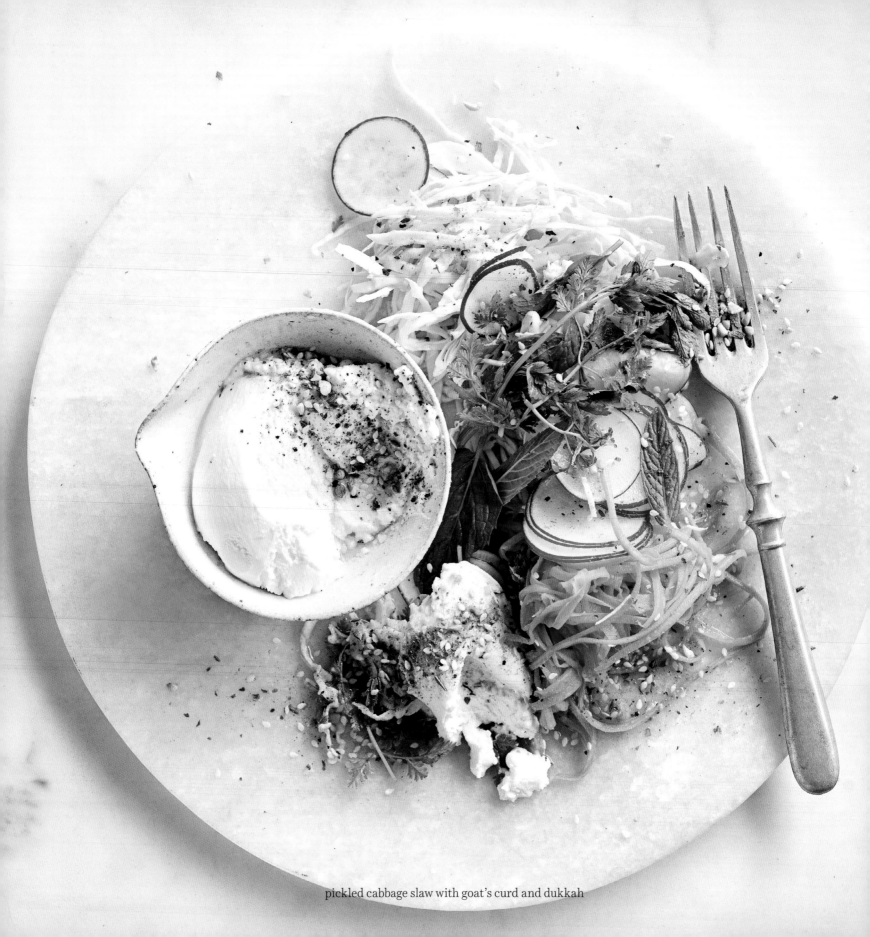

pickled cabbage slaw with goat's curd and dukkah

steamed barramundi parcels with crispy ginger

4 x 200g barramundi fillets, skin removed
¼ cup finely shredded ginger
2 tablespoons oyster sauce
⅓ cup (80ml) soy sauce
⅓ cup (80ml) mirin (Japanese rice wine)
⅓ cup (80ml) Shaoxing (Chinese cooking wine)
2 teaspoons sesame oil
2 tablespoons peanut oil
baby (micro) coriander (cilantro) leaves (optional), to serve
2 bunches baby bok choy (300g), blanched, to serve
200g snow peas (mange tout), trimmed, shredded
   and blanched, to serve
1 bunch broccolini (175g), blanched, to serve

Preheat oven to 180°C (350°F). Place each barramundi fillet on a sheet of non-stick baking paper and top with half the ginger. Place the oyster sauce, soy sauce, mirin, Shaoxing and sesame oil in a bowl and whisk to combine. Spoon the sauce mixture over the fish and fold in the edges of the paper to enclose. Carefully place the parcels on a baking tray and bake for 10 minutes or until the fish is just cooked.

While the fish is cooking, heat the peanut oil in a small non-stick frying pan over high heat. Add the remaining ginger and cook for 2–3 minutes or until crispy.

To serve, place the fish parcels on serving plates. Open the paper and top with the crispy ginger and coriander. Serve with the bok choy, snow peas and broccolini. **SERVES 4**

nori and sesame crusted tuna

1 sheet nori*, processed until coarsely chopped
2 tablespoons black sesame seeds, toasted
2 teaspoons sea salt flakes
400g sashimi-grade tuna
3 tablespoons mirin (Japanese rice wine)
2 tablespoons lemon juice
1 teaspoon finely grated fresh horseradish*
1 celery heart, thinly sliced
1 cup (25g) small celery leaves
1 cup (150g) shredded white radish (daikon)

Place the nori, sesame seeds and salt in a bowl and mix to combine. Press the tuna into the salt mixture to coat and refrigerate for 30 minutes or until chilled, reserving any remaining salt mixture.

Place the mirin, lemon juice and horseradish in a bowl and whisk to combine. Slice the tuna thinly. Divide the celery and radish between serving plates and top with the tuna and dressing. Sprinkle with the reserved salt mixture to serve. **SERVES 4**

pickled cabbage slaw with goat's curd and dukkah

1 small cabbage (400g), coarsely shredded
8 radishes (280g), trimmed and thinly sliced
2 carrots (240g), peeled and shredded
½ cup chervil sprigs
2 tablespoons store-bought dukkah
¼ cup mint leaves
200g soft goat's curd
pickling liquid
½ cup (125ml) apple cider vinegar
2 tablespoons rice malt syrup*
2 teaspoons juniper berries, lightly crushed
1 teaspoon sea salt flakes

Place the cabbage, radish, carrot and chervil in a bowl and set aside.

To make the pickling liquid, place the vinegar, rice malt syrup, juniper berries and salt in a small saucepan over high heat. Stir to combine and bring to the boil. Reduce the heat to medium and simmer for 4–5 minutes or until slightly reduced.

Pour the hot liquid over the cabbage mixture and toss to combine. Allow to cool for 5 minutes. Divide between serving plates and sprinkle with dukkah and mint. Serve with the goat's curd. **SERVES 4**

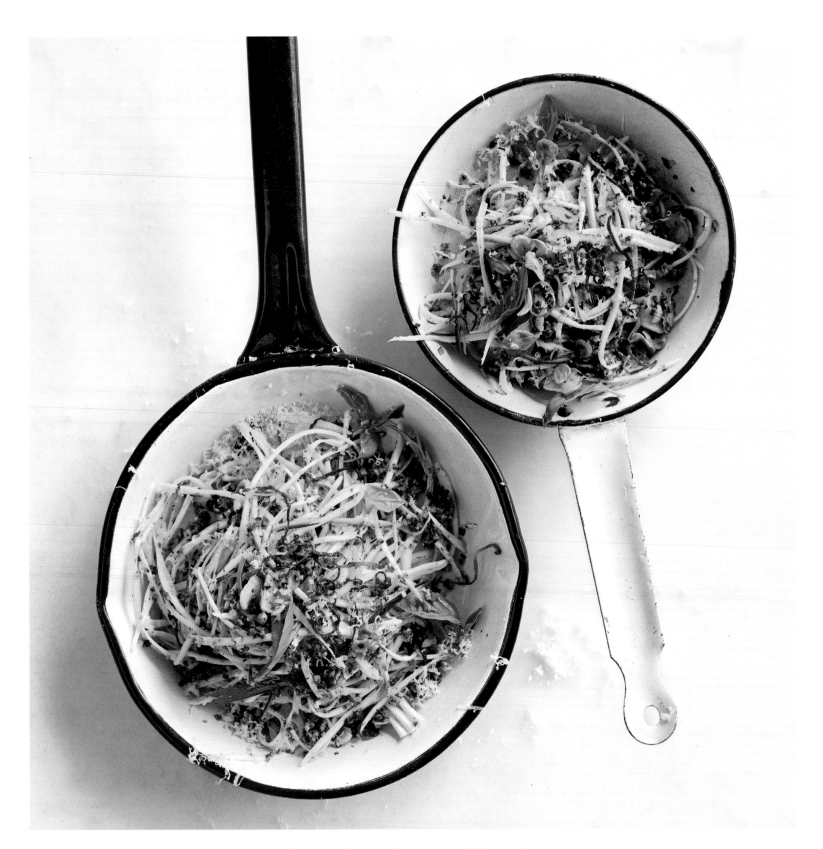

zucchini, parsnip and celeriac pasta with broccoli sauce

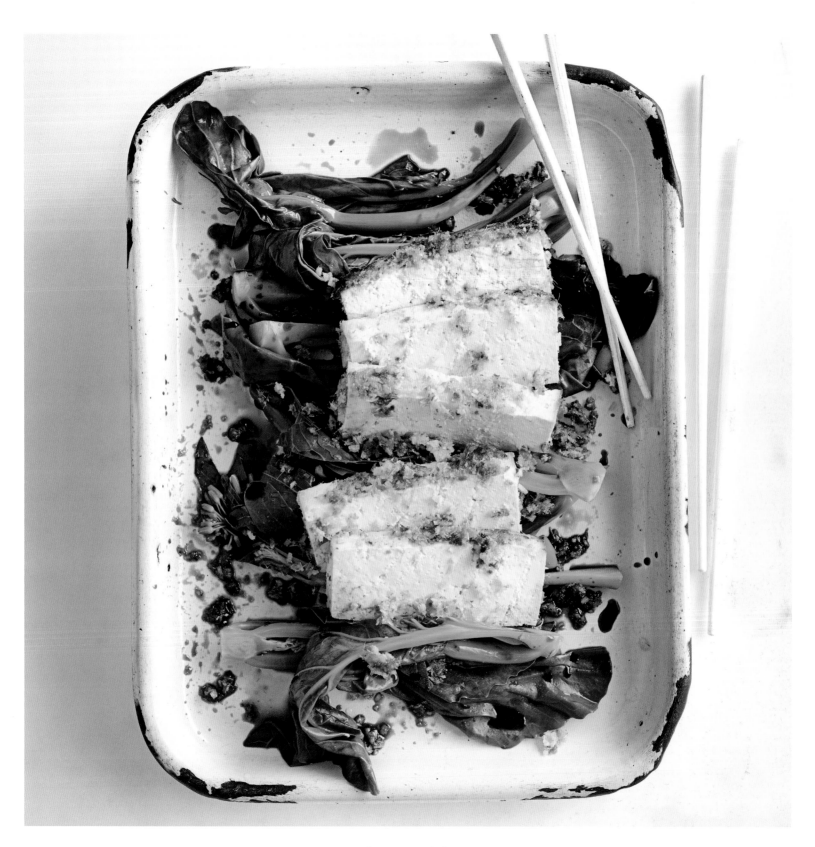

lemongrass tofu

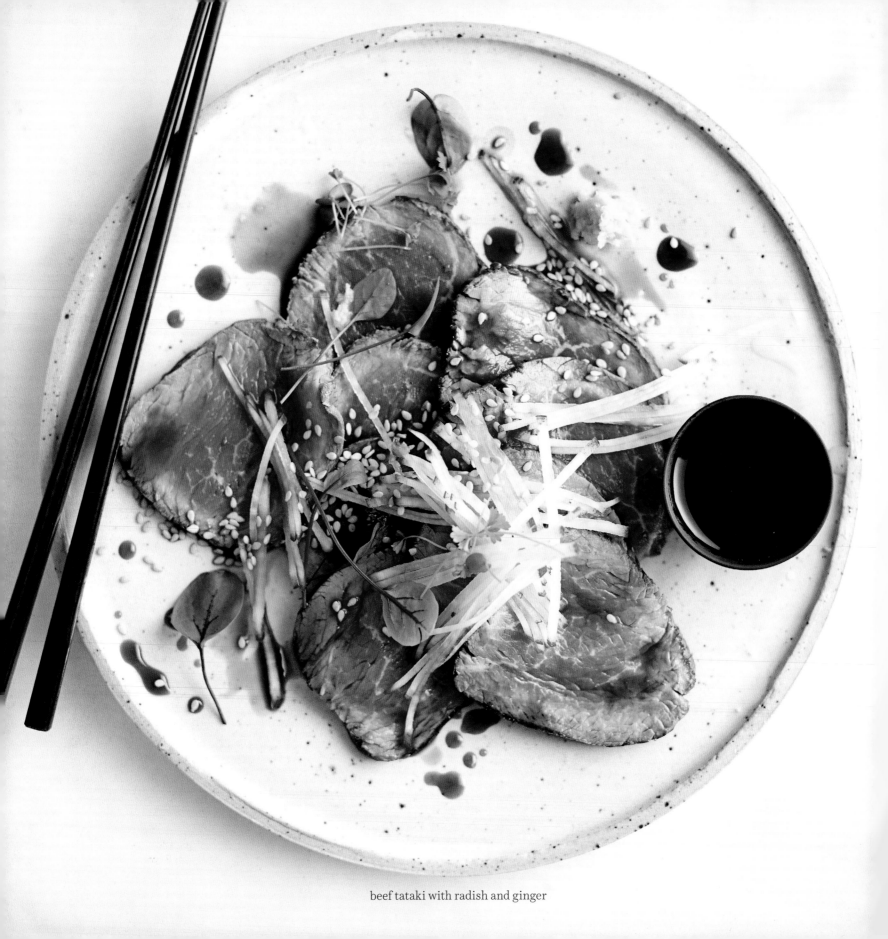

beef tataki with radish and ginger

zucchini, parsnip and celeriac pasta with broccoli sauce

3 medium zucchinis (courgettes) (390g), shredded
3 medium parsnips (750g), peeled and shredded
1 small celeriac (celery root) (250g), peeled and shredded
extra virgin olive oil, for drizzling
finely grated parmesan and small basil leaves, to serve
broccoli sauce
8 cups (480g) broccoli florets
½ cup (40g) finely grated parmesan
⅓ cup (55g) cashews
1 teaspoon sea salt flakes
¼ cup (60ml) extra virgin olive oil
4 cloves garlic, sliced
2 long red chillies, seeded and finely chopped
2 tablespoons lemon zest

To make the broccoli sauce, place the broccoli, parmesan, cashews and salt in a food processor and process until the mixture resembles fine crumbs. Heat the oil in a large non-stick frying pan over high heat. Add the garlic and chilli and cook, stirring, for 1–2 minutes or until soft. Add the lemon zest and broccoli mixture and cook, stirring, for 6–8 minutes or until golden.

Add the zucchini, parsnip and celeriac to the broccoli sauce and toss until combined. Divide between serving bowls, drizzle with oil and top with parmesan and basil to serve. **SERVES 4**

lemongrass tofu

3 stalks lemongrass, white part only, chopped
5 cloves garlic, chopped
1 x 6cm piece ginger, peeled and chopped
6 kaffir lime leaves*, sliced
3 long green chillies, seeded and chopped
1 tablespoon finely grated lime rind
¼ cup (60ml) rice malt syrup*
2 tablespoons rice wine vinegar
2 x 750g blocks firm tofu
2 tablespoons vegetable oil
kecap manis (sweet Indonesian soy sauce), to serve
gai lan (Chinese broccoli), blanched, to serve

Place the lemongrass, garlic, ginger, lime leaf, chilli, lime rind, rice malt syrup and vinegar in a small food processor and process to a paste. Spread the lemongrass paste onto the tofu to coat, place on a tray and refrigerate for 30 minutes to marinate.

Heat the oil in a large non-stick frying pan over medium heat. Cook the tofu for 2–3 minutes each side or until golden and crisp. Slice and serve with the kecap manis and gai lan. **SERVES 4**

beef tataki with radish and ginger

750g beef eye fillet
peanut oil, for brushing
sea salt flakes, for sprinkling
¼ cup (60ml) each soy sauce, mirin (Japanese rice wine) and sake
2 tablespoons lime juice
4 radishes (140g), trimmed and cut into matchsticks
1 tablespoon finely grated ginger
toasted sesame seeds, baby (micro) red-veined sorrel
    and coriander (cilantro) leaves (optional), to serve

Brush the beef with the oil and sprinkle with salt. Heat a large non-stick frying pan over medium heat. Add the beef and cook, turning, for 12 minutes or until browned on all sides. Allow to cool slightly, wrap tightly in plastic wrap and refrigerate for 2 hours.

Place the soy sauce, mirin and sake in a small saucepan over medium heat and simmer for 10–15 minutes or until slightly thickened. Remove from the heat and stir through the lime juice.

Unwrap the beef and slice thinly. Place on a serving plate and top with the radish, ginger, dressing, sesame seeds and herbs. **SERVES 4**

coconut poached chicken salad

1½ cups (375ml) coconut milk
2 tablespoons lime juice
6 kaffir lime leaves*
1 teaspoon sea salt flakes
3 x 200g chicken breast fillets, trimmed
1 green papaya (850g), peeled, seeded and shredded
2 cups coriander (cilantro) leaves
lime wedges, to serve
chilli lime dressing
1 teaspoon fish sauce
¼ cup (60ml) lime juice
2 teaspoons coconut sugar*
1 long green chilli, seeded and finely chopped
½ teaspoon sea salt flakes

Place the coconut milk, lime juice, lime leaves and salt in a large non-stick frying pan over very low heat and stir to combine. Add the chicken and cook, without simmering, for 12 minutes each side or until cooked through. Allow to cool slightly and refrigerate in the poaching liquid until chilled.

While the chicken is cooling, make the chilli lime dressing. Place the fish sauce, lime juice, sugar, chilli and salt in a bowl. Whisk to combine and allow the sugar to dissolve. Set aside.

Slice the chicken, reserving the poaching liquid. Place the papaya and coriander on a serving plate and top with the chicken. Drizzle with the reserved coconut poaching liquid and serve with the dressing and lime wedges. **SERVES 4**

hot-smoked salmon salad
with crunchy pickled cucumber

500g hot-smoked salmon, flaked
200g green beans, trimmed and blanched
1 white onion, thinly sliced
⅓ cup tarragon leaves
⅓ cup chervil sprigs
yoghurt dressing
¼ cup (60ml) extra virgin olive oil
2 tablespoons white balsamic vinegar
1 teaspoon Dijon mustard
1 anchovy fillet, finely chopped
2 tablespoons plain Greek-style (thick) yoghurt
sea salt and cracked black pepper
pickled cucumber
¾ cup (180ml) rice wine vinegar
⅓ cup (80ml) rice malt syrup*
1 tablespoon sea salt flakes
4 Lebanese cucumbers (520g), thickly sliced

you can swap the anchovy for a few finely chopped salted capers ← here, if you prefer

To make the pickled cucumber, place the rice wine vinegar, rice malt syrup and salt in a small saucepan over medium heat. Cook, stirring, for 1 minute or until the syrup has dissolved. Place the cucumber in a bowl, top with the pickling liquid and set aside to cool.

To make the yoghurt dressing, place the oil, balsamic vinegar, mustard, anchovy, yoghurt, salt and pepper in a bowl and mix to combine.

Divide the salmon between serving plates. Top with the beans, onion, tarragon and chervil. Drizzle with the yoghurt dressing, sprinkle with pepper and serve with the pickled cucumber. **SERVES 4**

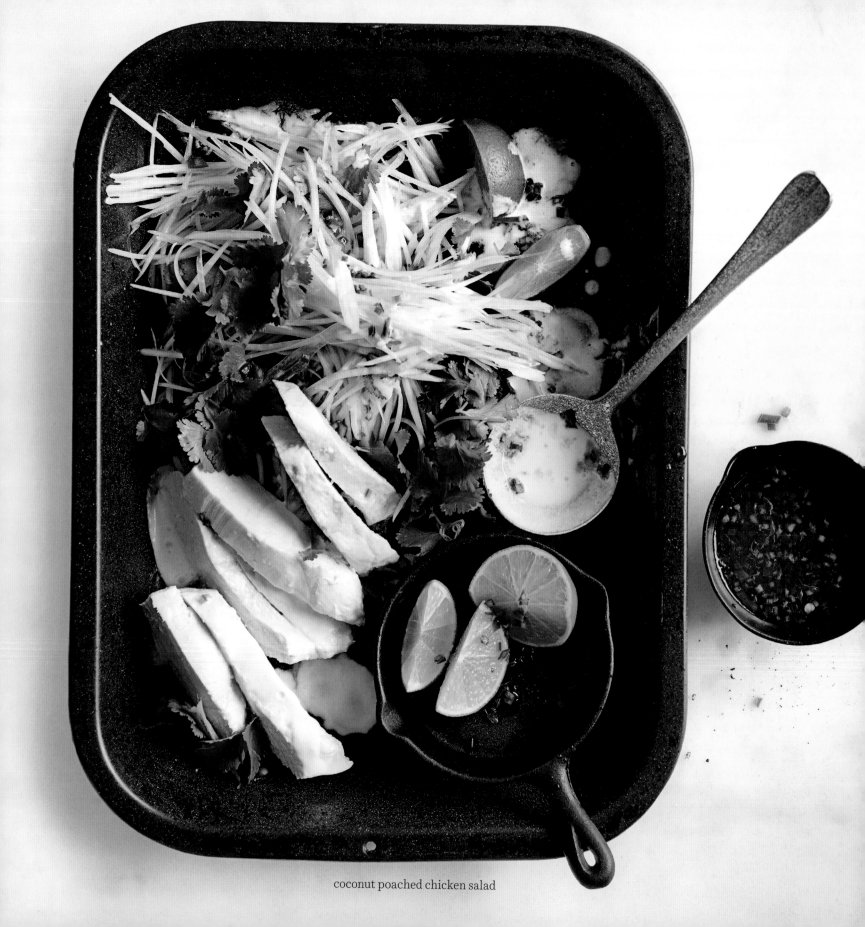

coconut poached chicken salad

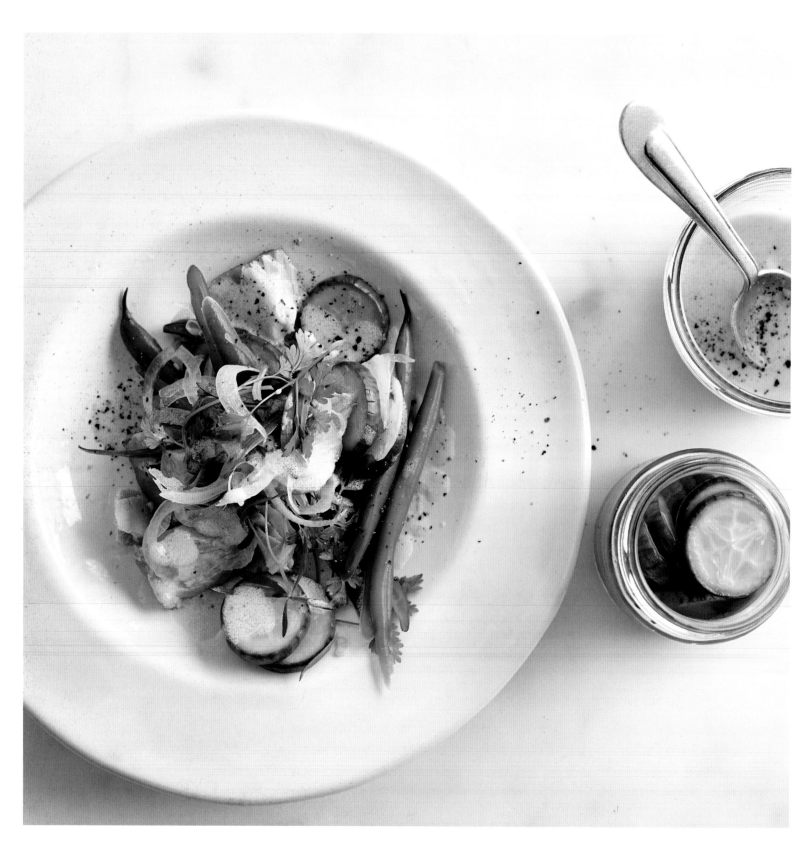

hot-smoked salmon salad with crunchy pickled cucumber

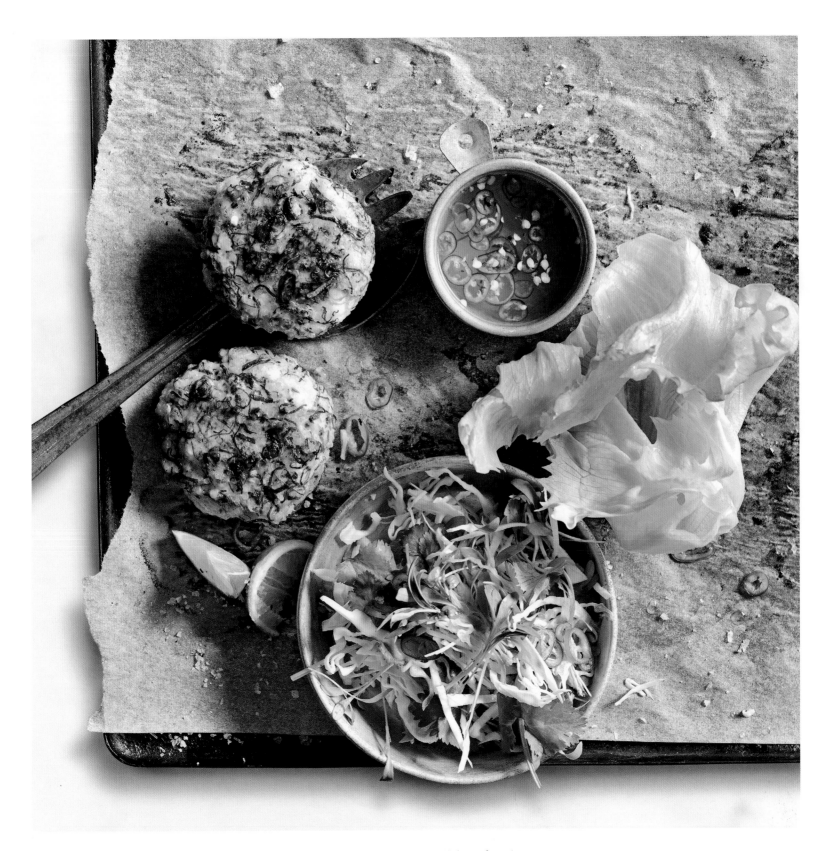

baked fish cakes with chilli lime dressing

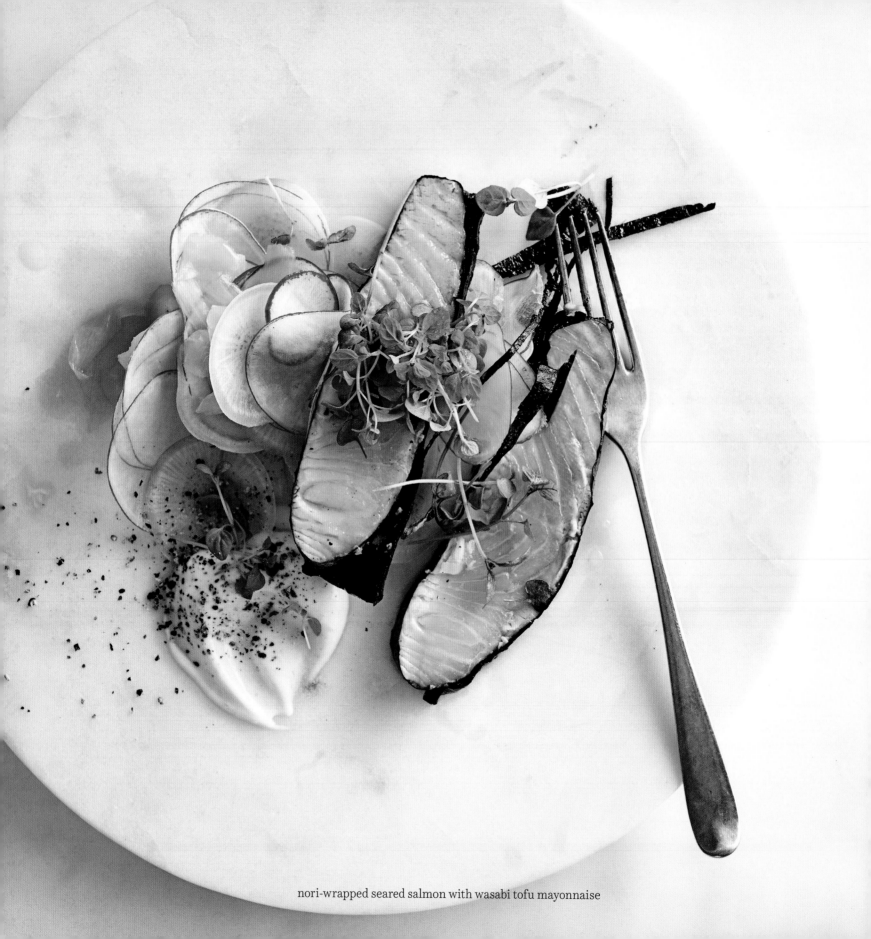

nori-wrapped seared salmon with wasabi tofu mayonnaise

baked fish cakes with chilli lime dressing

450g firm white fish fillets, chopped
1 cup (160g) cooked quinoa* (see *glossary*, page 230)
1 jalapeño chilli, finely chopped
2 cloves garlic, crushed
4 kaffir lime leaves*, finely shredded
½ cup each mint and coriander
    (cilantro) leaves, shredded
2 green onions (scallions), shredded
1 eggwhite
sea salt and cracked black pepper
vegetable oil, for brushing
½ cup (40g) shredded cabbage
1 cup coriander (cilantro) leaves, extra
baby (micro) coriander (cilantro) leaves
    (optional), to serve
4 iceberg lettuce leaves, to serve
lime wedges, to serve
chilli lime dressing
2 tablespoons mirin (Japanese rice wine)
2 tablespoons lime juice
1 long green chilli, sliced

buy fresh lime leaves from asian grocers — you can keep them in the freezer

To make the chilli lime dressing, place the mirin, lime juice and chilli in a bowl and whisk to combine. Set aside.

Preheat oven to 220°C (425°F). Place the fish in a food processor and process until finely chopped. Transfer to a large bowl and add the quinoa, chilli, garlic, lime leaf, mint, coriander, onion, eggwhite, salt and pepper. Mix until well combined. Divide and shape the mixture into ⅓-cup (80ml) patties, place on a baking tray lined with non-stick baking paper and brush both sides with oil. Bake for 8 minutes. Turn and cook for a further 8 minutes or until golden and crisp.

Place the cabbage and extra coriander in a bowl, toss to combine and top with baby coriander. Serve the fish cakes with the lettuce cups, cabbage salad, dressing and lime wedges. **SERVES 4**

nori-wrapped seared salmon with wasabi tofu mayonnaise

4 x 150g salmon fillets, skin removed
2 tablespoons vegetable oil
sea salt and cracked black pepper
4 sheets nori*
4 radishes (140g), trimmed and thinly sliced
2 tablespoons pickled ginger,
    plus 2 tablespoons pickling liquid
baby (micro) shiso (optional), to serve
wasabi tofu mayonnaise
300g silken tofu
1 tablespoon rice wine vinegar
1 teaspoon wasabi* paste

To make the wasabi tofu mayonnaise, place the tofu, vinegar and wasabi in a small food processor and process until smooth. Set aside.

Brush the salmon with half the oil and sprinkle with salt and pepper. Place a salmon fillet in the centre of a nori sheet and brush the edges with water. Fold the nori over the salmon and wrap to enclose. Repeat with the remaining salmon and nori. Heat the remaining oil in a large non-stick frying pan over high heat. Cook the salmon, in batches, for 1 minute each side or until seared. Set aside and keep warm.

Divide the radish between serving plates and top with the ginger and pickling liquid. Slice the salmon and place on the radish. Sprinkle with shiso and pepper, and serve with the mayonnaise. **SERVES 4**

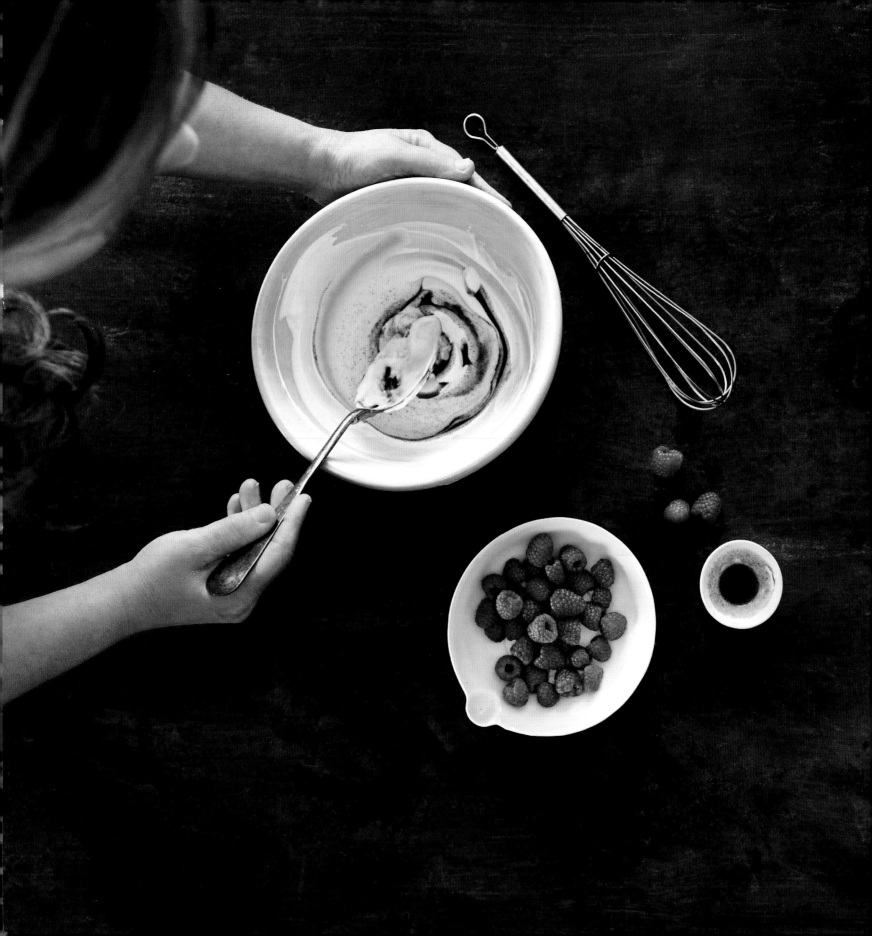

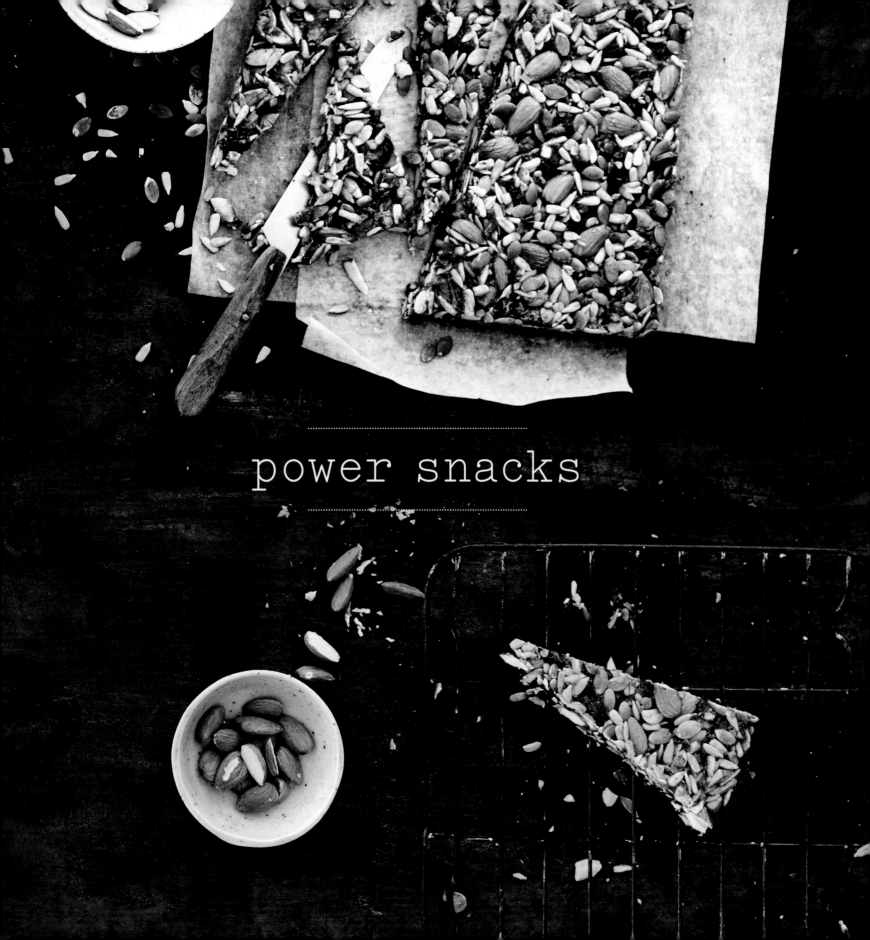

power snacks

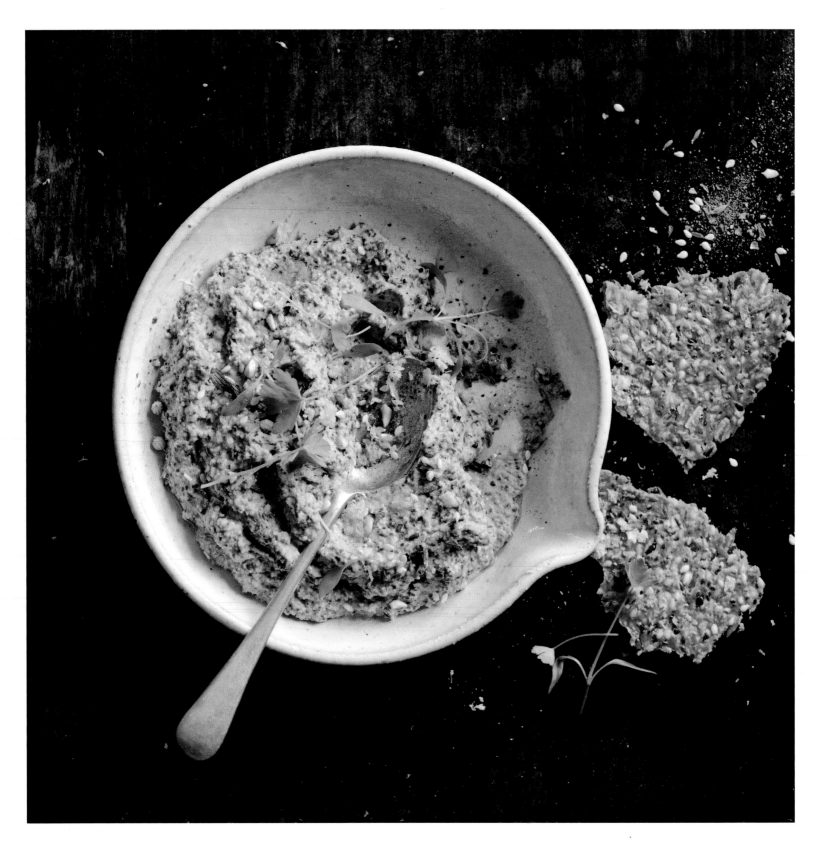

kale and cashew dip

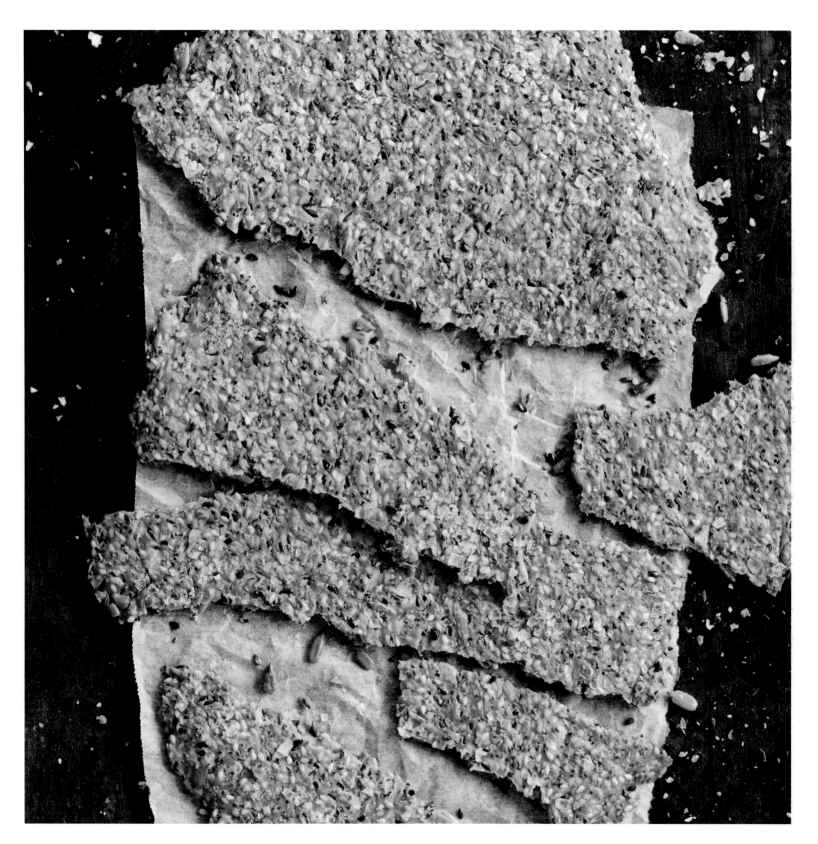

seeded crackers

kale and cashew dip

1 cup (160g) cashews
3 cups (750ml) warm water
2 cups (60g) shredded kale leaves
1 litre boiling water
¼ cup (60ml) extra virgin olive oil,
    plus extra to serve
½ clove garlic, chopped
2 tablespoons lemon juice
1 tablespoon tahini*
⅓ cup (80ml) cold water
sea salt and cracked black pepper
baby (micro) parsley leaves (optional), to serve
seeded crackers (see *recipe*, right) or vegetable chips, to serve

find crispy baked vegie chips at most supermarkets - try beetroot or parsnip

Place the cashews in a large bowl, cover with the warm water
and allow to soak for 1 hour. Drain and set aside.

Place the kale in a bowl, cover with the boiling water and allow
to stand for 1–2 minutes. Drain and pat dry with paper towel. Place
the cashews and kale in a food processor and process until finely
chopped. Add the oil, garlic, lemon juice, tahini, cold water, salt
and pepper and process until smooth. Refrigerate until chilled.

Drizzle the dip with extra oil, top with baby parsley and serve
with crackers or vegetable chips. **MAKES 2 CUPS**

seeded crackers

½ cup (80g) sunflower seeds*
¼ cup (45g) linseeds (flaxseeds)*
¼ cup (40g) sesame seeds
2 tablespoons chia seeds*
1 teaspoon sea salt flakes, plus extra for sprinkling
1 cup (130g) white spelt flour*
½ cup (125ml) water
⅓ cup (80ml) extra virgin olive oil

Preheat oven to 180°C (350°F). Place all the seeds, the salt and
flour in a large bowl and stir to combine. Add the water and oil
and mix to form a dough. Divide the dough in half and roll each
piece between 2 sheets of non-stick baking paper to 3mm thick.
Transfer to baking trays and remove the top sheets of paper.
Sprinkle with extra salt, pressing lightly to secure, and bake
for 15–20 minutes or until golden and crisp.

Allow to cool on wire racks and break into large pieces to
serve. Store in an airtight container for up to 2 weeks. **SERVES 6-8**

matcha yoghurt pops

1¼ cups (350g) plain Greek-style (thick) yoghurt
1 cup (250ml) coconut milk
⅓ cup (120g) honey
1 tablespoon matcha green tea powder*
finely chopped pistachios, to serve

finely ground green tea gives these creamy pops an antioxidant boost

Place the yoghurt, coconut milk, honey and matcha in a blender
and blend until smooth. Divide between 10 x ⅓-cup-capacity (80ml)
popsicle moulds, insert popsicle sticks and freeze for 4–5 hours or
until firm. Remove from the moulds and dip each pop in pistachio
to serve, pressing gently to secure. **MAKES 10**

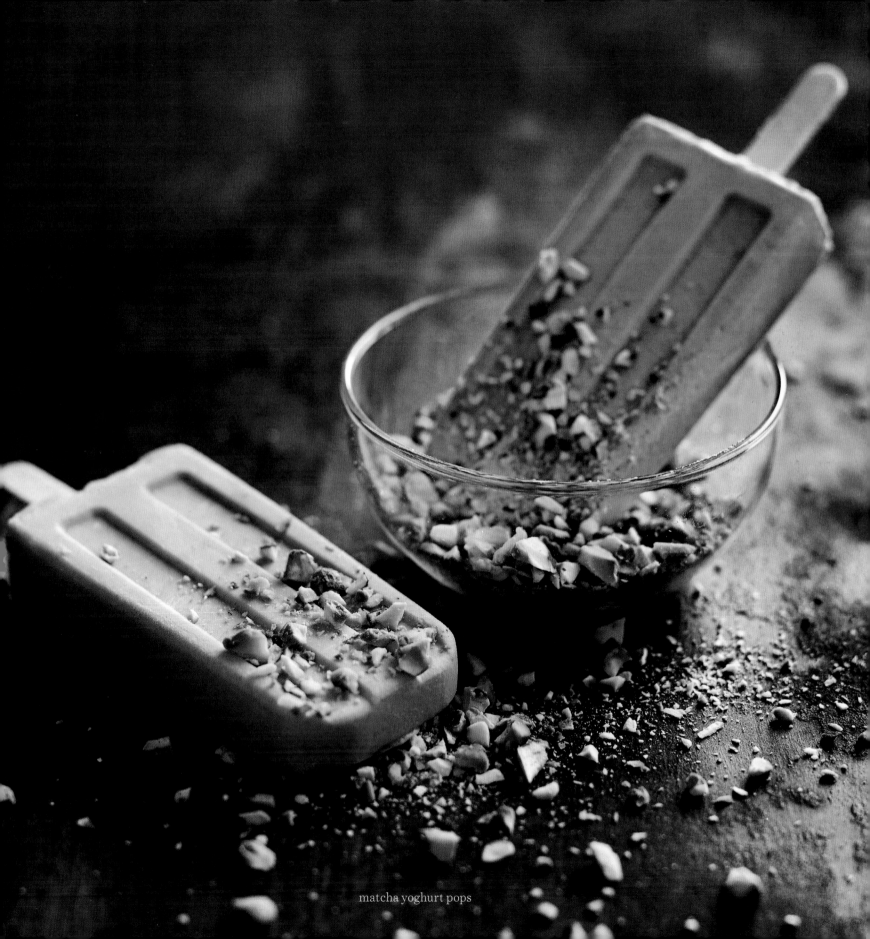

matcha yoghurt pops

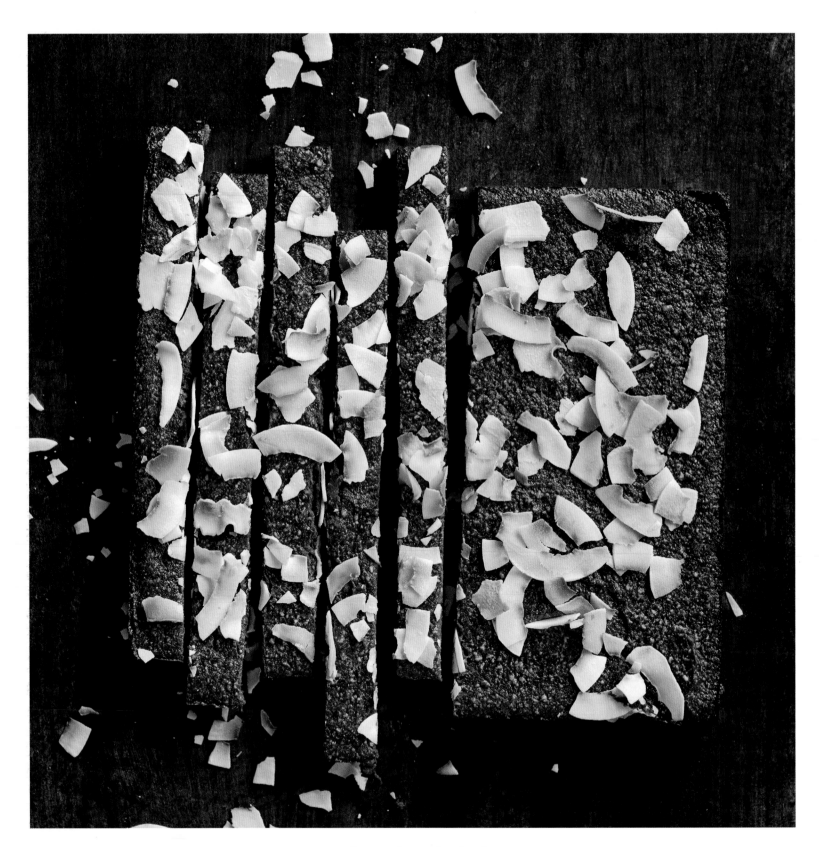

cacao, banana, date and cashew bars

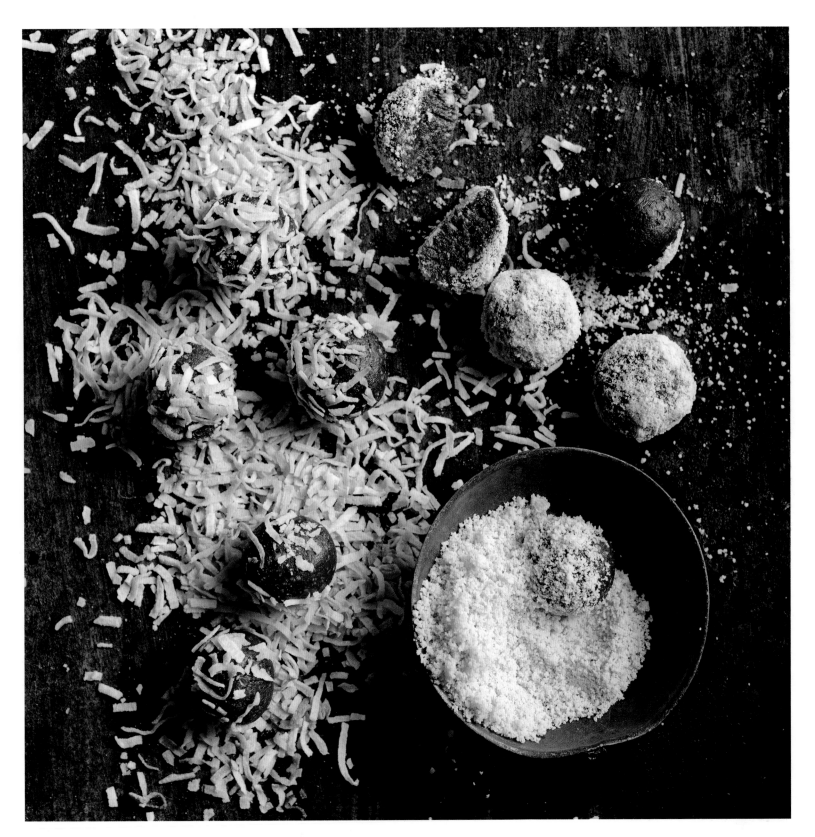

cacao date truffles

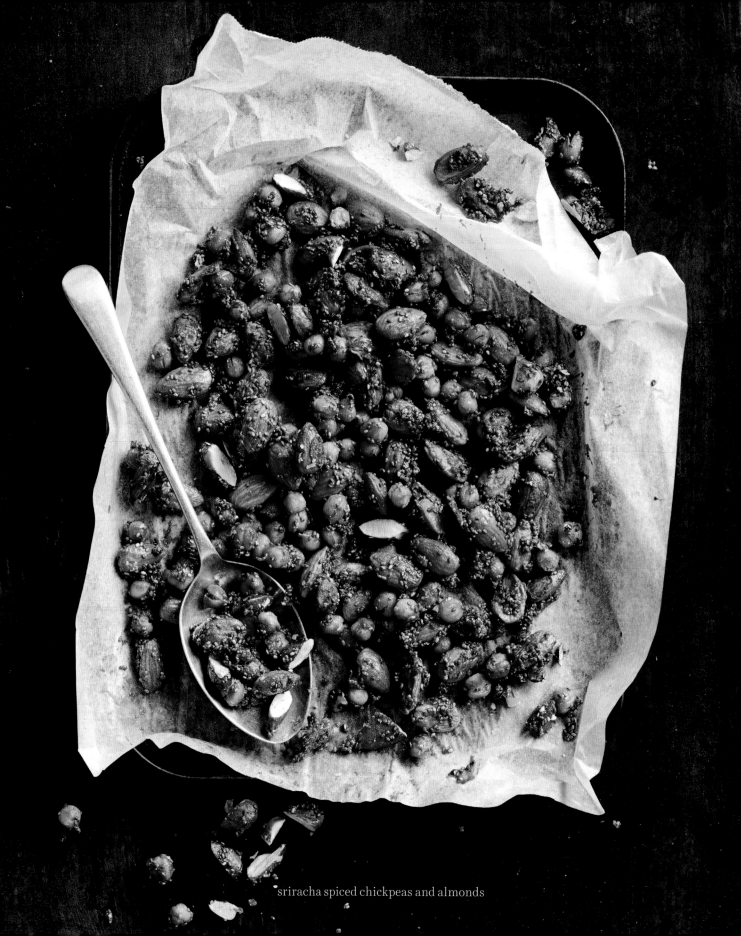

sriracha spiced chickpeas and almonds

cacao, banana, date and cashew bars

⅓ cup (35g) raw cacao powder*
¾ cup (180g) firmly packed chopped pitted
   fresh dates (about 10 dates)
¼ cup (60ml) vegetable, nut or coconut oil*
1½ cups (240g) cashews
1½ teaspoons vanilla extract
¾ cup (200g) mashed banana (about 3 bananas)
coconut flakes, for sprinkling

Preheat oven to 160°C (320°F). Line a 20cm square cake tin
with non-stick baking paper and set aside.
   Place the cacao, date, oil, cashews, vanilla and banana in a
food processor and process until smooth. Spoon the mixture
into the prepared tin, spread evenly and sprinkle with coconut.
Bake for 40 minutes or until firm to touch. Allow to cool in the
tin before slicing into bars to serve. Store bars in an airtight
container in the refrigerator for up to 1 week. **MAKES 12**

cacao date truffles

½ cup (80g) almonds
1 cup (250ml) warm water
24 fresh dates, pitted
¼ cup (25g) raw cacao powder*
2 tablespoons coconut oil*
toasted shredded coconut, almond meal (ground almonds)
   or extra raw cacao powder, to coat

Place the almonds in a bowl, cover with the water and allow
to soak for 20 minutes. Drain and place in a food processor.
Add the dates, cacao and oil and process until smooth. Divide
and shape the mixture into 2-teaspoon balls and toss in the
coconut to coat. Refrigerate for 2–3 hours or until firm
before serving. Store truffles in an airtight container in
the refrigerator for 10–14 days. **MAKES 50**

sriracha spiced chickpeas and almonds

1 x 400g can chickpeas (garbanzo beans), rinsed and drained
1 cup (160g) almonds
2 tablespoons black chia seeds*
½ cup (125ml) Sriracha chilli sauce*
2 tablespoons honey

Preheat oven to 160°C (320°F). Place the chickpeas on layers of
paper towel and dry well. Transfer to a bowl and add the almonds
and chia seeds. Place the Sriracha and honey in a small bowl and
mix well to combine. Add to the chickpea mixture and toss to coat.
Divide the mixture between 2 baking trays lined with non-stick
baking paper. Roast, turning occasionally, for 30–35 minutes or
until golden. Allow to cool on trays before serving. Store the mix
in an airtight container for up to 1 week. **MAKES 4 CUPS**

a pantry must have, sriracha hot sauce is the secret ingredient in this spicy snack

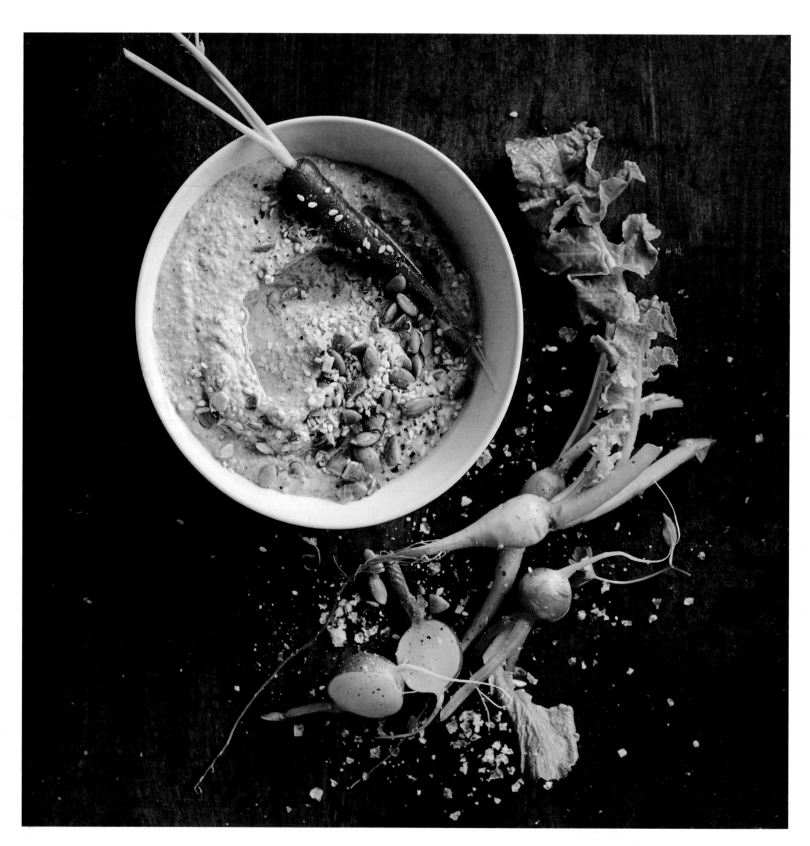

pepita dip

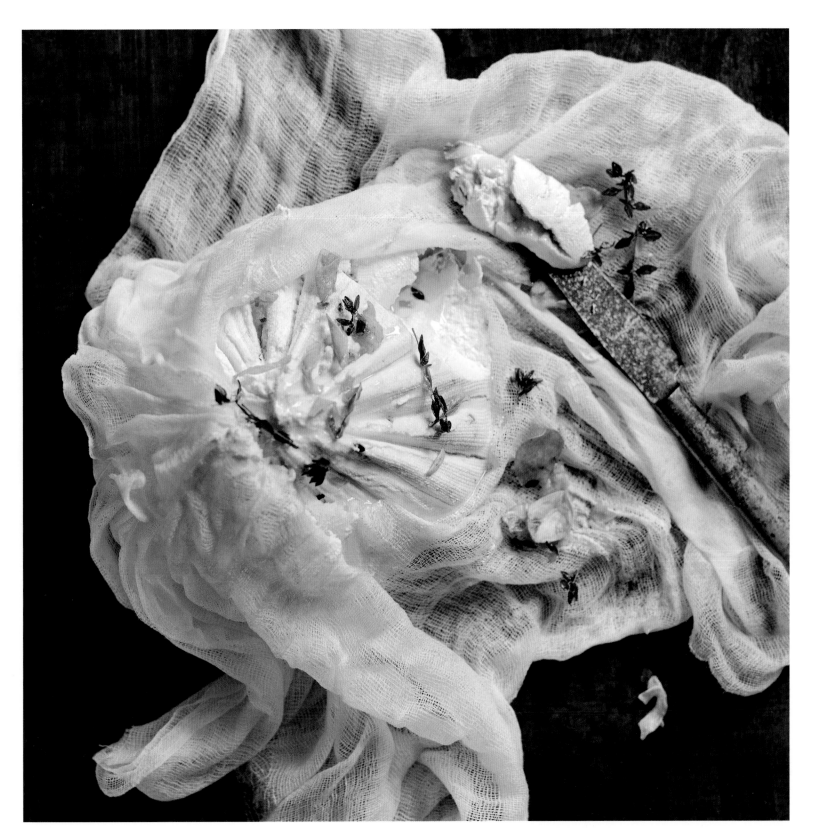

fast yoghurt cheese with preserved lemon

pepita dip

1 cup (160g) pepitas (pumpkin seeds)*,
  plus extra for sprinkling
¼ cup (60ml) extra virgin olive oil,
  plus extra for drizzling
1 tablespoon tahini*
¼ cup (60ml) lemon juice
½ cup (125ml) water
½ cup chopped flat-leaf parsley
sea salt and cracked black pepper
sesame seeds, to serve
vegetables or crackers, to serve

roasting the pepitas brings out their rich, nutty flavour

Preheat oven to 160°C (320°F). Place the pepitas on a baking tray and roast for 20 minutes or until light golden in colour. Place in a food processor and add the oil, tahini, lemon juice, water, parsley, salt and pepper. Process for 1–2 minutes or until the mixture resembles a thick paste. Refrigerate until chilled.

Drizzle with extra oil, sprinkle with sesame seeds and extra pepitas and serve with vegetables or crackers. MAKES 1¼ CUPS

fast yoghurt cheese with preserved lemon

2 tablespoons extra virgin olive oil
2 teaspoons finely chopped preserved lemon rind
3 cloves garlic, sliced
1 tablespoon sea salt flakes
2 teaspoons lemon thyme leaves
1¾ cups (500g) plain Greek-style (thick) yoghurt

Place the oil, lemon rind, garlic, salt and thyme in a saucepan over medium heat and cook, stirring occasionally, for 5 minutes or until the garlic is soft and golden. Reserve and set aside half the mixture and place the remaining half in a bowl. Add the yoghurt and mix to combine. Transfer to a bowl lined with a double layer of muslin and gather up the edges to enclose. Suspend the yoghurt from a shelf in the refrigerator, placing a bowl underneath to collect any moisture, for 4 hours or until the mixture is firm.

Unwrap the yoghurt cheese, place on a serving plate and top with the reserved preserved lemon mixture. Serve as a dip, spread or side to a salad or vegetables. SERVES 4–6

buckwheat and quinoa blueberry muffins

½ cup (50g) quinoa flakes*,
  plus extra for sprinkling
½ cup (125ml) milk
1 cup (140g) wholemeal spelt flour*
1 cup (160g) buckwheat flour*
3 teaspoons baking powder
½ teaspoon ground cinnamon
¼ cup (55g) raw or rapadura sugar*,
  plus extra for sprinkling
1 teaspoon vanilla extract
1 egg
¾ cup (180ml) vegetable, nut or coconut oil*
¾ cup (180ml) maple syrup
2 cups (300g) fresh or frozen blueberries

grab one of these on your way out the door for an easy breakfast on the go

Preheat oven to 180°C (350°F). Line 12 x ¼-cup-capacity (125ml) muffin tins with paper cases and set aside.

Place the quinoa flakes and milk in a large bowl, mix to combine and allow to soak for 20 minutes. Add both the flours, the baking powder, cinnamon, sugar, vanilla, egg, oil and maple syrup and mix to combine. Add the blueberries and fold to combine. Spoon the mixture into the cases and sprinkle with extra quinoa flakes and sugar. Bake for 20–25 minutes or until just cooked when tested with a skewer. Allow to cool in the tins for 5 minutes before transferring to a wire rack to cool completely. Store muffins in an airtight container for up to 3 days or wrap individually and freeze for up to 2 months. MAKES 12

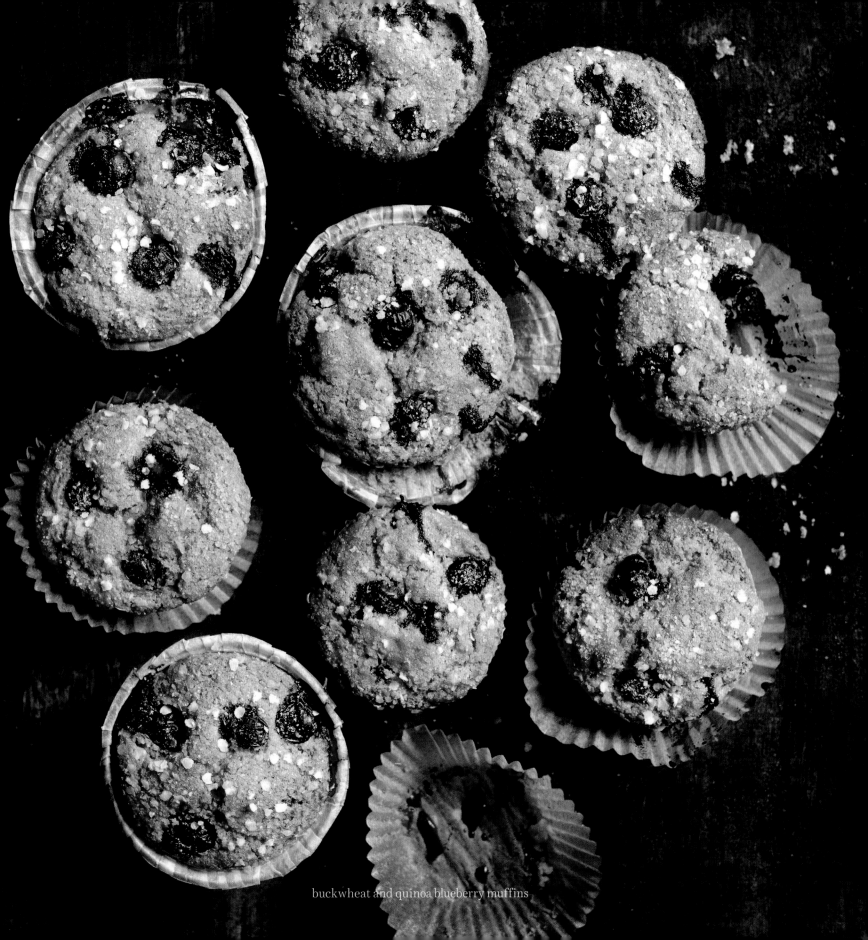

buckwheat and quinoa blueberry muffins

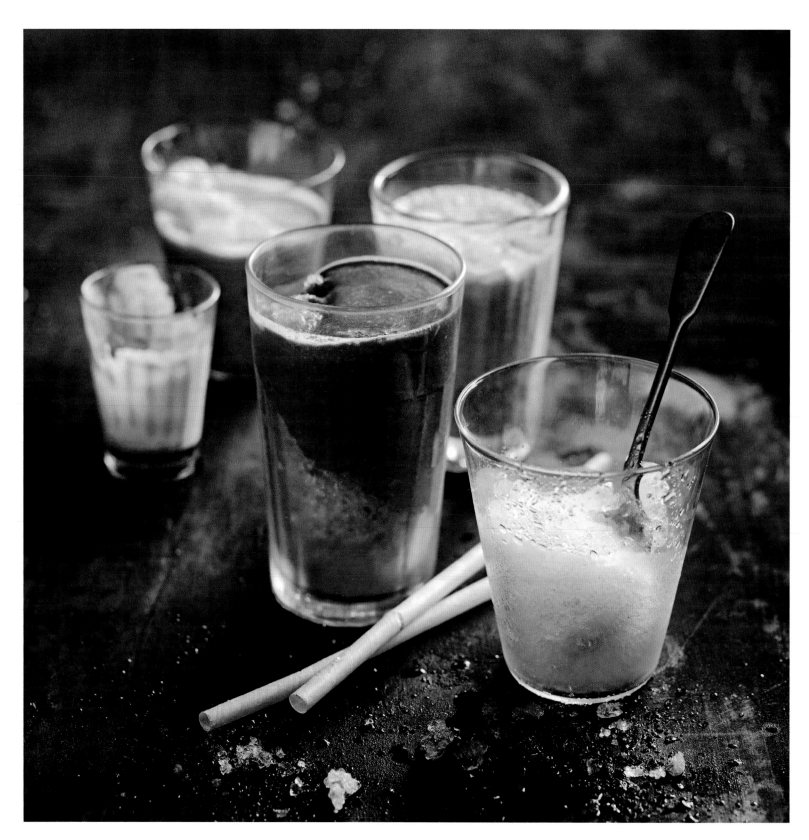

cacao almond shakes + espresso cashew shakes

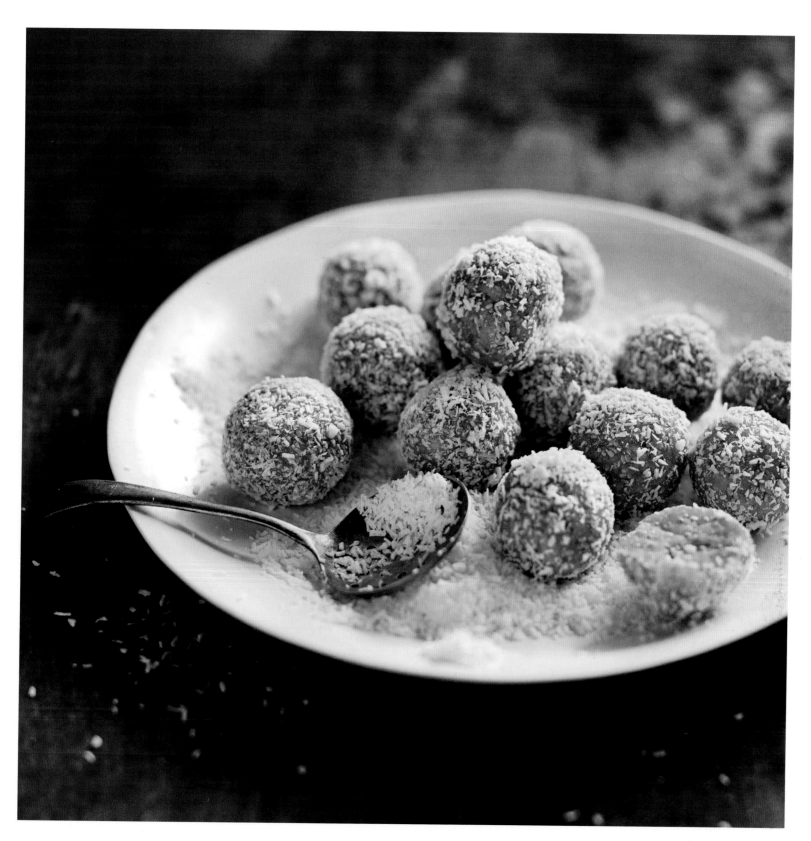

peach and coconut chia snacks

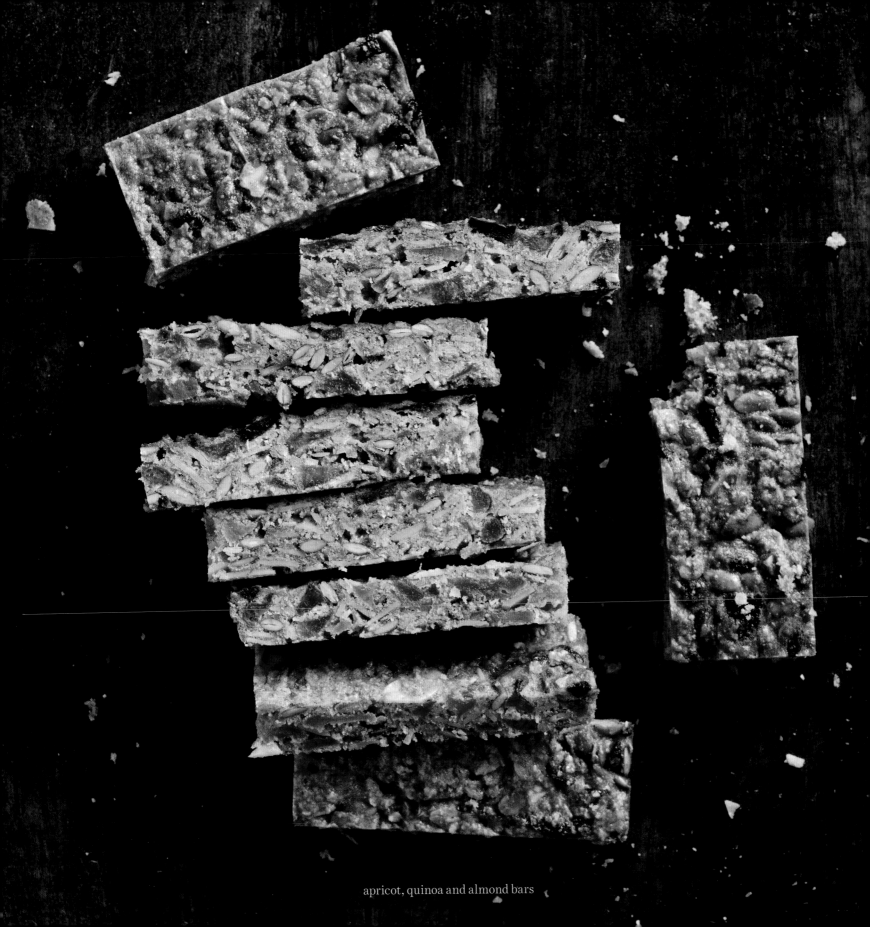

apricot, quinoa and almond bars

cacao almond shakes

⅓ cup (55g) almonds
2 cups (500ml) warm water
2 cups (500ml) cold water
8 fresh dates, pitted
¼ cup (25g) raw cacao powder*

a purer way to indulge, raw cacao has been cold-pressed to retain its goodness

Place the almonds in a bowl, cover with the warm water and allow to soak for 20 minutes. Drain, rinse well and place in a blender. Add the cold water, dates and cacao and blend until smooth. Divide between glasses, over ice, to serve. **SERVES 4**

espresso cashew shakes

¼ cup (40g) cashews
2 cups (500ml) warm water
2 cups (500ml) cold water
2 x 30ml shots espresso or strong brewed coffee
6 fresh dates, pitted

Place the cashews in a bowl, cover with the warm water and allow to soak for 30 minutes. Drain, rinse well and place in a blender. Add the cold water, espresso and dates and blend until smooth. Divide between glasses, over ice, to serve. **SERVES 4**

peach and coconut chia snacks

2 cups (280g) chopped dried peaches
¼ cup (60g) coconut oil*
¼ cup (60ml) rice malt syrup*
¼ cup (50g) white chia seeds*
2 tablespoons lemon juice
desiccated coconut, to coat

Place the peach, oil, rice malt syrup, chia seeds and lemon juice in a food processor and process for 2–3 minutes or until a soft dough forms. Divide and shape the mixture into 2-teaspoon balls and toss in the coconut to coat. Refrigerate for 1 hour or until firm before serving. Store snacks in an airtight container in the refrigerator for up to 2 weeks. **MAKES 30**

apricot, quinoa and almond bars

½ cup (50g) quinoa flakes*
½ cup (40g) flaked almonds
¼ cup (40g) pepitas (pumpkin seeds)*
½ cup (60g) rolled oats
1¼ cups (185g) chopped dried apricots
½ cup (40g) desiccated coconut
½ cup (70g) wholemeal spelt flour*
½ cup (125ml) vegetable or nut oil
¾ cup (180ml) maple syrup
1 teaspoon ground cinnamon

spelt is an ancient grain that's high in protein and easy to digest

Preheat oven to 160°C (320°F). Line a 20cm x 30cm slice tin with non-stick baking paper and set aside.

Place the quinoa flakes, almonds, pepitas and oats on a baking tray, toss to combine and bake for 10 minutes or until lightly toasted. Place in a large bowl, add the apricot, coconut, flour, oil, maple syrup and cinnamon and mix well to combine. Press the mixture firmly into the prepared tin and bake for 40–45 minutes or until the slice is golden and firm to touch. Allow to cool in the tin for 10 minutes before turning out onto a wire rack to cool completely. Slice into bars to serve. Store bars in an airtight container for up to 1 week. **MAKES 16**

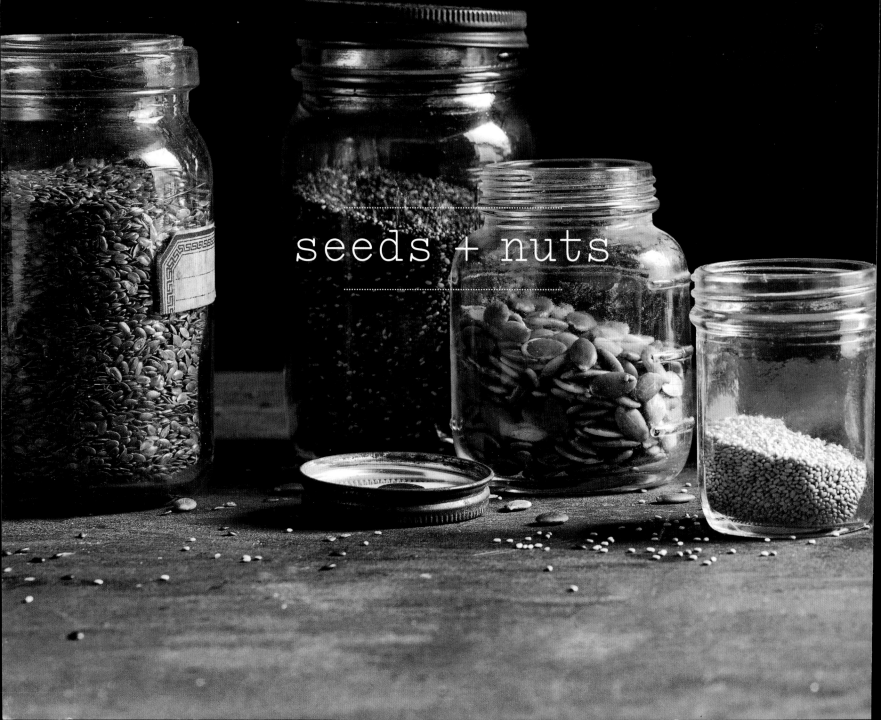

seeds + nuts

With just a handful of nuts thrown into my smoothie or a sprinkling of seeds through a sweet baked treat, I've brought these tiny power foods into my day — easy! Packed with minerals and nourishing oils, they're my cheat's path to a healthy glow. Here's what's in my pantry.

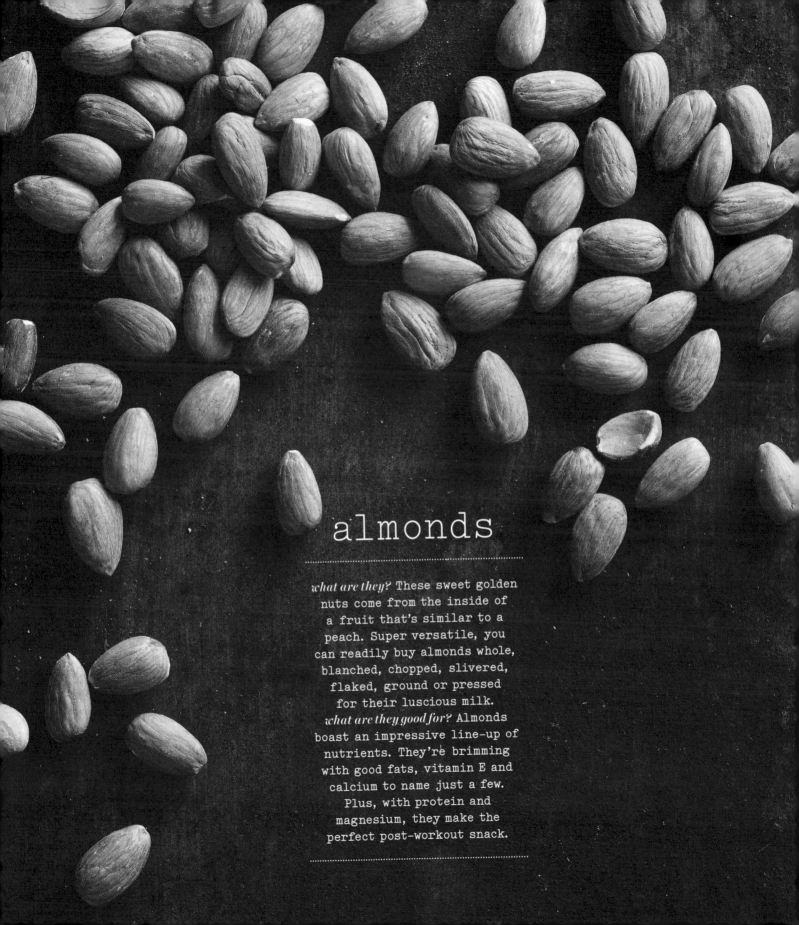

almonds

what are they? These sweet golden nuts come from the inside of a fruit that's similar to a peach. Super versatile, you can readily buy almonds whole, blanched, chopped, slivered, flaked, ground or pressed for their luscious milk.

what are they good for? Almonds boast an impressive line-up of nutrients. They're brimming with good fats, vitamin E and calcium to name just a few. Plus, with protein and magnesium, they make the perfect post-workout snack.

sesame seeds

what are they? Tiny with a mild, nutty flavour, these ancient seeds are widely used in the Middle East and Asia. You can find red, brown and black, but the glossy ivory colour is more common. Toss them into baking, onto salads, over seafood or grind them into tasty tahini.

what are they good for? Sesame seeds are rich in minerals like zinc, which is good for our immune systems. A source of calcium, iron and copper, too, they may be tiny but they're full of goodness!

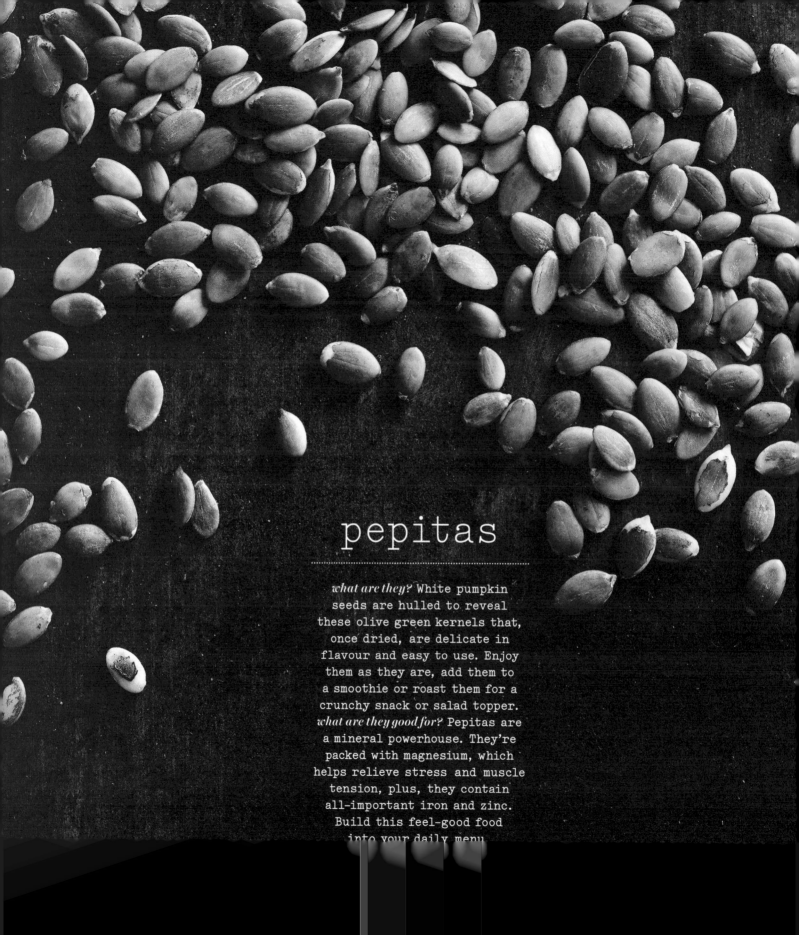

pepitas

what are they? White pumpkin seeds are hulled to reveal these olive green kernels that, once dried, are delicate in flavour and easy to use. Enjoy them as they are, add them to a smoothie or roast them for a crunchy snack or salad topper. *what are they good for?* Pepitas are a mineral powerhouse. They're packed with magnesium, which helps relieve stress and muscle tension, plus, they contain all-important iron and zinc. Build this feel-good food into your daily menu

cashews

what are they? Sweet, buttery
cashews grow at the base of
the cashew apple on a tropical
tree. Traditionally used in
Indian and Southeast Asian
cuisines, their creamy texture
has made them a popular snack.
They're also easy to blend into
milk as a dairy alternative.
what are they good for? Like most
nuts, cashews are high in good
fats, but they also contain
lots of iron and zinc. Enriched
with protein, too, a handful
of these crunchy kernels makes
for a satisfying raw treat.

linseeds

what are they? Also known as flaxseeds, these shiny brown seeds have a mild nutty flavour. They're most commonly pressed for their oil, but they can be baked into bread, sprinkled over cereal and blended into smoothies.

what are they good for? Linseeds are high in fibre, so can be helpful for our digestive systems. They're also enriched with plant-based omega-3 fatty acids (similar to those found in oily fish), which have numerous body benefits.

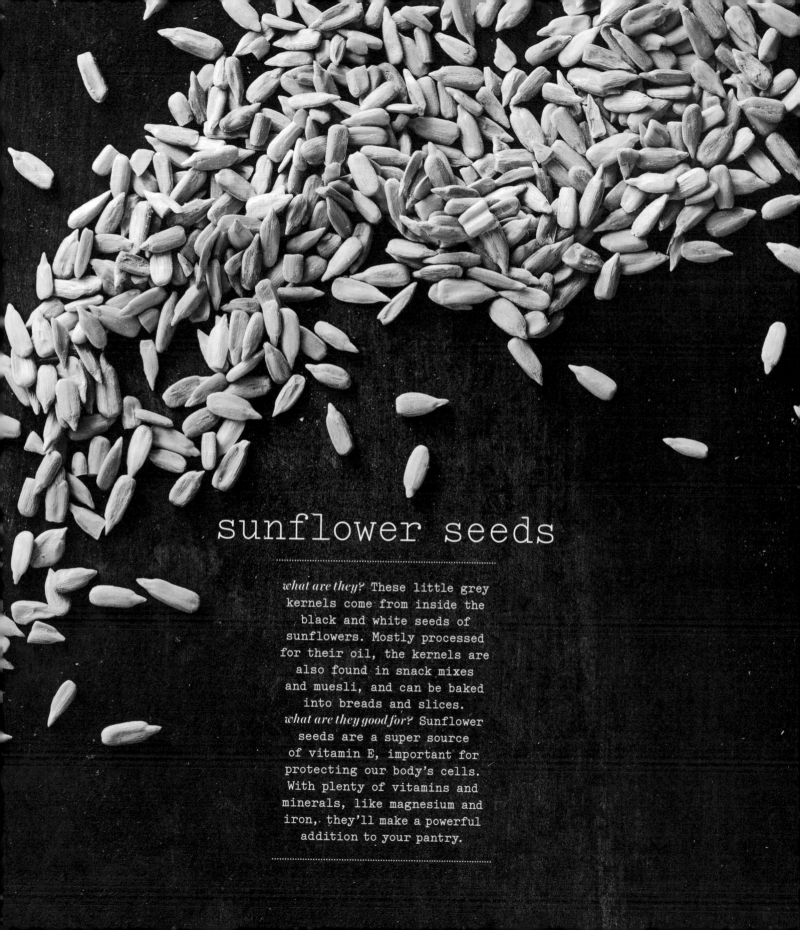

sunflower seeds

what are they? These little grey kernels come from inside the black and white seeds of sunflowers. Mostly processed for their oil, the kernels are also found in snack mixes and muesli, and can be baked into breads and slices.

what are they good for? Sunflower seeds are a super source of vitamin E, important for protecting our body's cells. With plenty of vitamins and minerals, like magnesium and iron, they'll make a powerful addition to your pantry.

chia seeds

....

what are they? This ancient seed, harvested from a desert plant, has made a comeback for its super qualities. Versatile in its whole form, chia also expands in water to be spooned as a pudding. You can buy both black and white chia seeds.

what are they good for? Like linseeds, chia seeds are one of the highest sources of plant-based omega-3s. They pack in plenty of antioxidants, plus fibre and protein. Keep them on-hand to enhance your cereal, smoothies and salads.

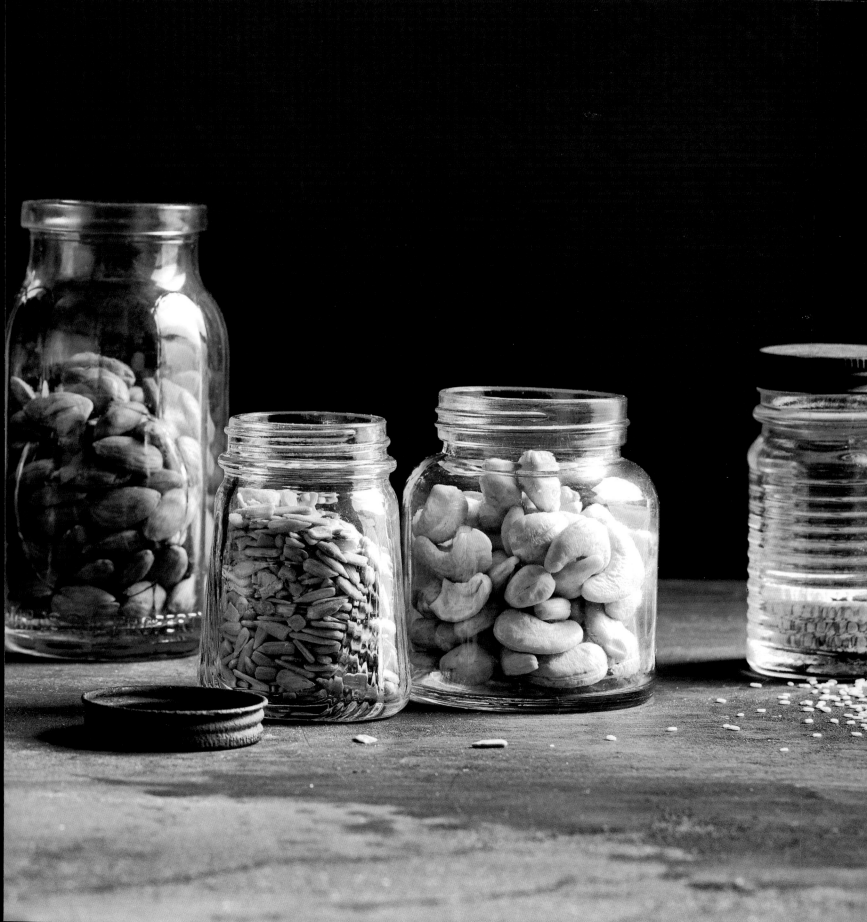

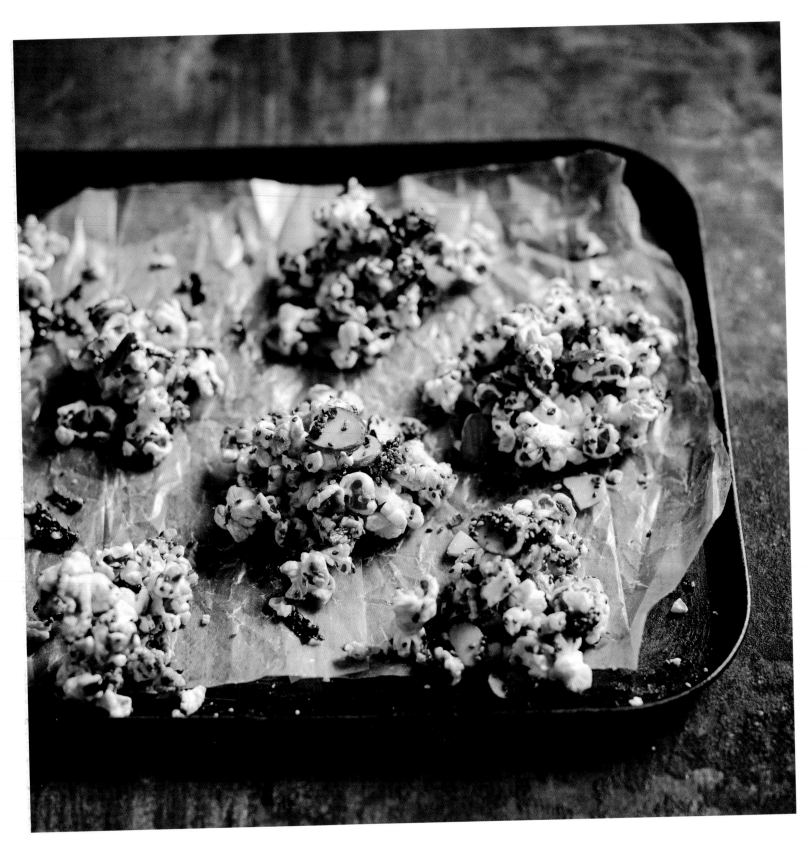

chilli caramel popcorn clusters

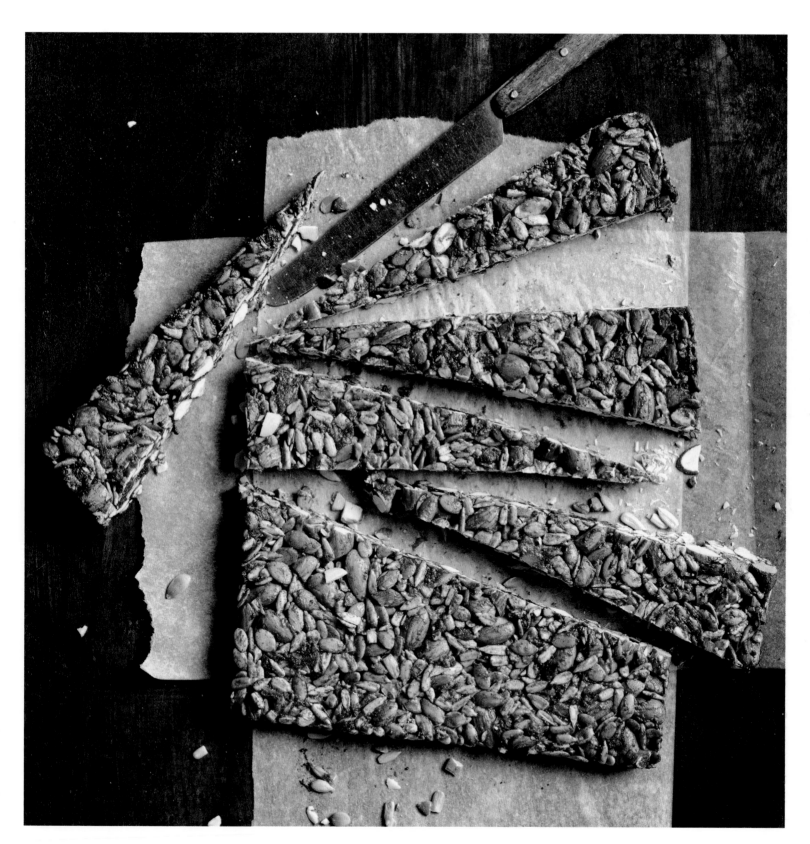

seed and date bars

chilli caramel popcorn clusters

6 cups (90g) popped popcorn
¼ cup (50g) black chia seeds*
⅓ cup (55g) almonds, chopped
¼ cup (5g) shredded nori*
chilli caramel
1 teaspoon dried chilli flakes
½ teaspoon sea salt flakes
½ cup (125ml) maple syrup
30g unsalted butter or coconut oil*

for a mild coconut flavour, swap butter for coconut oil here
↓

Preheat oven to 120°C (250°F). Place the popcorn, chia seeds, almonds and nori in a bowl, mix to combine and set aside.

To make the chilli caramel, place the chilli, salt, maple syrup and butter in a saucepan over low heat. Cook, stirring occasionally, for 5 minutes or until the butter has melted. Increase the heat to medium, bring to the boil and cook for 2 minutes or until the mixture has thickened slightly and is golden. Pour the caramel over the popcorn mixture and toss well to combine. Place heaped tablespoons of the mixture onto 3 baking trays lined with non-stick baking paper. Bake for 15 minutes or until crisp. Allow to cool on trays for 10 minutes before serving. MAKES 36

seed and date bars

1 cup (240g) firmly packed chopped pitted
   fresh dates (about 20 dates)
¾ cup (120g) chopped almonds
¾ cup (120g) sunflower seeds*
½ cup (80g) pepitas (pumpkin seeds)*
2 tablespoons honey
1 teaspoon ground cinnamon
1 teaspoon vanilla extract

Preheat oven to 160°C (320°F). Line a 20cm square cake tin with non-stick baking paper and set aside.

Place the date, almond, sunflower seeds, pepitas, honey, cinnamon and vanilla in a bowl and mix well to combine. Press the mixture firmly into the prepared tin and bake for 45 minutes or until crisp to touch. Allow to cool in the tin before slicing into bars to serve. Store in an airtight container for up to 10 days. MAKES 12

raspberry swirl yoghurt pops

2 cups (560g) plain Greek-style (thick) yoghurt
½ cup (125ml) rice malt syrup*
1 teaspoon vanilla bean paste
2 cups (300g) frozen raspberries
¼ cup (60ml) rice malt syrup*, extra

Place the yoghurt, rice malt syrup and vanilla in a bowl and mix to combine. Place ¼ cup (125ml) of the yoghurt mixture, the raspberries and the extra rice malt syrup in a blender and blend until smooth.

Layer alternate spoonfuls of the yoghurt and raspberry mixtures into 10 x ⅓-cup-capacity (80ml) popsicle moulds. Swirl gently using a butter knife, insert popsicle sticks and freeze for 4–5 hours or until firm. Remove the pops from the moulds to serve. MAKES 10

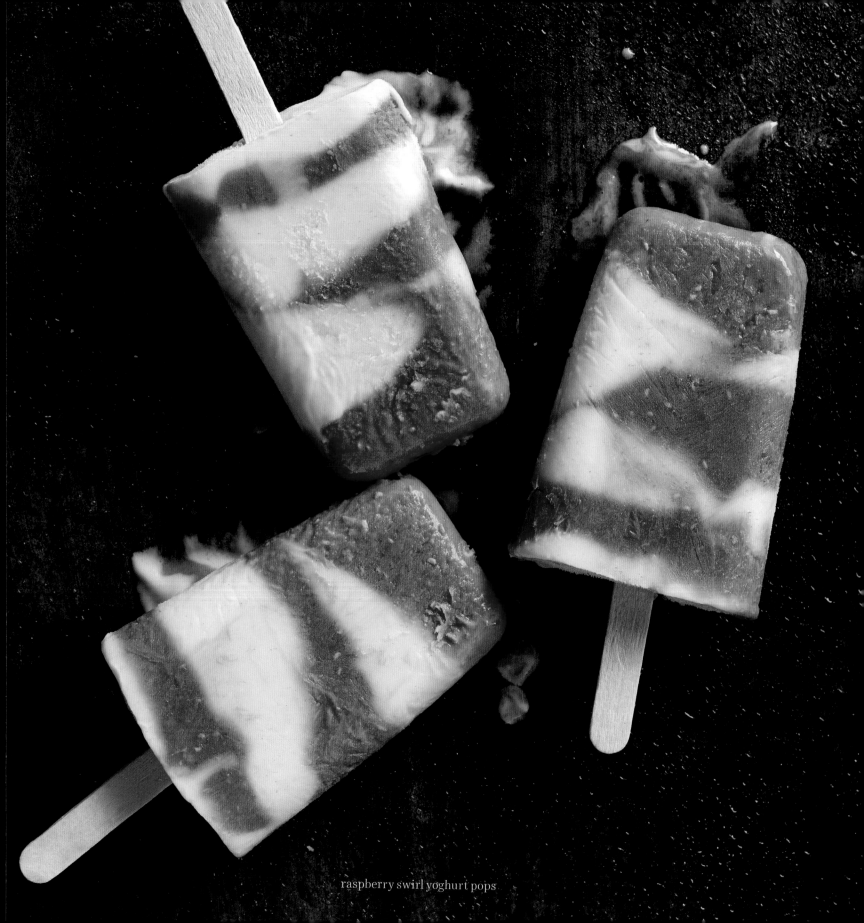

raspberry swirl yoghurt pops

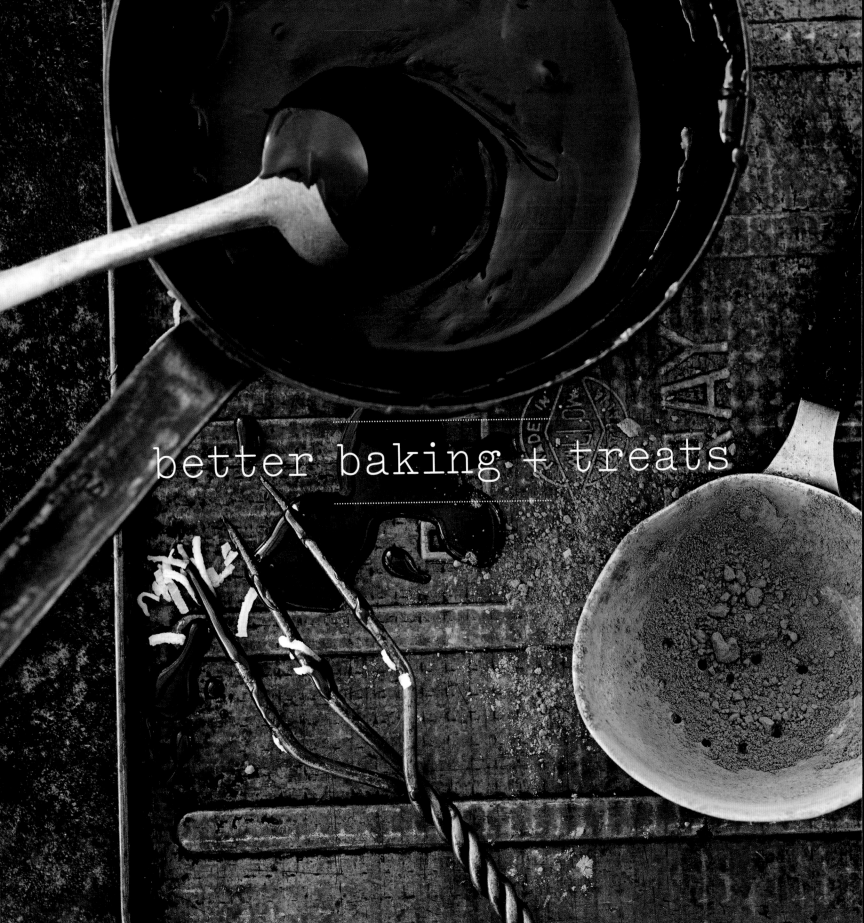

better baking + treats

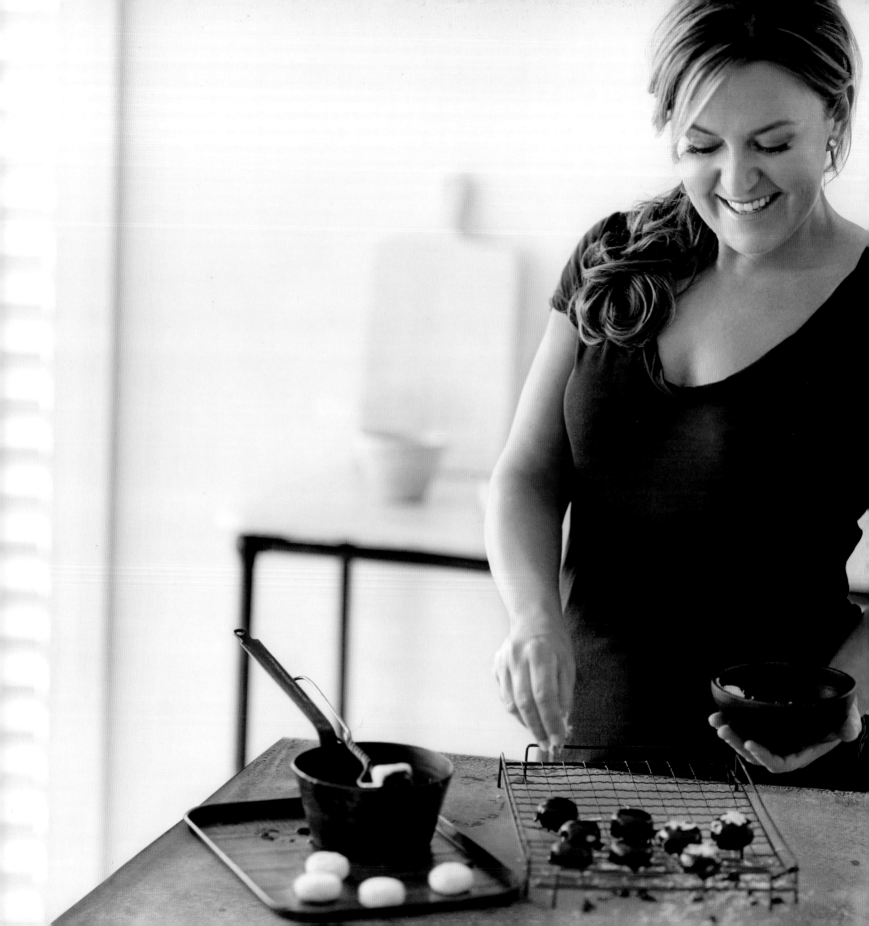

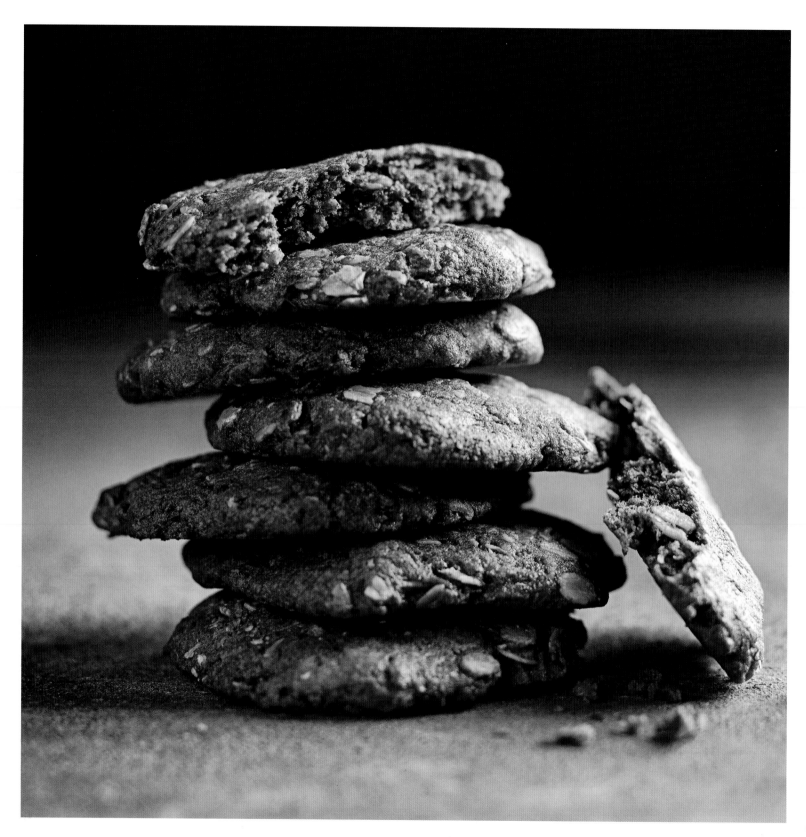

caramel sticky date cookies

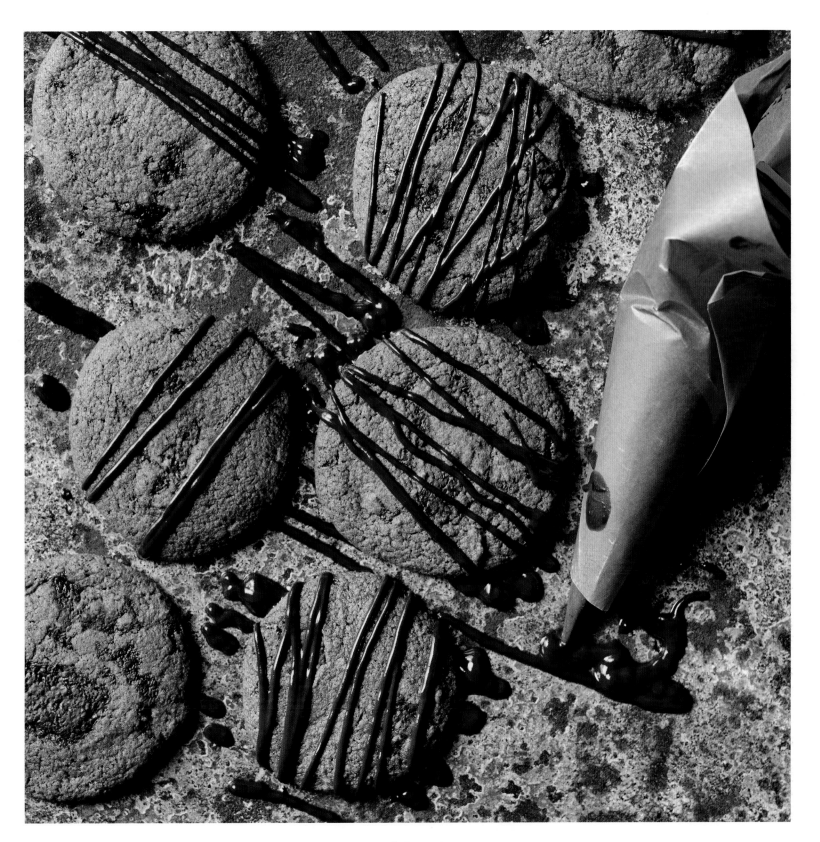

cacao fudge cookies

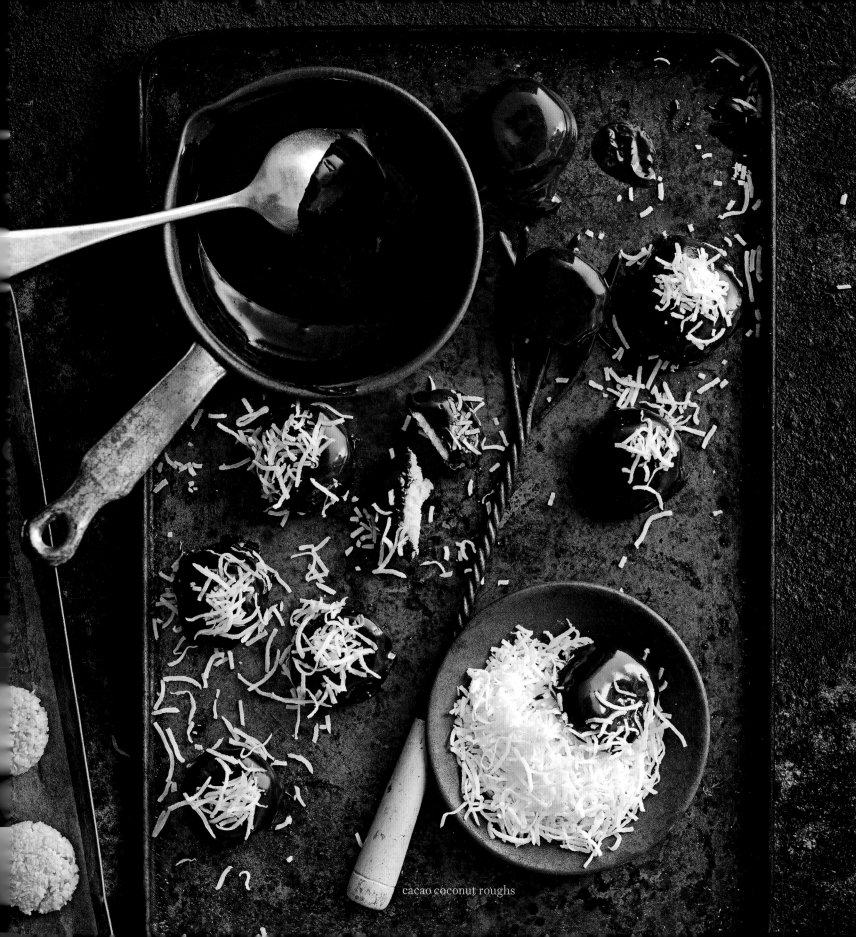

cacao coconut roughs

caramel sticky date cookies

Soft and chewy, these cookies make the perfect afternoon snack

1½ cups (360g) firmly packed chopped
    pitted fresh dates (about 15 dates)
½ cup (85g) brown sugar
125g unsalted butter or coconut oil*
1 teaspoon bicarbonate of (baking) soda
1 cup (140g) wholemeal spelt flour*
1 cup (80g) spelt flakes*
1 egg
1 teaspoon ground cinnamon
1 teaspoon vanilla extract

Preheat oven to 160°C (320°F). Place the dates, sugar and butter in a small saucepan over medium heat and stir until the butter is melted. Cook, stirring, for a further 5 minutes or until the dates are soft. Add the bicarbonate of soda, mix to combine and set aside to cool.

Place the flour, spelt flakes, egg, cinnamon and vanilla in a large bowl. Add the date mixture and mix to combine. Divide and shape the mixture into 2-tablespoon balls, flatten slightly and place on baking trays lined with non-stick baking paper. Bake for 12–14 minutes or until golden. Allow to cool on trays. Store cookies in an airtight container for up to 1 week. **MAKES 12**

Keep these bites on-hand in your freezer for an instant indulgent treat

cacao fudge cookies

1 cup (175g) brown sugar
100g unsalted butter or coconut oil*, slightly softened
½ cup (125ml) maple syrup
2 teaspoons vanilla extract
⅓ cup (35g) raw cacao powder*
1 cup (140g) wholemeal spelt flour*
½ cup (80g) buckwheat flour*
1 egg
150g raw cacao chocolate* or dark chocolate,
    roughly chopped, plus extra, melted, to serve

Preheat oven to 160°C (320°F). Place the sugar, butter, maple syrup and vanilla in a bowl and mix to combine. Add the cacao, both the flours, the egg and chopped chocolate and mix to combine. Roll tablespoons of the mixture into balls, flatten slightly and place on baking trays lined with non-stick baking paper. Bake for 12 minutes or until golden. Allow to cool on trays.

Drizzle cooled cookies with the extra melted chocolate to serve. Store in an airtight container for up to 1 week. **MAKES 24**

cacao coconut roughs

2 cups (150g) shredded coconut, plus extra to coat
⅓ cup (80ml) rice malt syrup*
chocolate topping
⅓ cup (80g) coconut oil*
½ cup (125ml) rice malt syrup*
½ cup (50g) raw cacao powder*

Place the coconut and rice malt syrup in a food processor and process for 30 seconds – 1 minute or until the mixture is roughly chopped and comes together. Shape teaspoons of the mixture into small patties and place on a tray lined with non-stick baking paper. Freeze for 15 minutes or until firm.

To make the chocolate topping, place the oil, rice malt syrup and cacao in a saucepan over low heat, stirring, until smooth.

Using two forks, dip each patty into the chocolate topping to coat, tapping to remove any excess. Place on a chilled tray lined with non-stick baking paper and sprinkle with the extra coconut. Return to the freezer for 10–15 minutes or until set. Store coconut roughs in an airtight container in the freezer for up to 4 weeks. **MAKES 30**

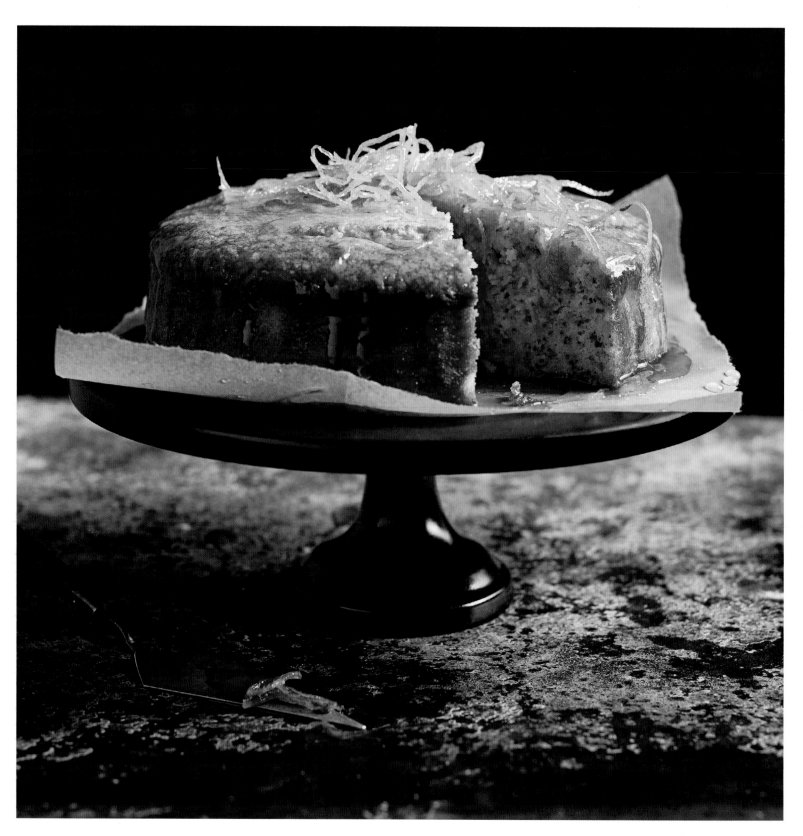

orange and chia seed syrup cake

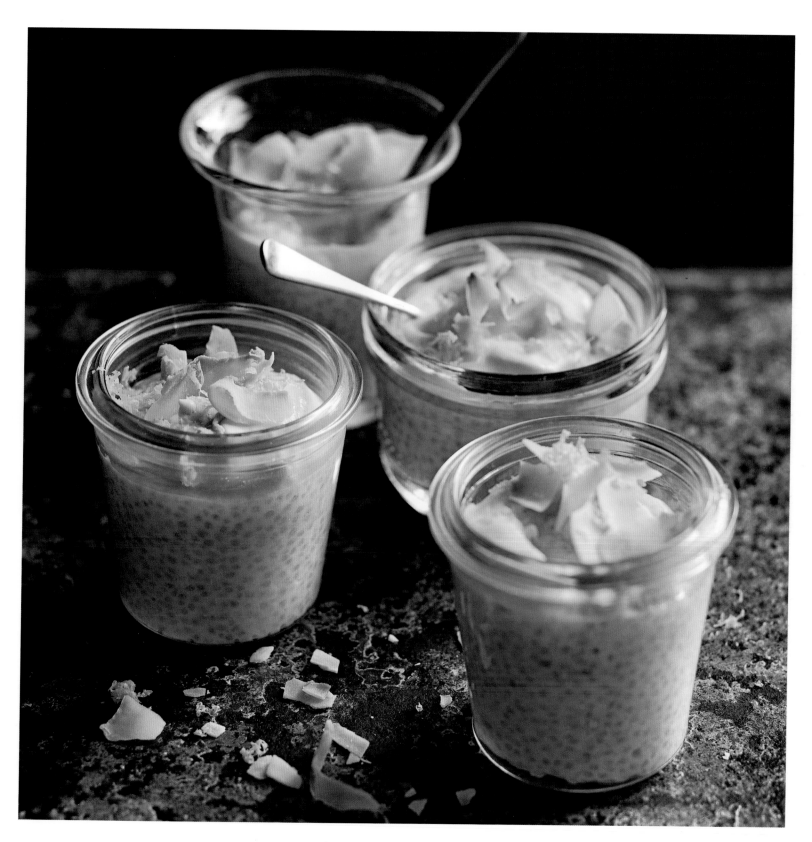

lemon delicious chia puddings

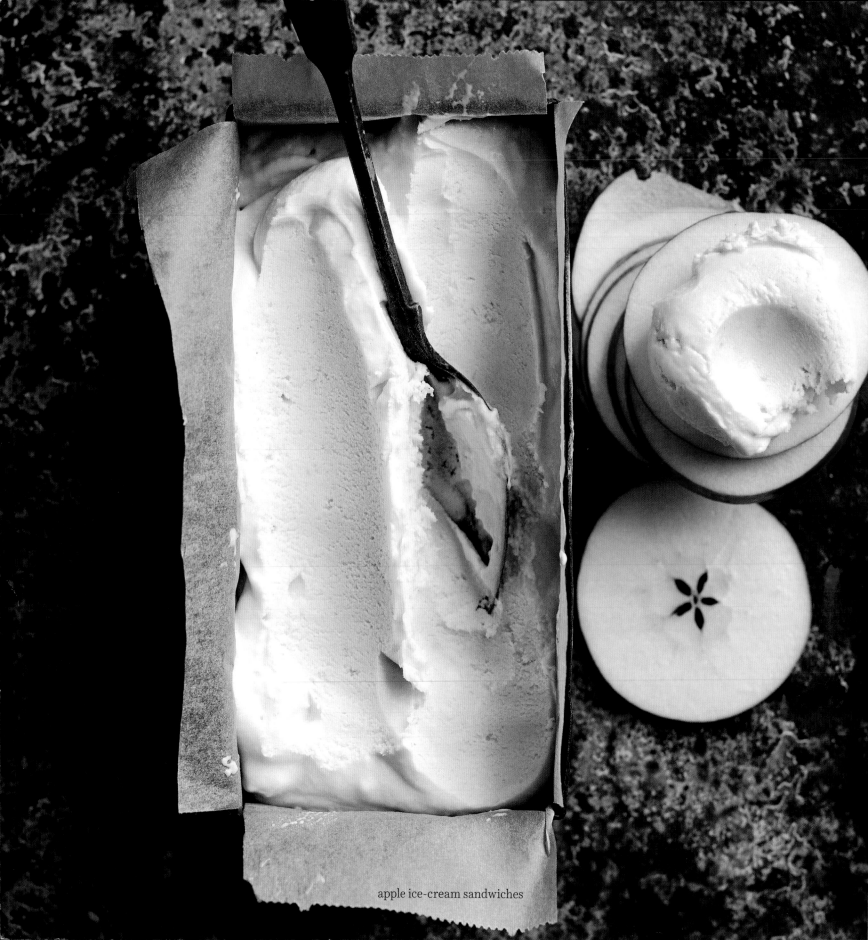

apple ice-cream sandwiches

orange and chia seed syrup cake

¼ cup (50g) black chia seeds*
½ cup (125ml) milk
125g unsalted butter, chopped
1 tablespoon finely grated orange rind
1 cup (220g) raw sugar
4 eggs
2 cups (240g) almond meal (ground almonds)
1 cup (130g) white spelt flour*
1½ teaspoons baking powder
orange syrup
½ cup (125ml) rice malt syrup*
2 tablespoons orange zest
½ cup (125ml) orange juice

Preheat oven to 160°C (320°F). Lightly grease a 20cm round cake tin, line with non-stick baking paper and set aside. Place the chia seeds and milk in a bowl and set aside to soak for 10 minutes.

Place the butter, orange rind and sugar in the bowl of an electric mixer and beat for 8 minutes or until light and creamy. Add the eggs and beat until well combined. Add the chia mixture, almond meal, flour and baking powder and fold to combine. Spoon the mixture into the prepared tin and bake for 1 hour – 1 hour 10 minutes or until cooked when tested with a skewer.

While the cake is baking, make the orange syrup. Place the rice malt syrup, orange rind and juice in a small saucepan over medium heat. Simmer for 12 minutes or until the syrup is reduced by half and thickened.

Invert the cake onto a cake stand and, while still hot, top with the syrup. Slice and serve warm. SERVES 12

lemon delicious chia puddings

½ cup (100g) white chia seeds*
¼ cup (60ml) lemon juice
2 cups (500ml) milk
½ cup (125ml) coconut cream
⅓ cup (80ml) rice malt syrup*
½ cup (140g) coconut yoghurt*, plus extra to serve
toasted shredded coconut and finely grated lemon rind, to serve

Place the chia seeds, lemon juice, milk and coconut cream in a bowl and whisk to combine. Set aside to soak for 20–30 minutes.

Add the rice malt syrup and yoghurt and stir to combine. Divide between glasses and top the puddings with extra yoghurt, toasted coconut and lemon rind to serve. SERVES 4–6

apple ice-cream sandwiches

2 cups (560g) plain Greek-style (thick) yoghurt
½ cup (180g) honey
¼ cup (60ml) rice malt syrup*
1 cup (260g) mashed banana (about 3 bananas)
1 cup (250ml) coconut cream
3 apples, nectarines or peaches, very thinly sliced

Place the yoghurt, honey, rice malt syrup, banana and coconut cream in a large snap-lock plastic bag. Seal, shake to combine and freeze for 3–4 hours or until solid.

Line a metal container with non-stick baking paper. Break up the ice-cream by bending and tapping the bag on a hard surface. Place the ice-cream in a food processor and process until smooth. Pour into the prepared tin and freeze for 2 hours or until firm.

Press scoops of the banana coconut ice-cream between slices of apple to make sandwiches. Place on trays lined with non-stick baking paper and freeze for 30 minutes or until firm. MAKES 20

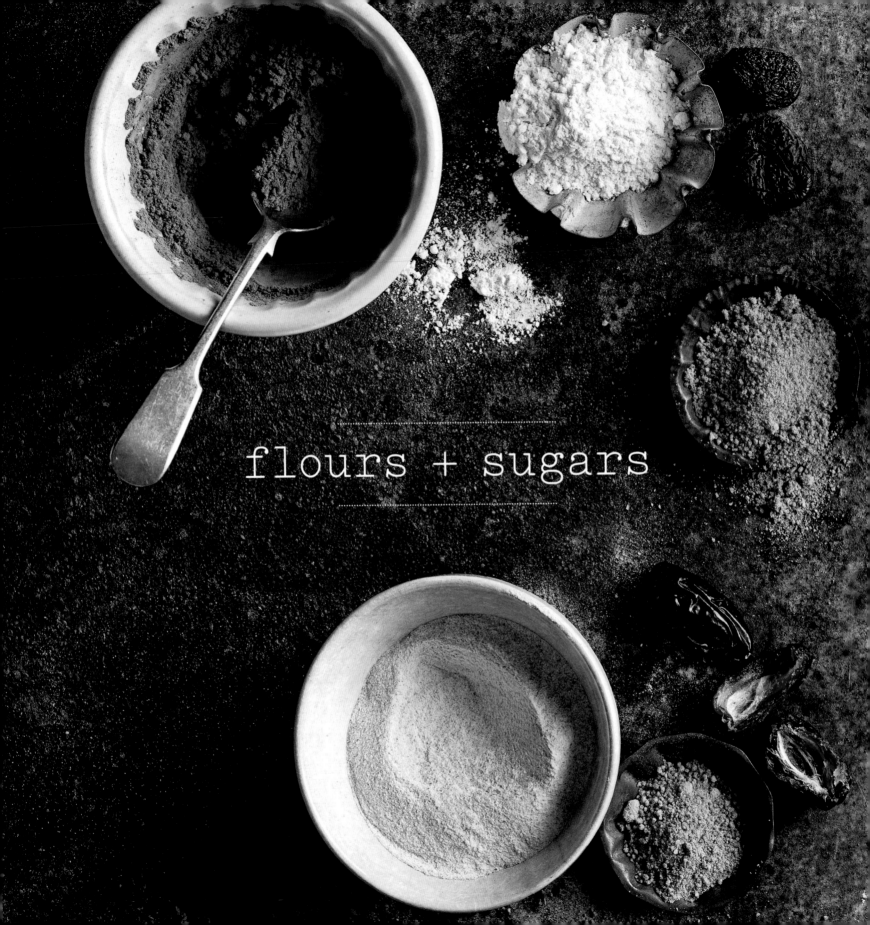

flours + sugars

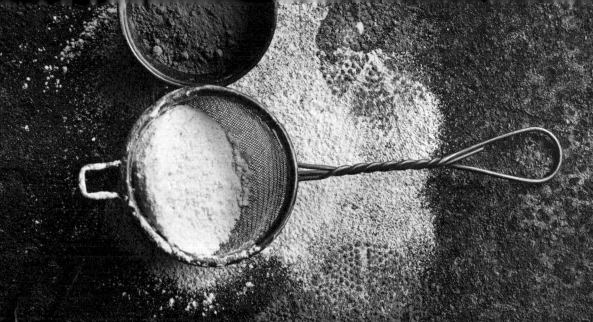

It's no secret I love to bake
(my therapy!) and I'm a firm
believer in treating oneself.
That being said, I'm always on the
lookout for smart ways to swap
in some goodness to my sweets.
These clever ingredients, from
rich caramel sugars to super raw
cacao, will help you make the
most of your every indulgence.

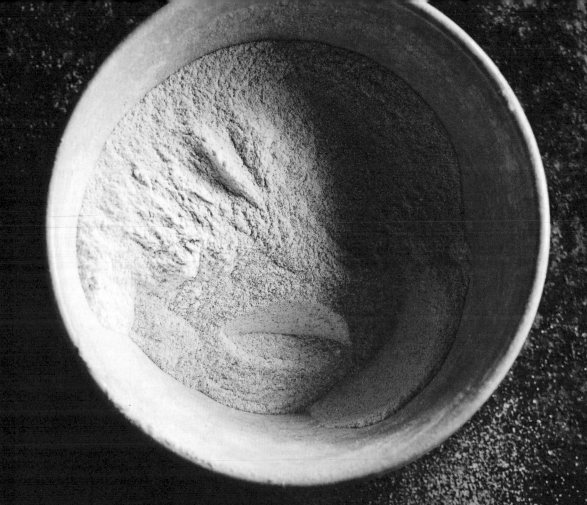

buckwheat flour

what is it? Despite its name,
buckwheat flour isn't
technically from a grain, but
milled from the seed of a plant
related to rhubarb and sorrel.
Often used in pancakes and
noodles for its rich, nutty
flavour and wholesome benefits,
it's also gluten free.
what is it good for? High in protein
and soluble fibre, buckwheat
flour has a lower glycaemic
index than regular wheat flour.
It also tends to stay moist
in baking, unlike some other
gluten-free flours.

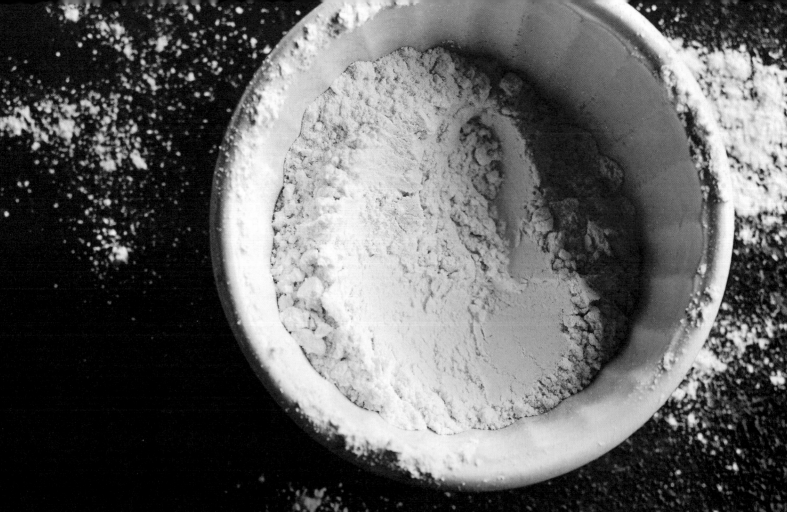

spelt flour

what is it? Spelt is an ancient cereal grain. Its flour (white or wholemeal) can often be used in place of regular wheat flour as it boasts more nutrients and can be tolerated more by some. It gives breads and pastas a mild nutty flavour and a caramel colour.

what is it good for? With fibre, protein and high water solubility, spelt flour can be easier to digest than some other flours. Additionally, it lends baked treats a slightly sweet, malted taste.

nut meals

what are they? Nut meals, or
simply ground nuts, give a
delicious richness to baking,
with the added benefits of good
fats and minerals. Often used
as alternatives to flour,
you can buy them or make
your own by processing nuts
like almonds or hazelnuts.
what are they good for? Nut meals
are gluten free and boast the
nutrients of whole nuts. They
help to keep baked goods super
moist, giving them a lovely
dense texture – without the
need for extra fats and oils.

unrefined sugars

what are they? Rapadura sugar, or panela, is extracted from the pure juice of sugar cane and evaporated over low heat. It has light to dark golden grains, depending on production, and a warm caramel flavour. Coconut sugar, with a more earthy, butterscotch taste, comes from the flowers of the coconut palm. *what are they good for?* Choosing these over more processed sugars can be a smarter way to sweeten, as some trace minerals are retained. They'll enrich the flavour of your baking, too.

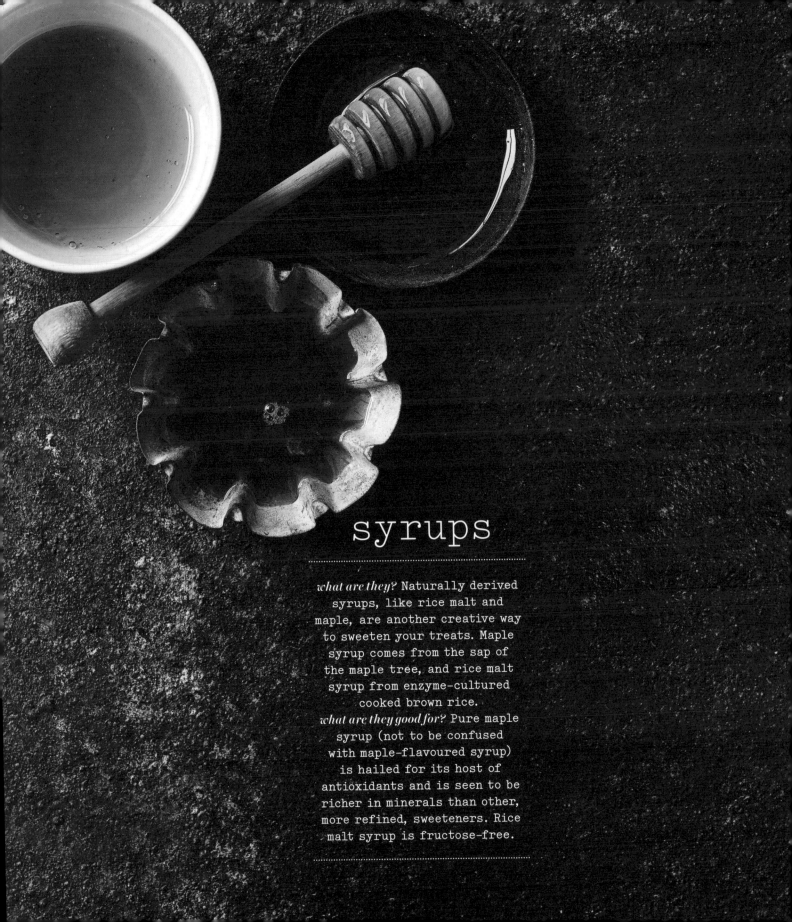

syrups

what are they? Naturally derived
syrups, like rice malt and
maple, are another creative way
to sweeten your treats. Maple
syrup comes from the sap of
the maple tree, and rice malt
syrup from enzyme-cultured
cooked brown rice.

what are they good for? Pure maple
syrup (not to be confused
with maple-flavoured syrup)
is hailed for its host of
antioxidants and is seen to be
richer in minerals than other,
more refined, sweeteners. Rice
malt syrup is fructose-free.

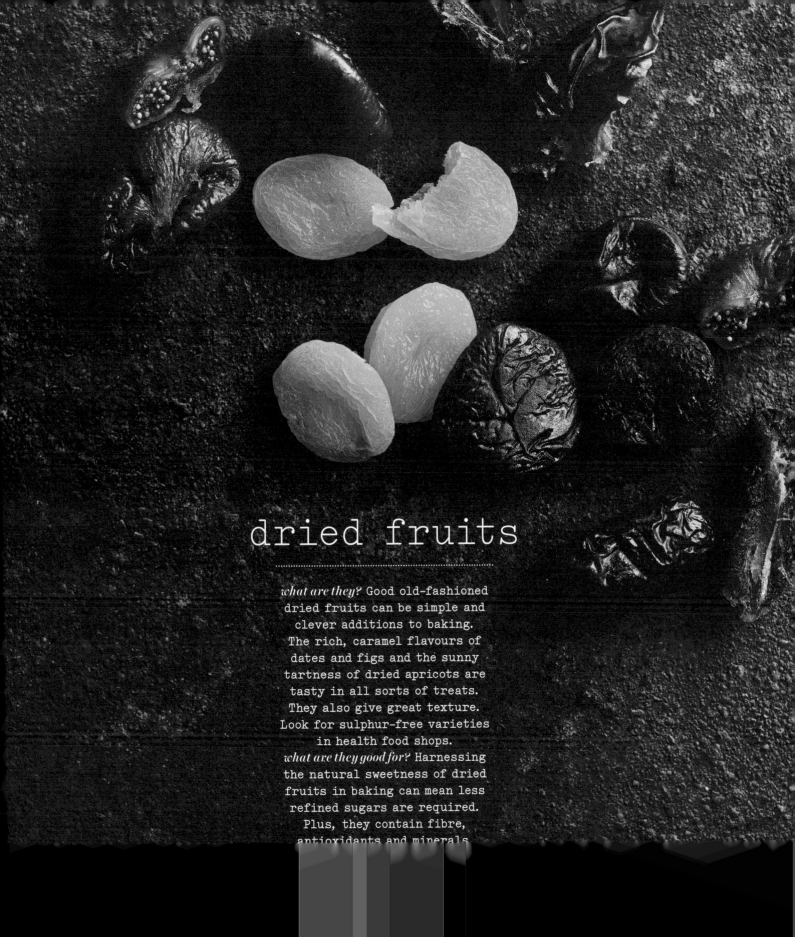

dried fruits

what are they? Good old-fashioned dried fruits can be simple and clever additions to baking. The rich, caramel flavours of dates and figs and the sunny tartness of dried apricots are tasty in all sorts of treats. They also give great texture. Look for sulphur-free varieties in health food shops.

what are they good for? Harnessing the natural sweetness of dried fruits in baking can mean less refined sugars are required. Plus, they contain fibre, antioxidants and minerals.

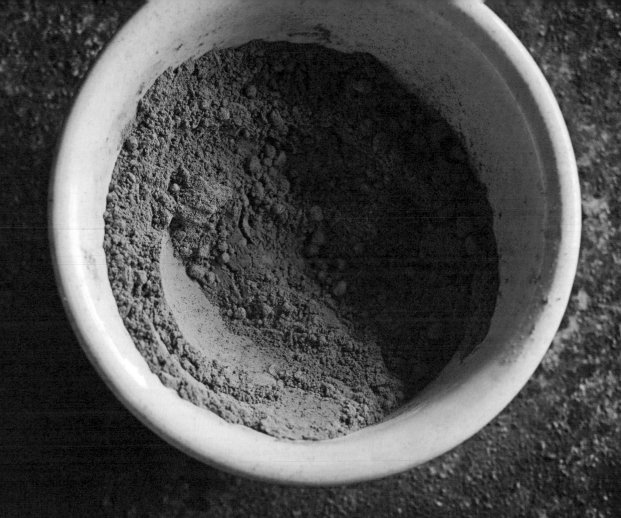

raw cacao

what is it? Available in nibs and powder form, raw cacao comes from tropical cacao beans that have been cold pressed. Rich, dark and pleasantly bitter, you can now buy raw cacao powder in most good supermarkets. *what is it good for?* Sourced from the same beans as regular cocoa, raw cacao retains more antioxidants and enzymes thanks to lower processing temperatures. Bake with it or dust it over truffles and cakes for a super way to get your chocolate fix.

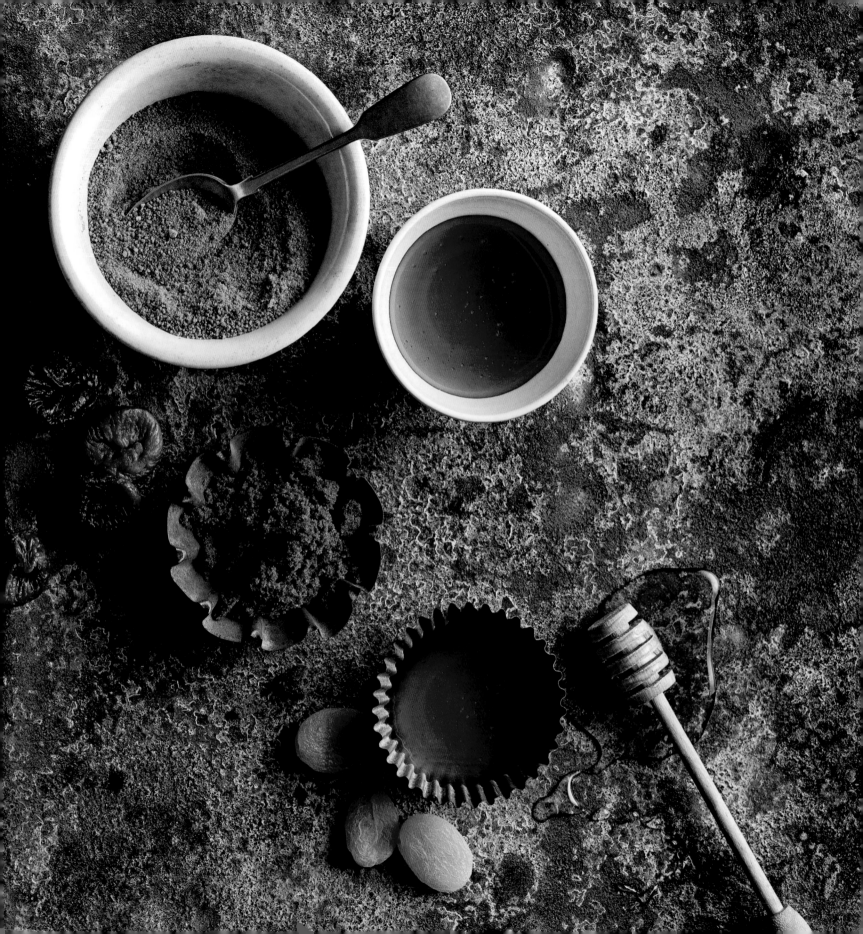

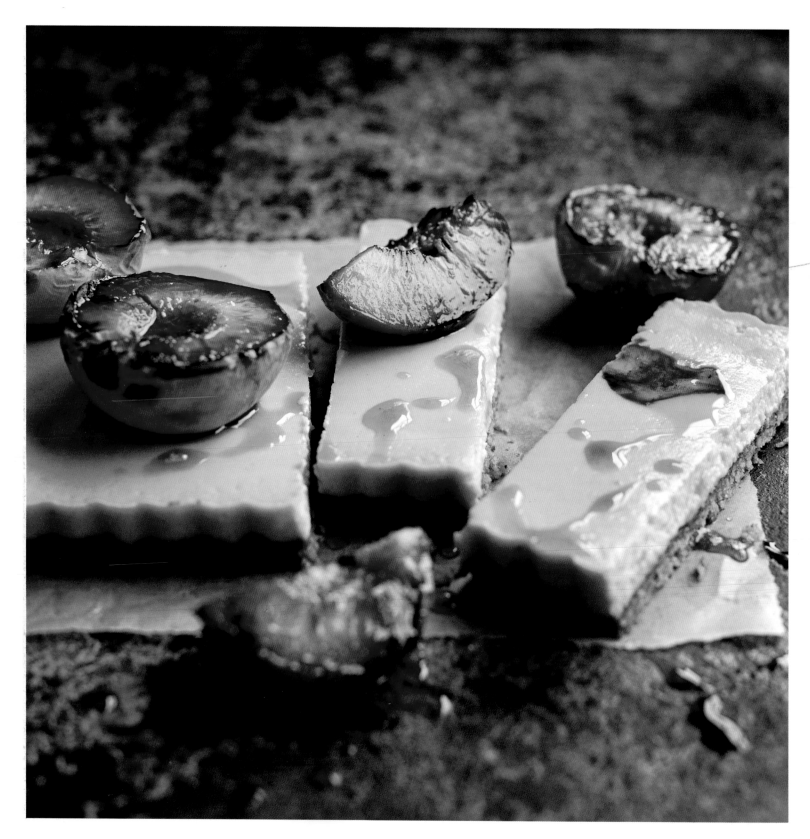

lemon cheesecake with blistered peaches

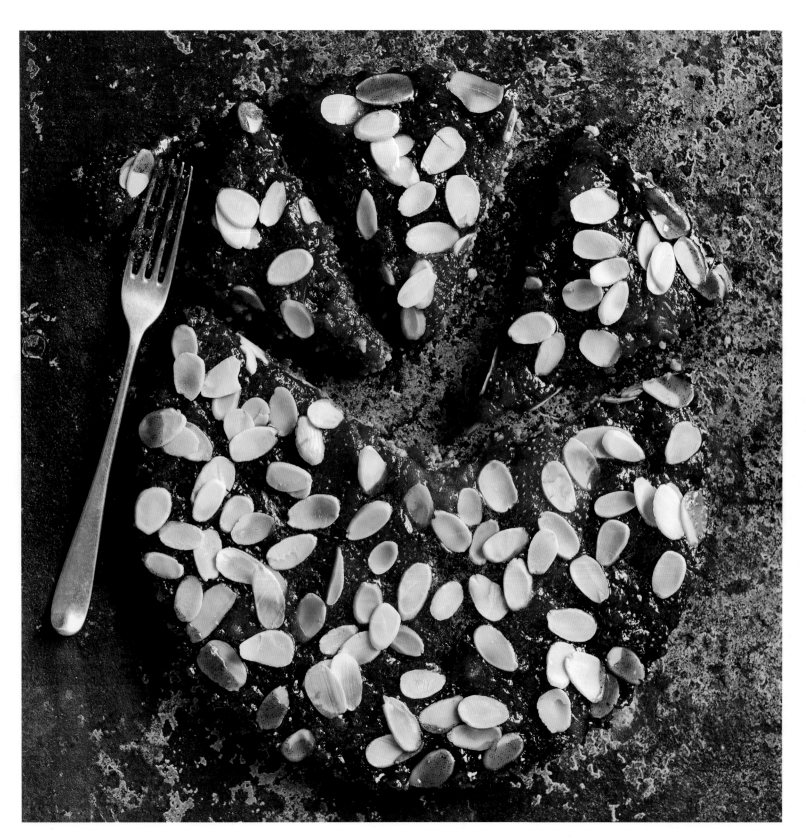

almond and jam tart

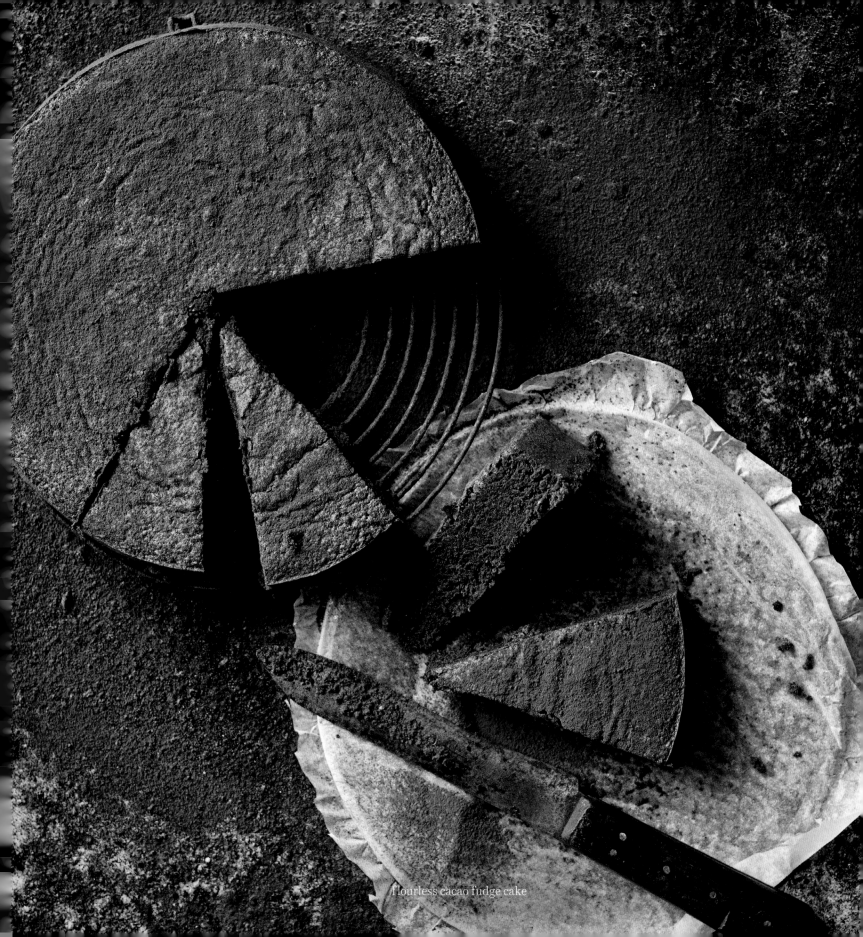

flourless cacao fudge cake

lemon cheesecake with blistered peaches

1 cup (160g) almonds
¼ cup (45g) white rice flour*
80g unsalted butter, chopped
2 tablespoons honey
2 peaches, halved and stones removed
2 tablespoons rapadura* or raw sugar
filling
1 cup (240g) fresh ricotta
150g cream cheese
2 egg yolks
1 teaspoon finely grated lemon rind
1 teaspoon vanilla extract
2 tablespoons white rice flour*
½ cup (125ml) maple syrup

Preheat oven to 160°C (320°F). Place the almonds in a food processor and process until fine. Add the flour, butter and honey and process until a sticky dough forms. Turn out the dough and press into the base of a 12cm x 35cm rectangular loose-based tart tin. Bake for 20 minutes or until golden. Remove from the oven and reduce the oven temperature to 150°C (300°F).

To make the filling, place the ricotta, cream cheese, egg yolks, lemon rind, vanilla, flour and maple syrup in a food processor and process until smooth. Spread the filling over the base and bake for 20 minutes or until just set.

Sprinkle the cut side of the peaches with the sugar and place on a baking tray. Place under a preheated hot grill (broiler) for 5 minutes or until golden and slightly blistered. Remove the cheesecake from the tin, slice and serve with the peaches. SERVES 6–8

You can swap almond meal for hazelnut meal here, if you prefer

almond and jam tart

1 cup (160g) almonds
10 fresh dates, pitted
80g cold unsalted butter, chopped
½ cup (90g) white rice flour*
1 teaspoon vanilla extract
2 teaspoons ground cinnamon
500g strawberries, hulled and halved
1 tablespoon lemon juice
2 tablespoons water
½ cup (125ml) rice malt syrup*
2 vanilla beans, split lengthways
¼ cup (20g) flaked almonds, for sprinkling

Preheat oven to 160°C (320°F). Lightly grease a 22cm springform cake tin and line the base with non-stick baking paper. Place the almonds in a food processor and process until finely chopped. Add the dates, butter, flour, vanilla and cinnamon and process until a soft dough forms. Press into the base of the prepared tin and bake for 20–25 minutes or until golden and crisp.

Place the strawberries, lemon juice and water in a large non-stick frying pan over medium heat. Bring to a simmer and cook, stirring, for 6 minutes or until soft. Stir in the rice malt syrup and vanilla beans, reduce the heat to low and simmer for 12 minutes or until thickened. Discard the vanilla beans. Spread the jam over the base and sprinkle with the flaked almonds. Bake for 20–25 minutes or until lightly golden. Allow to cool in the tin. Slice to serve. SERVES 8–10

flourless cacao fudge cake

200g unsalted butter, chopped
¾ cup (75g) raw cacao powder*, plus extra for dusting
6 eggs
1¼ cups (220g) brown sugar
1 cup (120g) almond meal (ground almonds)

Preheat oven to 160°C (320°F). Lightly grease a 22cm springform cake tin and line with non-stick baking paper. Place the butter and cacao in a saucepan over low heat and stir until smooth. Place the eggs and sugar in the bowl of an electric mixer and beat until doubled in volume. Add the cacao mixture and almond meal and gently fold to combine. Pour into the tin and bake for 35–40 minutes or until just set. Allow to cool in the tin. Turn out and dust with extra cacao to serve. SERVES 10–12

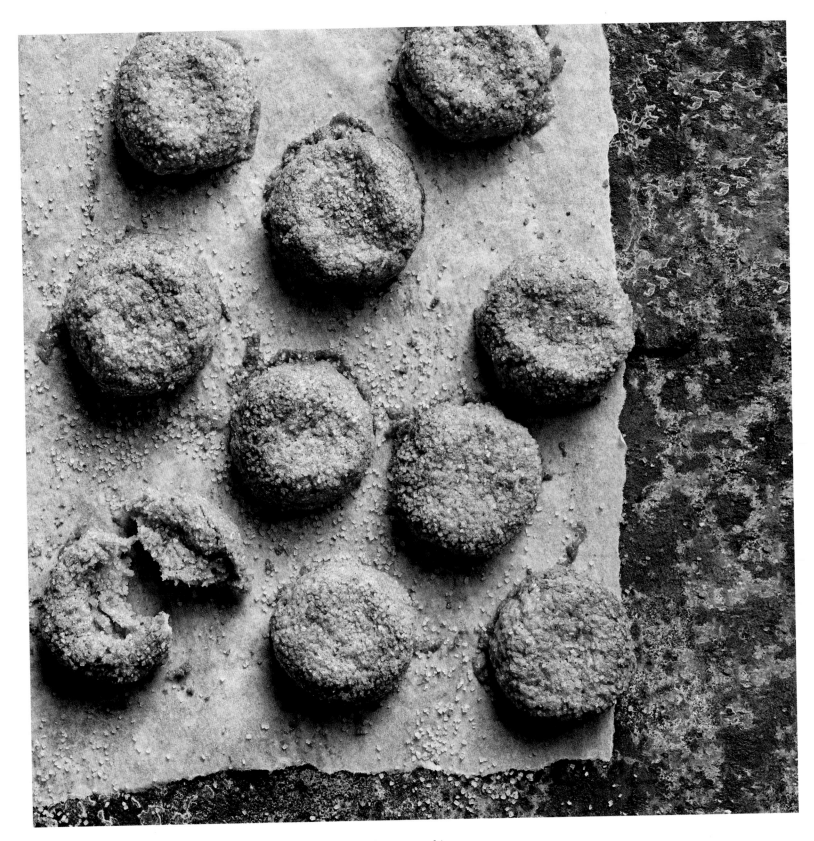

banana cookies

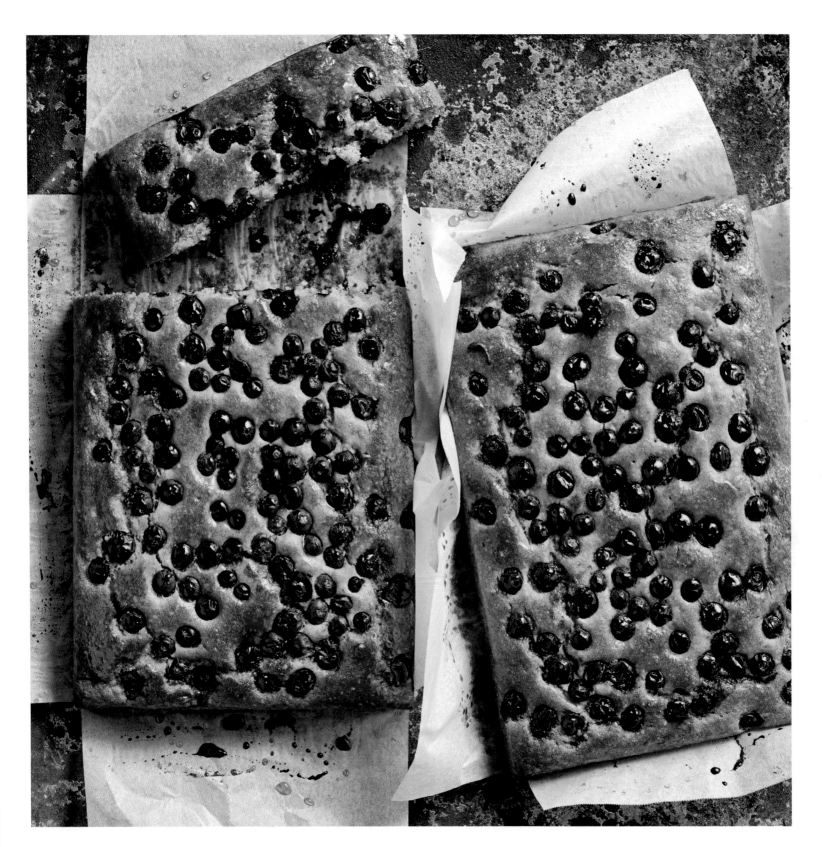

banana and berry tray cake

banana cookies

1 cup (260g) mashed banana (about 3 bananas)
2 cups (240g) almond meal (ground almonds)
⅓ cup (80ml) maple syrup
1½ teaspoons ground cinnamon
¼ cup (55g) demerara sugar*

Preheat oven to 160°C (320°F). Place the banana, almond meal, maple syrup and ¼ teaspoon of the cinnamon in a bowl and mix to combine. Place the sugar and remaining cinnamon in a separate bowl and mix to combine.

Roll tablespoons of the banana mixture into balls, flatten slightly and gently toss in the sugar mixture to coat. Place on baking trays lined with non-stick baking paper and bake for 35–40 minutes or until golden and crisp to touch. Allow to cool on trays. Store in an airtight container for up to 3 days. **MAKES 16**

banana and berry tray cake

1½ cups (390g) mashed banana (about 4 bananas)
⅓ cup (40g) oat bran
¼ cup (60ml) milk
½ cup (125ml) maple syrup, plus extra for brushing
1 cup (250ml) vegetable or coconut oil*
2 eggs
1 teaspoon vanilla extract
1 teaspoon ground cinnamon
1 cup (160g) buckwheat flour*
1 cup (130g) white spelt flour*
3 teaspoons baking powder
1 cup (150g) blueberries, raspberries or blackberries

find these flours in health food stores and most supermarkets

Preheat oven to 160°C (320°F). Lightly grease a 20cm x 30cm slice tin, line with non-stick baking paper and set aside.

Place the banana, oat bran, milk, maple syrup, oil, eggs, vanilla and cinnamon in a large bowl, mix to combine and allow to stand for 15 minutes.

Sift in both the flours and the baking powder and mix to combine. Pour into the prepared tin and sprinkle with the blueberries. Bake for 45 minutes or until just cooked when tested with a skewer. Turn out onto a serving plate and, while the cake is still hot, brush with extra maple syrup. Slice and serve warm. **SERVES 15**

hazelnut and chocolate cookie sandwiches

1 cup (160g) buckwheat flour*
¾ cup (75g) hazelnut meal (ground hazelnuts)
¼ teaspoon sea salt flakes
½ cup (125ml) maple syrup
⅓ cup (80ml) vegetable oil
filling
150g dark chocolate, melted
2 tablespoons almond butter*
¼ cup (60ml) maple syrup

Preheat oven to 180°C (350°F). Place the flour, hazelnut meal, salt, maple syrup and oil in a bowl and mix to combine. Roll teaspoons of the mixture into balls and flatten slightly. Place on baking trays lined with non-stick baking paper and bake for 14–16 minutes or until golden and crisp. Allow to cool on trays.

To make the filling, place the chocolate, almond butter and maple syrup in a bowl and mix until smooth. Spread half the cooled biscuits with the filling and sandwich with the remaining biscuits. Store unfilled biscuits in an airtight container for up to 1 week. **MAKES 20**

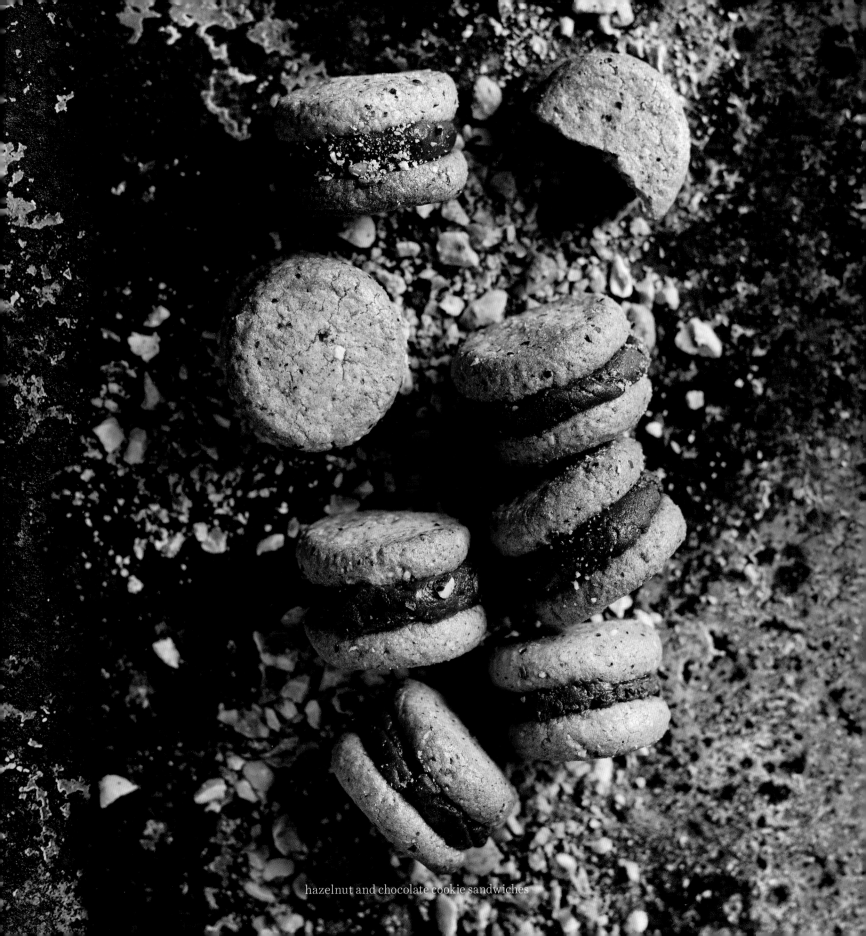

hazelnut and chocolate cookie sandwiches

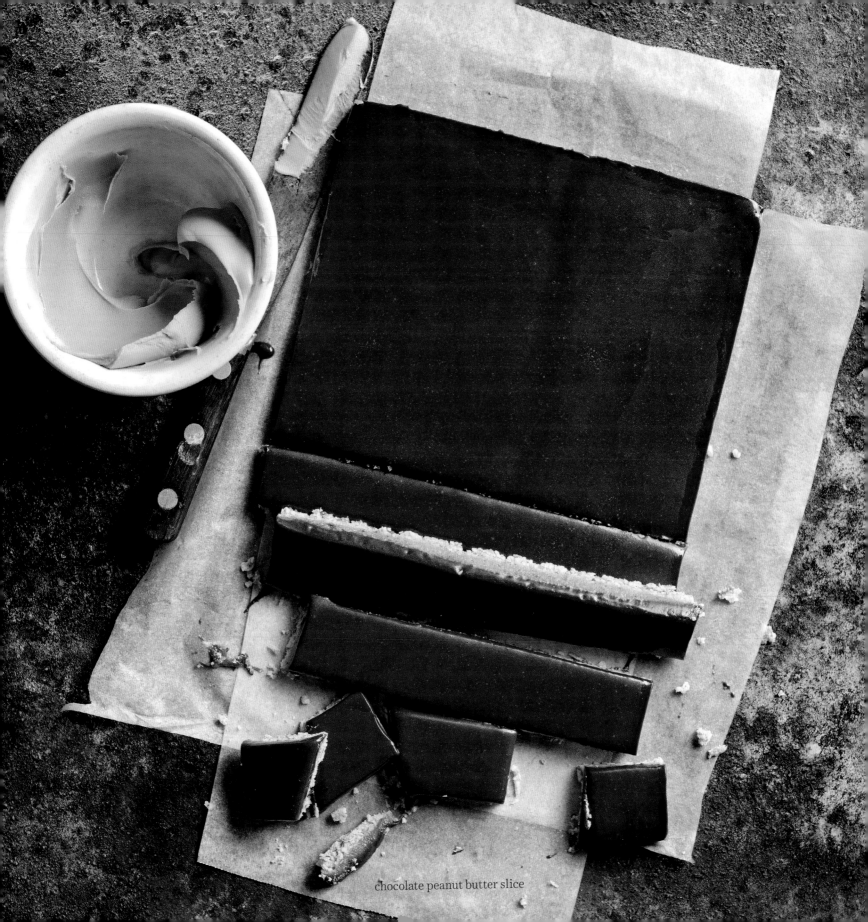

chocolate peanut butter slice

chocolate peanut butter slice

¾ cup (120g) almonds
½ cup (40g) desiccated coconut
6 fresh dates, pitted
¼ cup (60g) coconut oil*, melted
peanut butter filling
¾ cup (210g) smooth peanut butter
8 fresh dates, pitted
½ cup (125ml) rice malt syrup*
cacao topping
⅓ cup (35g) raw cacao powder*
¼ cup (60g) coconut oil*, melted
½ cup (125ml) rice malt syrup*

Lightly grease a 20cm x 30cm slice tin and line with non-stick baking paper. Place the almonds in a food processor and process until finely chopped. Add the coconut, dates and oil and process until well combined. Press the mixture into the base of the prepared tin and refrigerate for 30 minutes or until firm.

To make the peanut butter filling, place the peanut butter, dates and rice malt syrup in a food processor and process until smooth. Spread over the base and refrigerate for 1 hour or until firm.

To make the cacao topping, place the cacao, oil and rice malt syrup in a heatproof bowl over a saucepan of simmering water and stir until smooth. Remove from the heat and spoon over the peanut butter filling. Refrigerate for 3–4 hours or until set, remove from the tin and slice to serve. Store slice in an airtight container in the refrigerator for up to 1 week. **MAKES 24**

with nuts, dates, coconut and cacao, you'll need to sneak a second square of this heavenly slice

coconut cupcakes

1½ cups (195g) white spelt flour*
3 teaspoons baking powder
¾ cup (165g) raw sugar
⅔ cup (50g) desiccated coconut
⅔ cup (160ml) coconut milk
3 eggwhites
1 teaspoon vanilla extract
100g coconut oil*, melted
shredded coconut, to serve
coconut frosting
¾ cup (180ml) rice malt syrup*
3 eggwhites

this honey-like syrup is made from brown rice - it's a great natural sweetener

Preheat oven to 160°C (320°F). Place the flour, baking powder, sugar, desiccated coconut, coconut milk, eggwhites, vanilla and oil in a large bowl and mix until well combined. Spoon the mixture into 12 x ⅓-cup-capacity (80ml) cupcake tins lined with paper cases. Bake for 25 minutes or until just cooked when tested with a skewer. Turn out onto wire racks to cool.

To make the coconut frosting, place the rice malt syrup in a small saucepan over medium heat until it reaches 120°C (250°F) on a sugar thermometer. Place the eggwhites in the bowl of an electric mixer and whisk until soft peaks form. With the motor running, gradually add the hot syrup to the eggwhite in a thin steady stream and whisk until thick and glossy.

Spread the frosting over the cooled cupcakes and sprinkle with shredded coconut to serve. Store unfrosted cupcakes in an airtight container for up to 1 week. **MAKES 12**

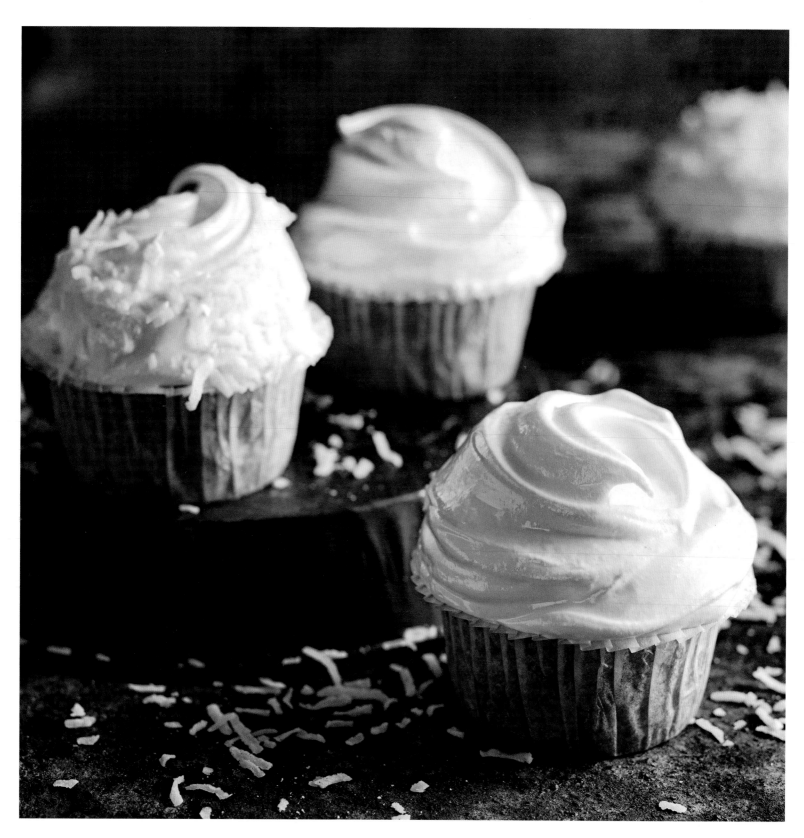

coconut cupcakes

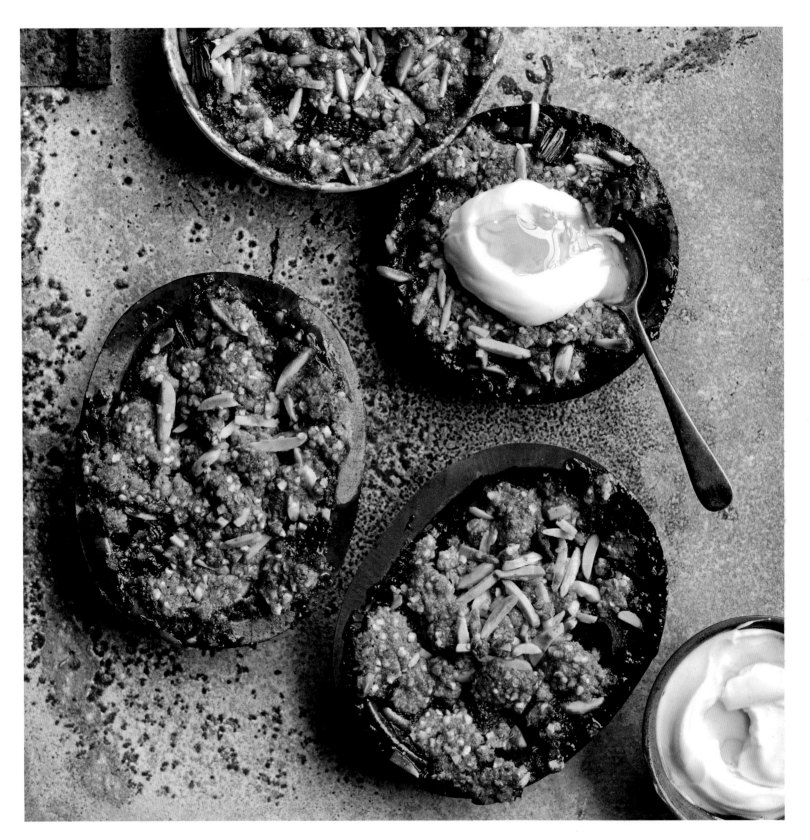

rhubarb, ginger and strawberry crumbles

rhubarb, ginger and strawberry crumbles

500g rhubarb, trimmed and chopped
300g strawberries, hulled and halved
1 tablespoon finely grated ginger
1 teaspoon vanilla extract
⅓ cup (80ml) maple syrup
plain Greek-style (thick) yoghurt and honey, to serve
crumble topping
¾ cup (75g) quinoa flakes*
½ cup (70g) slivered almonds
¼ cup (40g) buckwheat flour*
1 teaspoon ground cinnamon
⅓ cup (80ml) rice malt syrup*
¼ cup (60g) coconut oil*, melted
¼ cup (45g) brown sugar

Preheat oven to 180°C (350°F). Place the rhubarb, strawberries, ginger, vanilla and maple syrup in a bowl and toss to combine. Divide the fruit mixture between 4 x 1-cup-capacity (250ml) ovenproof ramekins. Place the ramekins on a baking tray and bake for 20 minutes or until the rhubarb is soft.

While the fruit is baking, make the crumble topping. Place the quinoa flakes, almonds, flour, cinnamon, rice malt syrup, oil and sugar in a bowl and mix to combine.

Spoon crumble topping onto the fruit in each ramekin and bake for a further 25 minutes or until golden. Serve crumbles warm, topped with yoghurt and honey. MAKES 4

coconut and summer fruit tart

3 white nectarines (500g), cut into wedges
3 peaches (450g), cut into wedges
1 cup (135g) raspberries
2 tablespoons maple syrup
⅓ cup (25g) desiccated coconut
1 cup (75g) shredded coconut
1 eggwhite
2 tablespoons raw sugar
pastry
1 cup (140g) wholemeal spelt flour*
¾ cup (120g) buckwheat flour*
125g unsalted butter, chopped
¼ cup (60ml) maple syrup
1 egg yolk
1 teaspoon vanilla extract

this tart gets its delicious nutty warmth from the wholesome pastry

To make the pastry, place both the flours and the butter in a food processor and process until the mixture resembles fine breadcrumbs. Add the maple syrup, egg yolk and vanilla and process until a soft dough forms. Turn out the dough and bring together to form a flat disc. Wrap in plastic wrap and refrigerate for 30 minutes or until firm.

Preheat oven to 190°C (375°F). Roll out the dough between 2 sheets of non-stick baking paper to form a 5mm-thick rough rectangle shape. Place on a baking tray, remove the top sheet of paper and bake for 10 minutes or until light golden.

Place the nectarine, peach, raspberries and maple syrup in a bowl and toss to combine. Sprinkle the pastry with the desiccated coconut and top with the fruit mixture, leaving a 1cm border. Place the shredded coconut, eggwhite and sugar in a bowl, mix to combine and sprinkle over the tart. Bake for 25–30 minutes or until the pastry is crisp and the coconut is golden. Slice and serve warm. SERVES 8

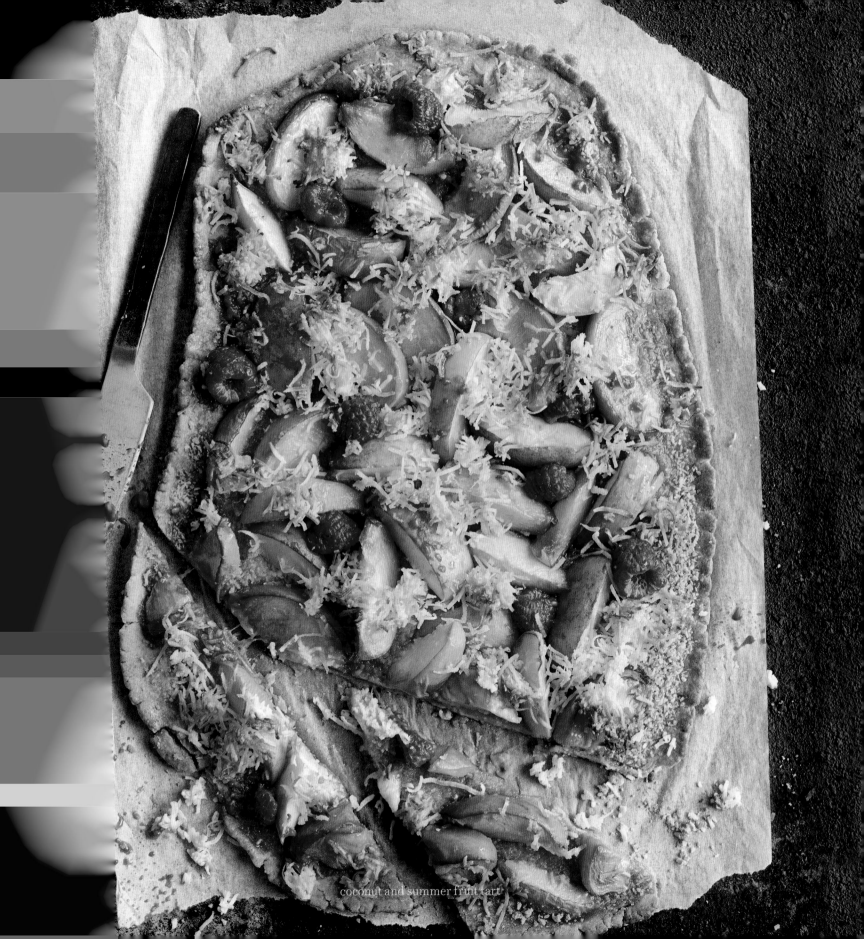

coconut and summer fruit tart

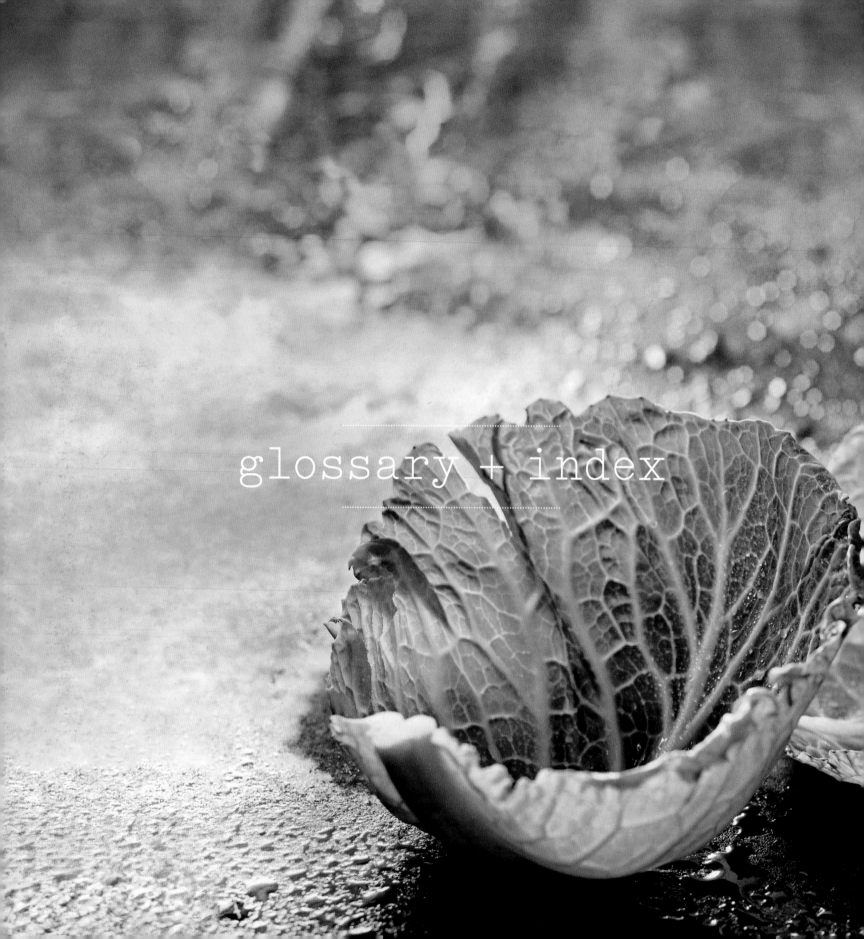

glossary + index

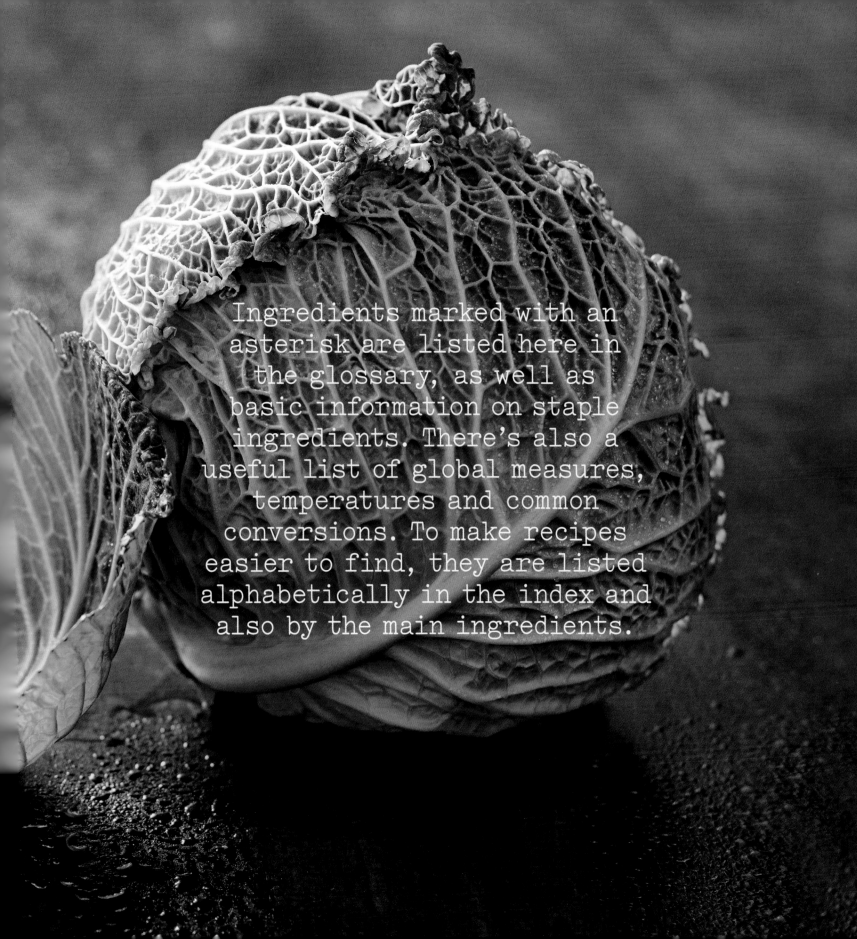

Ingredients marked with an asterisk are listed here in the glossary, as well as basic information on staple ingredients. There's also a useful list of global measures, temperatures and common conversions. To make recipes easier to find, they are listed alphabetically in the index and also by the main ingredients.

basics

almond meal

Also known as ground almonds, almond meal is available from most supermarkets. Make your own by processing whole almonds to a fine meal in a food processor or blender (125g almonds will give 1 cup almond meal).

asian chilli jam

Thai condiment made from ginger, chilli, garlic and shrimp paste, used in soups and stir-fries. It goes well with roasted meats, egg dishes and cheese and is often served in a dollop as a garnish.

barley, pearl

To make pearl barley, the barley husk and bran are removed and the grains are steamed and polished until smooth. When cooked, it's creamy and satisfying in soups, stews and wintry salads. *See also* **grains**, page 112. 1 cup cooked pearl barley weighs 185g. Directions for cooking pearl barley are as follows.

1 cup (210g) pearl barley
1¼ cups (310ml) water
sea salt flakes

Place the barley, water and a pinch of salt in a medium saucepan over high heat. Bring to the boil, immediately cover with a tight-fitting lid and reduce the heat to low. Simmer for 18 minutes or until almost tender. Remove from the heat and allow to steam for 10 minutes or until tender.
MAKES 2 CUPS (370G)

butter

Unless stated otherwise in a recipe, butter should be at room temperature for cooking. It should not be half-melted or too soft to handle.

cheese

burrata
An Italian stretched-curd cheese similar to mozzarella, burrata has a creamy, milky centre. It's best served simply with a tomato and basil salad. It's available from delicatessens and Italian grocery stores.

mozzarella
Italian in origin, mozzarella is the mild cheese of pizza, lasagne and tomato salads. It's made by cutting and spinning (or stringing) the curd to achieve a smooth, elastic consistency. The most prized variety is made from buffalo's milk. Available at delicatessens, specialty cheese shops and most supermarkets.

ricotta
A creamy, finely grained white cheese. Ricotta means 'recooked' in Italian, a reference to the way the cheese is produced by heating the whey leftover from making other cheese varieties. It's fresh, creamy and low in fat and there is also a reduced-fat version, which is lighter again.

chickpeas (garbanzo beans)

A legume native to western Asia and across the Mediterranean, chickpeas are used in soups, stews and are the base ingredient in the Middle Eastern dip, hummus. Dried chickpeas must be soaked before cooking, but you can also buy them canned.

chillies

There are more than 200 different types of chillies in the world. By general rule of thumb, long red or green chillies are milder, fruitier and sweeter, while small chillies are much hotter. Remove the membranes and seeds for a milder result in a dish.

coconut

cream
The cream that rises to the top after the first pressing of coconut milk. Coconut cream is both higher in energy and fat than regular coconut milk. A common ingredient in curries and Asian sweets, buy it in cans from the supermarket.

desiccated
Desiccated coconut is coconut meat that has been shredded and dried to remove the moisture. It's unsweetened and very powdery. Great for baking as well as savoury Asian sauces and sambals.

flakes
Coconut flakes have a large shape and chewier texture than the desiccated variety, and are often used for decorating and in cereals and baking.

milk
A milky, sweet liquid made by soaking grated fresh coconut flesh or desiccated coconut in warm water, and squeezing it through muslin or cheesecloth. Available in cans or freeze-dried from supermarkets, coconut milk should not be confused with coconut water, which is a clear liquid found inside young coconuts.

shredded
In slightly larger pieces than desiccated, shredded coconut is great for baking into slices, or for making condiments to accompany curries.

coriander (cilantro)

This pungent green herb is common in Asian and Mexican cooking. The finely chopped roots are sometimes incorporated in curry pastes. The dried seeds can't be substituted for fresh coriander.

dukkah

A Middle Eastern nut and spice blend available from some supermarkets, spice shops and specialty grocery stores. Great for sprinkling on meats and salads or using in a spice crust.

eggs

The standard egg size used in this book is 60g. It is important to use the right sized eggs for a recipe, as this will affect the outcome of baked goods. The correct volume is especially important when using eggwhites to make meringues. You should use eggs at room temperature for baking.

juniper berries

The aromatic and bitter dried berries of a hardy evergreen bush, juniper is used for pickling vegetables and flavouring sauces. It goes well with duck and pork.

lemongrass

A tall lemon-scented grass used in Asian cooking, particularly in Thai dishes. Peel away the outer leaves and chop the tender white root-end finely, or add in large pieces during cooking and remove before serving. If adding in larger pieces, bruise them with the back of a kitchen knife.

maple syrup

A sweetener made from the sap of the maple tree. Be sure to use pure maple syrup rather than imitation or pancake syrup, which is made from corn syrup flavoured with maple and does not have the same intensity of flavour. *See also* **flours + sugars**, page 206.

micro herbs

The baby version of edible herbs, these tiny leaves have a great intensity of flavour despite their size. Find them at farmers' markets and greengrocers.

marked ingredients

almond butter
A paste made from ground almonds, available at most supermarkets and health food stores. A popular alternative to peanut butter for those with peanut allergies (always check labels) or avoiding the additives in commercial blends.

amaranth
Similar to quinoa, amaranth is not a grain but a seed harvested from an annual plant. Gluten free and high in protein and minerals, it's available in health food stores and specialty grocers. 1 cup cooked amaranth weighs 285g. Directions for cooking amaranth are as follows.

1 cup (220g) amaranth
1 cup (250ml) water
sea salt flakes

Place the amaranth, water and a pinch of salt in a medium saucepan over high heat. Bring to the boil, immediately cover with a tight-fitting lid and reduce the heat to low. Simmer for 20 minutes or until tender. MAKES 2 CUPS (570G)

flakes
Amaranth seeds rolled into flakes make for a nourishing porridge or crispy addition to baked treats. Find amaranth flakes at health food stores.

puffed
Amaranth seeds that are heated and popped, or puffed, to become light and aerated. Perfect in cereals, bars or slices. Find puffed amaranth at health food stores.

buckwheat
Buckwheat is the seed of a plant related to rhubarb. Once cooked, it can be used like rice or pasta. Buy raw buckwheat at health food stores and some supermarkets. *See also* **flour** page 229; **grains** page 110. 1 cup cooked buckwheat weighs 100g. Directions for cooking buckwheat are as follows.

1 cup (200g) raw buckwheat, rinsed
    and drained

Place the buckwheat in a large saucepan of salted boiling water over high heat. Reduce the heat to low and simmer, stirring occasionally, for 8 minutes or until al dente. Drain well and rinse again if required. MAKES 2 CUPS (210G)

burghul
Burghul, or bulgur wheat, is wheat kernels that have been steamed, dried and crushed to give a tender, almost chewy texture. Used in Middle Eastern cooking, notably tabouli, find coarse burghul in most supermarkets. 1 cup cooked coarse burghul weighs 165g. Directions for cooking burghul are as follows.

1 cup (200g) coarse burghul

Place the burghul in a large saucepan of salted boiling water over high heat. Reduce the heat to low and simmer, stirring occasionally, for 18 minutes or until tender. Drain well. MAKES 3¾ CUPS (610G)

chia seeds
These ancient seeds come from a flowering plant and are full of protein, omega-3 fatty acids, minerals and fibre. You can use the black or white seeds interchangeably. They're available in supermarkets and health food stores and are great for smoothies, salads and baking. *See also* **seeds + nuts** page 184.

chilli bean paste
A Chinese sauce made from chillies and fermented beans. Available at Asian grocers.

coconut oil
Extracted from mature coconuts, coconut oil is sold in jars as a solid, so you may need to melt it before using. It adds a touch of tropical flavour to baked treats and slices and is sometimes used as a dairy-free alternative to butter. Look for virgin coconut oil in supermarkets and health food stores.

coconut yoghurt
Yoghurt made from coconut milk and probiotic cultures. Find this dairy alternative in specialty grocers and health food stores.

couscous, whole-wheat
Couscous made from whole-wheat durum flour, thus retaining more nutrients from the grain. Find it at specialty grocers. 1 cup cooked whole-wheat couscous weighs 140g. Directions for cooking whole-wheat couscous are as follows.

1 cup (160g) whole-wheat couscous
1 cup (250ml) boiling water or stock

Place the couscous in a large heatproof bowl. Add the water, stir to combine and immediately cover with plastic wrap or a tight-fitting lid. Allow to stand for 5 minutes or until the water is absorbed. Fluff up the grains with a fork to serve. MAKES 4 CUPS (560G)

crispy fried shallots (eschalots)
A popular Asian condiment, sprinkled on everything from soup to seafood. Eschalots (French shallots) are finely sliced and fried until crisp and crunchy. Buy them packaged from Asian grocers.

edamame

Immature soybeans in their pods. Find edamame in the freezer section of supermarkets or fresh from Asian grocers.

flours

buckwheat

Despite its name, buckwheat flour isn't from a grain, but milled from the seed of a plant related to rhubarb and sorrel. Often used in pancakes and noodles for its rich, nutty flavour and wholesome benefits, it's also gluten free. *See also* **flours + sugars** page 202.

rice

Fine flour made from ground rice. Available in white and brown varieties, it's often used as a thickening agent in baking and to coat foods when cooking Asian dishes, particularly those needing a crispy finish, such as tofu or chicken. It's gluten free and available in health food shops.

rye

Most commonly used to bake bread, rye flour is milled from the cereal grass rye. It contains less gluten than regular wheat flour, and produces dark, dense loaves when baked. Available in health food stores.

spelt

Milled from the ancient cereal grain, spelt flour (white or wholemeal) can often be used in place of regular wheat flour as it boasts more nutrients and can be tolerated more by some. It gives breads and pastas a mild nutty flavour and a caramel colour. Available in health food stores and specialty grocers. *See also* **flours + sugars** page 203.

whole-wheat

Different to wholemeal flour, in that whole-wheat flour is derived by grinding or mashing the whole grain of wheat. All of the grain (bran, germ and endosperm) is used, and aside from its nutritional value, it gives baked goods a unique body and flavour. Find it at health food stores.

freekeh, cracked

Immature or 'green' wheat grains that have been roasted. Can be used in place of cracked wheat in tabouli, or use as you would rice or pasta. Find it in supermarkets and health food stores. *See also* **grains** page 108. 1 cup cooked cracked freekeh weighs 170g. Directions for cooking cracked freekeh are as follows.

1 cup (165g) cracked freekeh
1¼ cups (310ml) water
sea salt flakes

Place the freekeh, water and a pinch of salt in a medium saucepan over high heat. Bring to the boil, immediately cover with a tight-fitting lid and reduce the heat to low. Simmer for 15 minutes or until almost tender. Remove from the heat and allow to steam for 10 minutes or until tender. MAKES 2¼ CUPS (380G)

harissa

A North African condiment, harissa is a hot red paste made from chilli, garlic and spices including coriander, caraway and cumin. It can also contain tomato. Available in jars and tubes from supermarkets and specialty food stores, harissa enlivens tagines and couscous dishes and can be added to dressings, sauces and marinades.

honey, raw

Unheated, unprocessed honey, said to retain more nutrients and have more beneficial properties than commercial honeys. It has sweet, rich and complex flavours. Buy raw honey at health food shops, specialty food stores and greengrocers.

horseradish

A pungent root vegetable that releases mustard oil when cut or grated. Used as a condiment, it's a perfect partner for pork and roast beef. It's available fresh from greengrocers, or substitute with pre-grated or creamed horseradish sold in jars at the supermarket.

kaffir lime leaves

Fragrant leaves from the kaffir lime tree, with a distinctive double-leaf structure. Commonly crushed or shredded and used in Thai dishes. Available fresh or dried from Asian food stores, the fresh leaves tend to have more flavour. Buy fresh leaves and store any extras in the freezer for next time.

linseeds (flaxseeds)

These small brown seeds, also known as flaxseeds, have a nutty flavour and are high in omega-3. They can be baked into bread, sprinkled in cereal and salads or used to make slices. Find linseeds at supermarkets and health food stores. *See also* **seeds + nuts** page 182.

matcha green tea powder

Green tea leaves, grown and selected for their superior flavour, are stone-ground to make this fine powder. High in nutrients with a malted, yet sharp, tea-like flavour, find matcha in health food stores and specialty tea shops.

miso paste

A traditional Japanese ingredient produced by fermenting rice, barley or soy beans to a paste. It is used for sauces, spreads and mixing with dashi stock to serve as miso soup. Yellow miso paste is more robust and earthy in flavour, while white miso paste is more delicate. Available from supermarkets and Asian food stores.

molasses

A by-product of sugar cane in the production of refined sugar, this syrup varies in colour and sweetness. Usually, darker molasses is more nutrient-dense, with a complex, slightly bitter flavour. Find molasses in supermarkets and health food stores.

nori

Thin sheets of dried seaweed, commonly used for making sushi rolls. High in protein and minerals, nori can also be toasted, chopped, added to soups or used as a garnish. Find nori in supermarkets and Asian grocers.

pepitas (pumpkin seeds)

Pumpkin seeds are hulled to reveal these olive green kernels that, once dried, are nutty in flavour and easy to use in smoothies, baking and salads. Find them in supermarkets. *See also* **seeds + nuts** page 180.

pomegranate molasses

A concentrated syrup made from pomegranate juice, with a sweet, tart flavour. It's available from Middle Eastern grocery stores and specialty food shops.

psyllium husk powder

The finely ground husks of psyllium seeds, available in health food shops and some supermarkets. Super-rich in fibre and often used in gluten-free baking as a binding ingredient.

quinoa

Packed with protein, this grain-like seed has a chewy texture, nutty flavour and is fluffy when cooked. Use it as you would couscous or rice. Red and black varieties are also available is supermarkets. *See also* **grains** page 111. 1 cup cooked quinoa weighs 160g. Directions for cooking quinoa are as follows.

1 cup (180g) white quinoa
1¼ cups (310ml) water
sea salt flakes

Place the quinoa, water and a pinch of salt in a medium saucepan over high heat. Bring to the boil, immediately cover with a tight-fitting lid and reduce the heat to low. Simmer for 12 minutes or until almost tender. Remove from the heat and allow to steam for 8 minutes or until tender.
MAKES 2¼ CUPS (440G)

black, red

Black or red varieties of quinoa are available in supermarkets and greengrocers. Mostly selected for their colour, they can vary slightly from regular white quinoa in texture when cooked, but all three are essentially interchangeable. *See also* **grains** page 111. 1 cup cooked black or red quinoa is 170g. Directions for cooking black or red quinoa are as follows.

1 cup (200g) black or red quinoa
1¼ cups (310ml) water
sea salt flakes

Place the quinoa, water and a pinch of salt in a medium saucepan over high heat. Bring to the boil, immediately cover with a tight-fitting lid and reduce the heat to low. Simmer for 15 minutes or until almost tender. Remove from the heat and allow to steam for 10 minutes or until tender. **MAKES 2¼ CUPS (460G)**

flakes

Simply quinoa that has been steamrolled into flakes. They can be used in breakfast cereals, pancakes or baked goods. Available from health food stores and some supermarkets.

ras el hanout

A North African spice mix, literally translating as 'top of the shop'. Ras el hanout can contain over 20 different spices, most commonly cinnamon, cardamom, cloves, coriander, chilli, paprika and turmeric. Find it at spice shops and most greengrocers.

raw cacao

powder

Available in nibs and powder form, raw cacao comes from tropical cacao beans that have been cold pressed. Rich, dark and pleasantly bitter, find raw cacao in most supermarkets. *See also* **flours + sugars** page 208.

chocolate

Bars or blocks of chocolate that have been made with raw cacao (see above). Available in select grocers and health food shops.

rice malt syrup

Made by culturing cooked brown rice with enzymes to break down the starches, this honey-like syrup is a great sweetener. It contains no fructose (unlike honey and maple syrup). Find it in some supermarkets and health food stores. *See also* **flours + sugars** page 206.

ricotta salata

Made by pressing, salting, drying and aging fresh ricotta. It's firm and salty and can be grated and shaved. Find ricotta salata in most Italian delicatessens.

shichimi togarashi

A common Japanese spice mixture made from ground chilli, orange peel, sesame seeds and more. It is often sprinkled on soups and noodles. Find it at Asian supermarkets and grocery stores.

spelt

This ancient cereal grain is part of the wider wheat family. It has a mild, nutty flavour and when cooked it becomes plump and chewy. Add cooked spelt to salads and soups, or use it as a wholesome alternative to rice or pasta. *See also* **flour** page 229; **grains** page 106. 1 cup cooked spelt weighs 200g. Directions for cooking spelt are as follows.

1 cup (200g) spelt
1¼ cups (310ml) water
sea salt flakes

Place the spelt, water and a pinch of salt in a medium saucepan over high heat. Bring to the boil, immediately cover with a tight-fitting lid and reduce the heat to low. Simmer for 20 minutes or until almost tender. Remove from the heat and allow to steam for 10 minutes or until tender.
MAKES 2 CUPS (400G)

oats, rolled
Like regular rolled oats, use spelt oats to make porridge or in baking. Find spelt oats at health food shops.

sriracha chilli sauce

A hot sauce containing chilli, salt, sugar, vinegar and garlic, Sriracha is both the brand name of a popular American blend, as well as the generic name for the Southeast Asian sauce. Available in supermarkets.

sugar

demerara
A coarse-grained golden cane sugar, with a mild molasses flavour. Like raw sugar, it's delicious stirred into coffee or sprinkled over baked treats for a sweet caramel crust.

coconut
With an earthy, butterscotch taste, coconut sugar, or coconut palm sugar, comes from the flowers of the coconut palm. It gives a lovely depth to baked goods. Find it in specialty food shops, Asian grocers and health food stores. *See also* **flours + sugars** *page 205.*

palm
Produced by tapping the sap of palm trees, palm sugar is allowed to crystallise and is sold in cubes or round blocks, which you can shave and add to curries, dressings and Asian desserts. Available from supermarkets, Asian food stores and specialty grocers.

rapadura
Extracted from the pure juice of cane sugar, rapadura (or panela) is evaporated over low heat, which means some minerals and vitamins in the cane are retained. Find it at specialty food shops and health food stores. *See also* **flours + sugars** *page 205.*

sumac

These dried berries of a flowering plant are ground to produce an acidic, vibrant crimson powder that's popular in the Middle East. Sumac has a lemony flavour and is great sprinkled on salads, dips or chicken. Find it at specialty spice shops, greengrocers and some supermarkets.

sunflower seeds

Small grey kernels from inside the black and white seeds of sunflowers. Mostly processed for their oil, the kernels are also found in snack mixes and muesli, and can be baked into breads and slices. Buy sunflower seeds in supermarkets and health food stores. *See also* **seeds + nuts** page 183.

tahini

A thick paste made from ground sesame seeds, used in Middle Eastern cooking. It's available in jars and cans from supermarkets and health food shops. It's used, along with chickpeas, as an ingredient in the popular dip, hummus.

vincotto

Translating literally as 'cooked wine', vincotto is a syrup made from grapes with a sharp, sweet-sour flavour. Use it as you would balsamic vinegar. Find it in supermarkets and specialty grocers.

wakame

A deep-green edible seaweed, commonly used in Japanese soups and salads. Wakame is available fresh and dried in Asian grocers.

water chestnuts

Popular in Asian stir-fries, water chestnuts are the crunchy white tuber of a water-plant native to Southeast Asia. They're available canned in the supermarket, or buy them fresh from Asian grocers and peel before use.

wasabi paste

A very hot Japanese paste, characterised by its powdery green colour. Similar to horseradish, wasabi is used in making sushi and as a condiment. It's available from Asian food stores and supermarkets.

global measures

Measures vary from Europe to the US and even from Australia to NZ.

metric and imperial

Measuring cups and spoons may vary slightly from one country to another, but the difference is generally not sufficient to affect a recipe. All cup and spoon measures are level. An Australian measuring cup holds 250ml (8 fl oz).

One Australian metric teaspoon holds 5ml, one Australian tablespoon holds 20ml (4 teaspoons). However, in North America, New Zealand and the UK they use 15ml (3-teaspoon) tablespoons.

When measuring liquid ingredients remember that 1 American pint contains 500ml (16 fl oz), but 1 Imperial pint contains 600ml (20 fl oz).

When measuring dry ingredients, add the ingredient loosely to the cup and level with a knife. Don't tap or shake to compact the ingredient unless the recipe requests 'firmly packed'.

liquids and solids

Measuring cups and spoons and a set of scales are great assets in the kitchen.

liquids

cup	metric	imperial
⅛ cup	30ml	1 fl oz
¼ cup	60ml	2 fl oz
⅓ cup	80ml	2½ fl oz
½ cup	125ml	4 fl oz
⅔ cup	160ml	5 fl oz
¾ cup	180ml	6 fl oz
1 cup	250ml	8 fl oz
2 cups	500ml	16 fl oz
2¼ cups	560ml	20 fl oz
4 cups	1 litre	32 fl oz

solids

metric	imperial
20g	½ oz
60g	2 oz
125g	4 oz
180g	6 oz
250g	8 oz
500g	16 oz (1 lb)
1kg	32 oz (2 lb)

made to measure

Equivalents for metric and imperial measures and ingredient names.

millimetres to inches

metric	imperial
3mm	⅛ inch
6mm	¼ inch
1cm	½ inch
2.5cm	1 inch
5cm	2 inches
18cm	7 inches
20cm	8 inches
23cm	9 inches
25cm	10 inches
30cm	12 inches

ingredient equivalents

bicarbonate of soda	baking soda
capsicum	bell pepper
caster sugar	superfine sugar
celeriac	celery root
chickpeas	garbanzo beans
coriander	cilantro
cos lettuce	romaine lettuce
cornflour	cornstarch
eggplant	aubergine
green onion	scallion
plain flour	all-purpose flour
rocket	arugula
self raising flour	self-rising flour
snow pea	mange tout
zucchini	courgette

oven temperature

Setting the oven to the right temperature can be critical when making baked goods.

celsius to fahrenheit

celsius	fahrenheit
100°C	200°F
120°C	250°F
140°C	275°F
150°C	300°F
160°C	325°F
180°C	350°F
190°C	375°F
200°C	400°F
220°C	425°F

electric to gas

celsius	gas
110°C	¼
130°C	½
140°C	1
150°C	2
170°C	3
180°C	4
190°C	5
200°C	6
220°C	7
230°C	8
240°C	9
250°C	10

butter and eggs

Let 'fresh is best' be your mantra when it comes to selecting dairy goods.

butter

For baking we generally use unsalted butter as it lends a sweeter flavour. Either way, the impact is minimal. Salted butter has a longer shelf life and is preferred by some people. One American stick of butter is 125g (4 oz). One Australian block of butter is 250g (8 oz).

eggs

Unless otherwise indicated we use large (60g) chicken eggs. To preserve freshness, store eggs in the refrigerator in the carton they are sold in. Use only the freshest eggs in recipes such as mayonnaise or dressings that use raw or barely cooked eggs. Be extra cautious if there is a salmonella problem in your community, particularly in food that is to be served to children, the elderly or pregnant women.

the basics

Here are some simple weight conversions for cups of common ingredients.

common ingredients

almond meal (ground almonds)
1 cup | 120g
brown sugar
1 cup | 175g
white sugar
1 cup | 220g
caster (superfine) sugar
1 cup | 220g
icing (confectioner's) sugar
1 cup | 160g
plain (all-purpose)
or self raising (self-rising) flour
1 cup | 150g
fresh breadcrumbs
1 cup | 70g
finely grated parmesan cheese
1 cup | 80g
uncooked white rice
1 cup | 200g
cooked white rice
1 cup | 165g
uncooked couscous
1 cup | 200g
cooked shredded chicken, pork or beef
1 cup | 160g
olives
1 cup | 150g

thank you

··

When it comes to star performing teams, I consider myself to have one of the best,
and in turn, to be one of the luckiest girls in the world.

My bigger than biggest of thank yous goes to the amazingly talented Chi Lam.
Art director and master of attention to detail, you are the calmest and kindest of souls.
You have guided this book smoothly and creatively from beginning to end.

To my always incredible photography team, William Meppem and Chris Court,
you have such talent in your craft. Thank you both for your beautiful images and
your innate ability to capture all things fresh and delicious.

To the über-brilliant styling and food team, Justine Poole and Hannah Meppem,
thank you for taking the reins and producing such a beautiful and totally scrumptious
book with me. And for testing the recipes to perfection, thank you Samantha Coutts
and Hayley Dodd.

Lovely, lovely words Abby Pfahl – thank you for your perfect turn of phrase
and for truly understanding my sentiment and vision for this book.

To Tony Houssarini in prepress production, thank you for your commitment
to making every image so beautiful.

Thank you to the amazing Shona Martyn and Catherine Milne, along with the rest of
the team at HarperCollins*Publishers*. I feel so lucky to have your unwavering support.

I can never thank my talented magazine team enough. Always willing to lend a
hand, you keep everything running smoothly while I'm immersed in my book projects
(with just a few practical jokes along the way!) and I so appreciate it.

Lastly, to my family and friends, thank you for your wisdom and love, for making
me laugh and for keeping me grounded. To my beautiful boys, Angus and Tom,
you make my world so fun, rich, inspiring and balanced – thank you both for that!

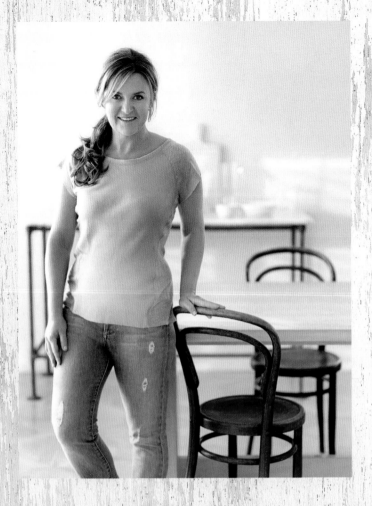

bio

....

Donna Hay is Australia's favourite and most trusted home cook, and an international food-publishing phenomenon. Donna's 24 books have sold more than 4 million copies worldwide, been translated into 10 different languages, and her television cooking shows have brought her signature style to life for viewers in more than 14 countries. In Australia, her recent books have dominated the bestseller charts, with *Fresh and Light* (2012) selling 185,000 copies to date and *the new classics* (2013) selling 150,000 copies to date.

Donna Hay is a household name. She is editor-in-chief of *donna hay magazine* (with more than 730,000 readers), creator of the number one magazine iPad app in Australia, and her column in the Sunday papers is read by 4 million readers in Australia every week. In addition, she is the creator of the donna hay for Royal Doulton collection, including homewares, and her food range is stocked in supermarkets nationally. She is also the working mum of two beautiful boys.

Books by Donna Hay include: *the new easy*; *the new classics*; *Fresh and Light*; *simple dinners*; *a cook's guide*; *fast, fresh, simple.*; *Seasons*; *no time to cook*; *off the shelf*; *instant entertaining*; and *the simple essentials collection*.

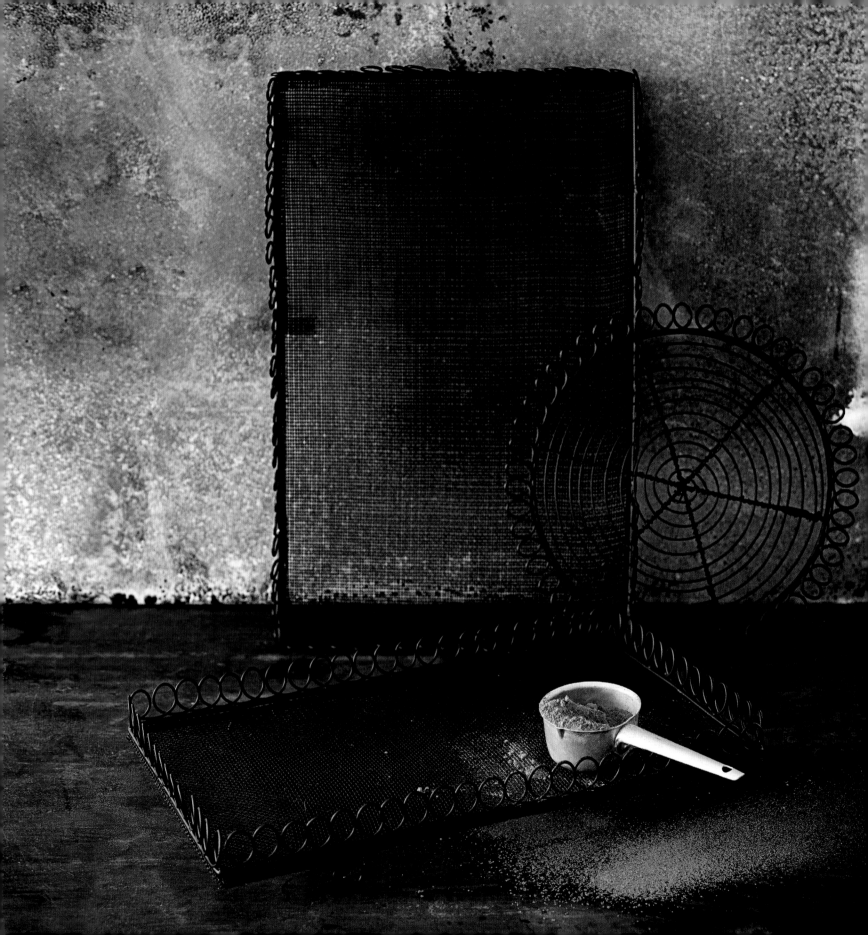

donnahay.com

For more of my cookbooks and simple recipes for weeknights and weekends, visit donnahay.com. You can explore my online store of gifts, hampers, beautiful homewares and my collection for Royal Doulton, plus create a gift registry for your next special occasion. Follow me on social media for all my news, inspiration, the latest on the magazine and my new blog.

Connect with Donna on Facebook, Twitter, Instagram and Pinterest

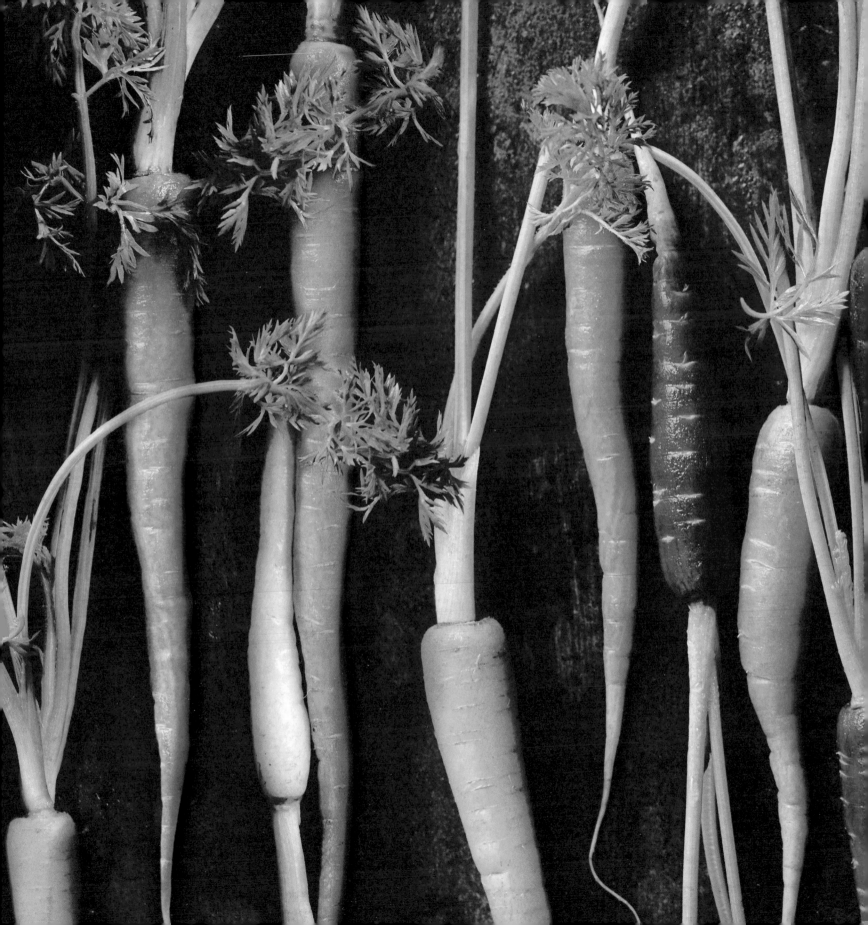